A Practical Handbook for Community Health Nurses

Working with Children and their Parents

Edited by

Katie Booth

Director, Macmillan Practice Development Unit, University of Manchester

and

Karen A. Luker

*Professor of Nursing, School of Nursing, Midwifery
and Health Visiting, University of Manchester*

**Blackwell
Science**

First published 1999

Set in 10 on 11.5pt Ehrhardt
by DP Photosetting, Aylesbury, Bucks
Printed and bound in Great Britain by
The Alden Press Ltd, Oxford and Northampton

The Blackwell Science logo is a
trade mark of Blackwell Science Ltd,
registered at the United Kingdom
Trade Marks Registry

DISTRIBUTORS

Marston Book Services Ltd
PO Box 269
Abingdon
Oxford OX14 4YN
(*Orders:* Tel: 01235 465500
         Fax: 01235 465555)

USA
Blackwell Science, Inc.
Commerce Place
350 Main Street
Malden, MA 02148 5018
(*Orders:* Tel: 800 759 6102
         781 388 8250
         Fax: 781 388 8255)

Canada
Login Brothers Book Company
324 Saulteaux Crescent
Winnipeg, Manitoba R3J 3T2
(*Orders:* Tel: 204 837-2987
         Fax: 204 837-3116)

Australia
Blackwell Science Pty Ltd
54 University Street
Carlton, Victoria 3053
(*Orders:* Tel: 03 9347 0300
         Fax: 03 9347 5001)

A catalogue record for this title is available from
the British Library

ISBN 0–632–04246–X

Library of Congress
Cataloging-in-Publication Data
is available

For further information on
Blackwell Science, visit our website:
www.blackwell-science.com

Contents

Contributors

David Barrett CQSW, MA, PhD, is Head of the Department of Applied Social Studies at the University of Luton.

Anthony S. Blinkhorn BDS, MSc, PhD, FDS is Professor of Oral Health at the University Dental Hospital, Manchester.

Isabelle Brodie MA is a Research Fellow in the Department of Applied Social Studies, University of Luton.

Kate Cernik BSc (Hons), RGN, RHV, Cert.Ed. is a Nurse Practitioner and Nurse Education Advisor with the Warrington Community Trust.

Karen I. Chalmers RN, BSc, MSc(a), PhD is Associate Professor and Associate Dean, Graduate Program, in the Faculty of Nursing, University of Manitoba, Canada.

Brian Corby BA, Dip.Soc.Admin., Dip.Applied Soc. Studies, CQSW is Senior Lecturer in Applied Social Studies at the University of Liverpool.

Barbara Elliott MSc, BNurs, RGN, RHV, NDNcert. is a Lecturer in the School of Nursing at the University of Hull.

Carmel Mary Flanagan BSc (Hons), MPH is Researcher in Public Health and Project Co-ordinator at the University of Liverpool.

Catherine Gaskell is a qualified mental health nurse with ENB 970 Principles of Child Protection, and is an Executive Nurse with City and Hackney Community Services NHS Trust.

Lynne Kennedy BSc (Hons), MPhil, RPhn is a Lecturer in Public Health Nutrition at the University of Liverpool.

Sean P.M. Magennis BDS, MB, ChB, FRCGP is a General Practitioner and Community Clinical Teacher at the University of Liverpool.

Soraya Meah MSc, BSc (Hons), RGN, RM is a Lecturer in Nursing and Clinical Effectiveness Manager at the University of Liverpool.

Pam Pritchard MA, RHV, RGN, Dip.Counselling is a Clinical Nurse Specialist with the Rhondda NHS Trust.

Steve Ryan MD is Consultant Paediatrician at Alder Hey Children's Hospital, Liverpool.

Sam Warner BA (Hons) Psychology, MClin.Psychology is a clinical psychologist and freelance consultant, training and researching in child and forensic psychology.

Jane Willock BSc, MSc, PGDE, RGN, RSCN is Senior Lecturer in Nursing and Senior Nurse in Paediatric Nephrology at the School of Nursing and Midwifery, University of Glamorgan.

Preface

This book is intended for all practising community health nurses or student nurses undertaking a community placement. The focus is normal, healthy children, and we have taken common areas of practice as it relates to children (especially those under five years of age) and their families. This work historically relates to health visiting practice, but it is acknowledged that today this work is conducted by a variety of nurses working in the community or health centres. The aim of the text is to provide community health nurses and their students with an up-to-date reference source, which brings together the available evidence on a range of issues central to their work with children and their parents.

The organisation of the text reflects three major themes from this area: enhancing child wellbeing and development in the family context, maintaining optimal family nutrition, and managing common childhood problems.

Part 1, 'The Child and the Family' highlights important facets of the present-day social and emotional framework within which children grow and develop. The six chapters in this section cover families and social policy, caring for the developing child, promoting psychological health, the impact of post-natal depression and the profound issues surrounding children at risk.

Part 2, 'The Child and Nutrition', has four chapters in all. The first three are intended to bring together issues concerning food and families, information on breast feeding, feeding with formula milks, weaning, and family nutrition in society today. The last chapter in Part 2 considers the impact of eating habits on dental health.

Part 3, 'Common Problems in Childhood', is designed to assist nurses in their advice to parents facing common health-related situations. As the overall emphasis is on prevention, it is fitting that the first chapter should look at the role of immunisation in the battle against disease in childhood. The remaining four chapters were chosen to explore topics which frequently face nurses working with children and their parents: infections and infestations, eczema, toilet training, and the family disruption which can surround child sleep disorders.

Throughout this book the issues are considered from a practical point of view. We hope community health nurses and their students find our choice of topics helpful and relevant.

Introduction: The Changing Context of Community Health Nursing

Karen A. Luker and Katie Booth

The re-structuring of the NHS to reflect market place values (HMSO 1990; NHS Executive 1995) has inspired nurses to identify more clearly their contribution to the health care agenda. The need to care for more patients and clients using limited resources has challenged managers and practitioners alike. The purchaser/provider dichotomy in the provision of health and social care services has encouraged both purchasers and practitioners to explore imaginative and different ways to make the same resources go further. During the 1990s there have been many challenges and changes for community health nurses to embrace. In particular we consider that three major issues will be pivotal in their influence on roles and practice:

(1) the movement towards a primary care led NHS;
(2) the demands for consumer participation;
(3) the increasing calls for health care practice to be evidence-based.

PRIMARY CARE LED NHS

The policy imperative which underpins the quest for a primary care led NHS is to encourage as many people as possible to receive treatment and care in the community. Early discharge from hospital and day case surgery are commonplace and community nurses have been required to extend their skill base to keep up with patient and client needs and demands. According to Wilkin *et al.* (1997), the publication of the green paper *Primary Care: The Future* initiated the process of moving away from fragmented networks of professionals, towards a more integrated framework of service delivery. The government's white papers *Choice and Opportunity* (DoH 1996a), and *Delivering the Future* (DoH 1996b) form the cornerstone for local policy developments by stressing flexibility of service provision.

A major plank of health policy for the next ten years was set out in the 1997 white paper *The New NHS – Modern, Dependable*. This paper upholds the original NHS principle of equality of access, healthcare being available on the basis of need (not ability to pay), and funded from general taxation. It outlines an increasing reliance in the future upon the effectiveness of a restructured primary health care system. Butler and Rowland (1998) go as far as to argue that the delivery of a health strategy will depend largely on the success of new primary care groups (PCGs) to deliver local health improvement programmes in partnership with Health Authorities. From April 1999, 500 of these new groups (typically serving populations of 100,000) will replace nearly 4000 existing commissioning organisations, including general practice fundholders. These primary care groups will be led by GPs and take over commissioning of all health care except specialist services.

The emphasis is on evolution during a ten year time-span, with pilot sites leading the way to enable others to learn from successful initiatives, and for the PCGs to have the opportunity to develop in four stages where necessary. It is envisaged that PCGs will:

- contribute to the Health Authority's health improvement programme;
- promote the health of the local population;
- commission health services;
- monitor performance against service agreements with NHS Trusts;
- develop primary care;
- better integrate primary and community health services and work more closely with social services.

Butler and Rowland (1998) consider that the success of this bold initiative will depend to a considerable degree upon the support of people working in primary care and its ability to demonstrate local accountability. One group of professionals mentioned specifically in the 1997 white paper, in terms of partnership, are community nurses.

Here the white paper opens up new horizons for community nurses; for the first time nurses will be members of PCGs and thus part of the decision making and commissioning processes. There will, however, be limits to this power. As the process of setting up these groups is decided it looks certain that GPs will both nominate the chair and hold the majority of seats (O'Dowd 1998; Willis 1998), and the members of the professions allied to medicine feel almost ignored (Gould 1998). Despite these reservations there is now a real opportunity for community nurses to make a difference by influencing health care and health promotion at local level.

Enshrined in current statements of policy is the acknowledgement that health and social care needs are intertwined. *Our Healthier Nation* (DoH 1998) is a green paper (and therefore a consultation document) concerned with public health policy. It was published in February 1998 and accepts explicitly that social disadvantage must be addressed in order to tackle inequalities in health. Air pollution, poverty, low wages, unemployment, poor housing, crime and disorder are all cited as problems requiring wide-ranging action, involving partnerships between the public, private and voluntary sectors. Whilst the paper has been welcomed as a serious attempt to shift the policy agenda from health care towards health, there are concerns about the breadth of the strategy (Hunter 1998) and the lack of attention to the details of implementation (Peckham *et al.* 1998).

However, this is an important document because much of the work of community health nurses,

especially health visitors, takes place on the boundaries between health and social care. Indeed, there have been recent media reports that health visitors (perhaps under the wing of the Home Office) might play a lead role in an initiative to promote positive parenting and prevent social exclusion amongst disadvantaged sections of society (*Nursing Times* 1998a and 1998b). Whilst many would welcome official recognition of the positive impact that long-term preventative work can have health visitors will have to consider the profound implications of this proposal. Not the least of these is how such a radical extension of their work might affect public acceptance of their more traditional activities.

Fundholding by GPs was heralded as the cornerstone of the 1990 NHS reform, and 60% of patients are registered with a fundholding GP. To date, evaluations of the fundholding schemes have focused on prescribing practices, budget control and waiting list times, and the differential between non-fundholding and fundholding practices in terms of the range of services offered. Thistlethwaite (1997) suggested that:

> 'In fact, progress in intersectoral collaboration may well be a better test of the theory and practice of fundholding than any of the more obvious issues which have been brought to public attention.'

In the new NHS structures it is envisaged that PCGs will be involved with Health Authorities and NHS Trusts in a national performance framework which is designed to reflect health improvement, fair access, effective delivery of appropriate health care, efficiency (value for money), the patient's experience and health outcomes. In addition, there is the intention to set up a National Institute for Clinical Excellence in order to produce and disseminate effective strategies to underpin these aspects of evaluation (DoH 1997a, p. 66 and p. 58).

These movements in policy (PCGs, wider types of service evaluation, an acceptance of the impact of social factors on health, and the involvement of nurses in the commissioning of care) could herald a period of positive change in community nursing, or perhaps just be remembered as a false dawn. It is as yet too early for community nurses to make their judgements. However, it is with hope and some optimism that we wait to see the unfolding of new models of service delivery and their impact on patients and clients.

Patients and clients have not remained untouched by the structural and policy changes experienced by the NHS. The Patients' Charter (DoH 1992), and media debates on the provision of health and social care have increased the public's awareness of health-related matters. The emphasis on patients and clients as consumers or service users, with expectations that deserve to be respected, has focused the minds of many nurses on issues of quality of care. There have been numerous attempts to capture consumer views and to measure satisfaction with services (Poulton 1997), and a new national survey of patient and user experience forms an important part of the proposals contained in *The New NHS*. The white paper also states that it expects health authorities 'to play a strong role in communicating with local people and ensuring public involvement' (p. 29).

Central commitment to the consumer view is further evidenced by the fact that the National Health Service Executive finances the National Association of Patient Participation (NAPP). The prime purpose of NAPP is to help in the setting up of patient participation groups. The functions of the groups vary, but the greatest challenge is to devise ways to encourage patients and clients to become more involved and to play an active role in decisions which affect their treatment and care. This idea fits very comfortably with the current thinking on health policy. However, a review of the literature on this subject, 'Partnerships with patients: the pros and cons of shared clinical decision making' (Coulter 1997), reminds us that the origins of the ideas on partnership come primarily from the academic community.

There is now a very deliberate attempt to bring objectivity into service planning and delivery, and research has a key role to play in this. Since 1991 we have had an NHS central Research and Development Committee in England which has the explicit goal of working towards a 'knowledge based health service'. Against this policy background, a number of serious questions are being asked concerning how we make best use of health care resources, and how we ensure a high quality of care for our customers. Health economists are now centre stage and are asking questions which take us back to basics: which treatment works and how do

you change the behaviour of health care providers and make them more aware of the most effective treatments? (Maynard 1993).

The widespread variation in medical practice noted amongst doctors highlights the weakness of the scientific basis of clinical practice, and the same variation is observable within nursing practice too. If patients and clients are to be offered choice it is important for all concerned that the choices offered reflect the best available care and treatment.

During the last five years the evidence-based practice movement has been gaining momentum. The aspiration is to provide care and treatment based upon the best available evidence. Much of the literature in this field focuses upon medical decision making, primarily because of the high costs of drugs and medical treatments and the stronger research base. However the ideology of the movement is very much in tune with debates at the centre of nursing practice. Since the 1970s the Royal College of Nursing has claimed the quality of patient care could be improved through the implementation of nursing research, and this belief may now be attracting powerful support. For instance, speaking at a conference in December 1997, Baroness Jay said concerning evidence-based care (DoH 1997b):

'The aim of this government is to improve the health and well-being of the population. Research is a powerful and essential way of achieving this objective. Research provides the basis for prioritising problems and identifying solutions. It is integral to good patient care and delivery of effective health services. It is essential to any strategy to improve health and health care. We all recognise the need for research which:

- develops the evidence base for nursing interventions
- identifies effective nursing practice in different settings
- considers the human resources issues around nurse training, continuing education and workforce planning'.

Although there is an accepted need for a strong body of evidence to underpin the practice of nursing little is known about some aspects of nursing practice. Community health nursing and primary health care in general are very under-researched areas. Despite the absence of scientific evidence underpinning many practices, care and treatment still have to be provided to patients and clients. It may help to think of evidence in a hierarchical way. At the top of the hierarchy is the evidence generated from well conducted, randomised, controlled trials (RCTs), although these are almost non-existent in community health nursing. At the bottom of the hierarchy is an individual practitioner's opinion. Much nursing practice is informed by consensus, that is the opinions of a range of well informed individuals, and sometimes this opinion is formalised into protocols or guidelines. Similarly, practice may be informed by research which is observational, or of a more qualitative kind. As scientific evidence is valued at all levels of the health service as the basis for decision making, it is particularly important for purchasers and managers as well as clinicians to grasp the principles involved in evaluating evidence; a particularly helpful text is *Evidence-based health care* (Muir Gray 1997).

Whilst practice based on strong evidence is the ideal, where the evidence exists there are often barriers to its implementation. We can take as an example the case of a high volume, high cost activity where good evidence exists to guide practice: the management of leg ulcers. There are many constraints to employing best practice, and lack of knowledge on the part of community health nurses is only a small part of the problem. In a study conducted by Luker and Kenrick (1995) patient non-compliance was cited as the most common constraining factor on best practice. Understaffing, consultant's instructions, inability to obtain preferred products were other reasons offered for not using the best available treatment, and only 15% of respondents in this study cited their own lack of knowledge as a constraint. It is clearly important to address the knowledge-related needs of community health nurses, but it must be remembered that education alone is not a panacea. The organisational context of the work plays a major role in promoting a climate for good practice in community health nursing.

REFERENCES

Butler, T. & Roland, M. (1998) How will primary care groups work? *British Medical Journal*, **316**, 214.

Coulter, A. (1997) Partnerships with patients: the pros and cons of shared clinical decision making, *Journal of Health Services Research and Policy*, **12** (2), 112–21.

Department of Health (1992) *The Patients' Charter*. HMSO, London.

Department of Health (1996a) *Primary care: The future – choice and opportunity*. Department of Health, London.

Department of Health (1996b) *Primary care: Delivering the future*. Department of Health, London.

Department of Health (1997a) *The New NHS – Modern, Dependable*. HMSO, London.

Department of Health (1997b) *NURSES WILL MAKE A MASSIVE CONTRIBUTION TO THE NEW NHS*. Press Release 97/391 Department of Health, London.

Department of Health (1998) *Our Healthier Nation: A Contract for Health*. HMSO, London.

Gould, M. (1998) Absent friends. *Health Service Journal*, **108** (5614), 13.

HMSO (1990) *NHS and Community Care Act*. HMSO, London.

Hunter, D. (1998) Cruel illusions of progress. *Health Service Journal*. **108** (5598), 22.

Luker, K.A. & Kenrick, M. (1995) Towards knowledge based practice, an evaluation of a method of dissemination. *International Journal of Nursing Studies*. **32** (1), 59–67.

Maynard, A. (1993) A suitable case for treatment. *Times Higher Educational Supplement*, 15 January, (1054), 11.

Muir Gray, J.A. (1997) *Evidence-based health care*. Churchill Livingstone, Edinburgh.

NHS Executive (1995) *Priorities and planning guidance for the NHS 1996/97*, NHSE, Leeds.

Nursing Times (1998a) Comment. *Nursing Times*, **94** (27), 3, 5.

Nursing Times (1998b) This Week. *Nursing Times*, **94** (29), 7.

O'Dowd, A. (1998) 'Stagnation' looms as PCG's sideline nurses. *Nursing Times*, **94** (26), 10.

Peckham, S., Turton, P. & Taylor, P. (1998) The missing link. *Health Service Journal*, **108**, 22–24.

Poulton, B.C. (1997) Consumer feedback and determining satisfaction with services. In: *Achieving Quality in Community Health Care Nursing* (ed. C. Mason), pp. 31–54. Macmillan, London.

Thistlethwaite, P. (1997) (ed.) *Finding common cause: Impressions of links between GP fundholders and five social services departments in England*. Association of County Councils, London, p. 3.

Wilkin, D., Butler, T. & Coulter, A. (1997) *New Models of Primary Care: Developing the Future.* National Primary Care Research and Development Centre, Manchester.

Willis, J. (1998) Last among equals. *Nursing Times*, **94** (26), 16.

Part 1

The Child and the Family

1

Families and Social Policy
Isabelle Brodie and David Barrett

1.1 INTRODUCTION

Whilst historical evidence suggests that there has always been considerable variety in the way in which families are organised, more recent changes such as the increased number of single parent households, and a rise in the number of marriages ending in divorce, require further shifts in our understanding of the many forms families may take.

However, in the UK it continues to be expected that children will be brought up and cared for within families. Furthermore that parents are responsible for their children, and that parents should ensure children behave in a way that is acceptable to the community and society at large. Consequently, many of the concerns which are expressed about, for example, disruptive behaviour in the classroom or delinquency within the community, are followed by criticisms concerning parental irresponsibility. When it is considered that children are not being appropriately cared for, or when relationships between parents and children break down, then the state – via professional agencies such as social services – will intervene to look after children and young people.

The relationship between parents, children and the state is a complex one, informed by the interaction of demographic, economic and cultural conditions. The purpose of this chapter is to examine evidence concerning the relationship between government policy and legislation relating to different patterns of family life in the UK today. It begins by considering the way in which 'families', and specifically the relationships between parents and their children, are defined and the meanings which are attached to them. The vary-

ing perceptions of children, who are central to our understanding of family life, according to the social, political and economic context are considered. The chapter then examines how the positive and negative meanings attached to different family forms are reflected in social policy aimed at families. It will be argued that such policies do not always take sufficient account of the social, cultural and economic changes which affect the nature of family life.

It is important to emphasise that within the present space it is impossible to cover the details of every aspect of social policy. Particular attention will be given to the experiences of children and families who are defined as being 'in need', and also to the area of antidiscriminatory practice.

1.2 DEFINING 'THE FAMILY'

Gittings (1993) argues that there is no such thing as 'the' family, and that no single form of the family has ever existed. Not only have death, disease and separation afflicted families in all periods of history, but the way in which families are constituted is inextricably linked to wider social, economic and cultural relationships. The biological link which exists between parents and their children is subject to social and cultural interpretation which will vary in different historical circumstances.

Notwithstanding the historical evidence, however, the *belief* that there is such a thing as 'the' family, and that it is essentially good, has exercised a powerful influence in social life and in the development of

9

social policy. Furthermore, this belief centres around a particular kind of family structure. As Frost and Stein (1989) comment, policies have typically been designed 'around the concept of two parents and their children sharing a discrete family home' (p. 4). It is also associated with a particular structuring of gender roles within a household, namely that men should provide financially for the household while women carry out domestic and caring roles. This model continues to be perceived favourably. One research study, examining perceptions of family life, found that two coherent groups could be identified. The larger group expressed support for conventional marriage and a division of labour within the home in which women were primarily responsible for domestic work and child care. However, the second group, described as 'alternative', diverged from this by emphasising persona; choice and the negotiation of roles within the home, including the rejection of the view that men should be the main economic providers. Support for this second model was greatest among African-Caribbeans brought up in the UK, and least among other non-European ethnic groups (Dench 1996). As the evidence outlined below will demonstrate, despite its dominance, the nuclear family model is very far from being the experience of all children and parents living in the UK today.

Changes during the twentieth century

During the twentieth century huge changes in social life have taken place. Especially important are changes in the pattern of employment, for example, the high proportion of women now working and the sustained high levels of unemployment. Such changes might have been expected to affect the nature of economic and gender roles within the home. Ferri and Smith's research (1996) has suggested that fathers in households where both partners work full-time are more likely than those in other employment situations to share child care and domestic work. However, the balance of evidence suggests that women continue to be responsible for most of the work associated with childrearing (Halsey 1993). Similarly social policy has tended to reinforce the position of women as carers within the home.

Another major shift has been in the number of people of different ethnic groups who live in the UK. The 1991 census showed that people of minority ethnic origin form 5.5% of the population of the UK

as a whole, and the majority of these live in England. In terms of family size, for example, the census showed that of the white ethnic group, almost 30% of families are childless couples, while 33% of Bangladeshi families are in large families containing three or more adults plus one or more child (Butt & Mirza 1996). This has important implications for our understanding of families, however the diversity of ethnic groups often goes unrecognised or is poorly understood by policy makers.

Many other changes have also taken place. Fertility rates have declined in 30 years from a post-war peak of 2.9 to 1.8 per woman. Rates of marriage have reduced dramatically, with a concomitant increase in cohabitation, and since 1961 there has been a six-fold increase in the rate of divorce. During the same period there has been a rapid increase in the number of births occurring outside marriage; in 1993 around a third of births were to unmarried women (OPCS 1995). However, a higher proportion of such births are to unmarried couples living at the same address who are assumed to be cohabiting.

An important consequence of these changes has been an increase in the number of lone parent families. One in five families with dependent children are headed by a lone parent compared to one in twelve in 1971. The majority of lone parent families are headed by mothers, just over half are divorced and a further third single. The number of single (never married) mothers has grown fastest, from 23% in 1981 to 35% in 1990. About one in thirteen lone parent families are of minority ethnic origin. Of these, about one in two is of West Indian origin, one in eight of Indian, Pakistani/Bangladeshi and mixed origin, and one in nine of African origin (Haskey 1991).

It is important, when discussing the family, to place such information in perspective: for example, seven out of ten families with dependent children continue to be headed by both birth parents. We must, therefore, be cautious of any over-enthusiastic attempts to underplay the importance of the 'nuclear' family. However, the evidence does emphasise the wide variation in family experience, and suggests that families are much more liable to undergo changes in structure through divorce and separation. The family life cycle has also been altered by demographic changes which mean that there are many more elderly people. Although there are a significant number of male carers, it is most often the female members of a family who will be called upon to undertake the work of caring for elderly or unwell relatives (Thompson, in Dean 1995). The dilemmas associated with such responsibilities have been exacerbated by legislation placing increased emphasis on care in the community. The assumption that there is a pool of available carers stands at odds with the increased number of women who work on a full- or part-time basis, and with the changing perceptions regarding the nature of gender roles. The acceptance that care provided by kin is a 'good thing' can also obscure the complex – and sometimes abusive – nature of familial relationships.

1.3 THE SOCIAL CONSTRUCTION OF CHILDHOOD

Most recent feminist analyses have drawn attention to the importance of gender relationships in understanding families, but such work has been criticised for the fact that children are frequently absent in feminist descriptions of family relationships. It is therefore important to examine the way in which children are defined in UK society, specifically in relation to the family. Changes in family structure, especially the rise in the number of births outside marriage and increased rate of divorce, mean that parenthood, specifically fatherhood, is often a transitory or part-time experience. It has been argued that one consequence of this is a greater investment in children and childhood (Jenks 1996). Certainly, it is now taken for granted that childhood is an important stage in the life cycle, and separate consideration must therefore be given to the way in which this is currently constructed. In the same way that images and ideologies of families vary historically, socially and culturally, so our understanding of childhood is equally variable.

The point in history when childhood became viewed as a part of life which was qualitatively different to that of adults remains debatable (Pinchbeck & Hewitt 1973; Aries 1996). Generally, it is agreed that from the seventeenth century childhood became imbued with special meaning, and increasingly it was felt that children were possessed of special characteristics and needed to be cared for and nurtured in a particular way. With this change in thinking came an increase in the attention given to childhood by philosophers and policy-makers. In the late nineteenth century and throughout the twentieth century, children have been a major focus of social policy, and a wide range of professionals are now responsible for safeguarding children and ensuring that they have the best possible social and educational experience.

Diversity in family life

As there is immense diversity in family life, so there are multiple experiences of childhood. Childhoods vary according to a range of factors including class, age, gender and ethnicity, urban or rural location and disability or ill-health (Frost & Stein 1989; James & Jenks 1996). However, an ideology of childhood, based on a perception of children as being essentially innocent and dependent, continues to be projected through the media and also through social policy. Indeed, the importance attached to childhood as a time of innocence is reflected in public horror at the murder of James Bulger by two young children (James & Jenks 1996). The relative powerlessness of children in relation to adults is reflected in legislation which prevents children from participating in aspects of public life which are defined as 'adult' – for example, employment, voting and so on. Contradictions which persist in our understanding of childhood are highlighted by the variations in the age limits set for different types of behaviour; for example, many young people leave school and begin work at the age of 16 but cannot hold a driving licence until they are aged 17, or marry without parental consent until they are 18. Many younger children actually perform 'adult' roles, for example in caring for sick or disabled parents.

Increasingly, however, a discourse has emerged within social policy which focuses upon 'children's rights'. This is a wide-ranging concept, which is most comprehensively defined within the United Nations Convention on the Rights of the Child. The Convention covers the four broad themes of survival, development, protection and participation, and emphasises that the welfare of the child is paramount (Lindsay 1992). These principles are also embedded in the 1989 Children Act in England and Wales, which also places a duty on local authorities to consult children, taking account of their age and level of understanding, when making decisions which concern them.

Inevitably, the experience of children within families has been affected by other changes in family life. In 1991 the General Household Survey estimated that 8% of all families with dependent children (whether married or cohabiting) contained at least one stepchild. If children were to continue to become stepchildren at the same rate, then about one in eight would live at some stage of their lives in a family where their birth parent had either remarried or formed a new partnership (Haskey 1993). The effects of parental divorce and single parenthood on children, provoke disagreement but there is some evidence that children who experience the breakdown of parental relationships are at risk of adverse behavioural, educational and health outcomes in comparison with children whose families remain intact (Cockett & Tripp 1994). Such outcomes are not inevitable for all children who experience such disruption.

1.4 IDEOLOGIES OF THE FAMILY

As Frost and Stein (1989) have pointed out, the importance of the nuclear family is not lessened because it is not the lifestyle of most people in our society, and it continues to have considerable ideological and political significance. Politicians on both the Left and the Right have promoted the nuclear family as the 'best' context for parents to bring up their children (Dean 1995). Some, most notably Charles Murray, have argued that there is a direct link between the demise of the nuclear family and the growth of a social and economic 'underclass' (Murray 1996). Under the Conservative governments of Margaret Thatcher and John Major, nuclear families were perceived to promote traditional values. Such analysis is often rooted in the idea of a golden age of family life, and does not take account of the way in which family structure is mediated by historical, cultural and economic circumstances. This family ideal is underpinned by a view of the family as a safe place where children are brought up by responsible parents. When problems occur, these are attributed to the deficiencies of individuals rather than the policies of the state.

Non-conforming families

Families which do not conform to the nuclear family have been subject to considerable criticism, for

example Dennis and Erdos (1993) claim that the absence of fathers from many households can be directly linked to an increase in antisocial behaviour. Many important social problems, such as crime and substance misuse, have been blamed by politicians and the media on the *irresponsibility* of parents towards their children, and a number of policies have placed increasing emphasis on the role of the parent for ensuring that children and young people do not cause trouble in local communities. In some areas, 'curfews' have been introduced, requiring parents to ensure that young children are at home after a certain time. Attempts have also been made to reinforce the law concerning the financial responsibilities of absent parents – usually fathers – for their children. The Child Support Act 1992 established a formula to assess the extent of an absent parent's liability to support a dependent child with whom he or she does not live, while the Child Support Agency (CSA) was given the power to assess, collect and enforce child maintenance payments (Dean 1995). While most people agree that parents have ongoing responsibilities for their children, the introduction of the CSA is problematic when an individual has responsibilities to a second family and to stepchildren.

Education legislation, beginning with the Education Reform Act 1988, has also tended to emphasise the importance of the parents' role in relation to their child's schooling. For example, the policy of 'parental choice' aimed to allow parents to select the school that their child attends – contrary to the idea of children's rights, especially as there is no requirement within the legislation that children should be consulted about such decisions. The tensions which exist between different aspects of social policy as it affects families are thus highlighted. At the same time as such policies appear to promote parents' rights, research evidence suggests that some parents and children will be advantaged more than others. Parents with access to more information about schools – what is sometimes termed 'cultural capital' – and with more resources to meet travel and other costs are ultimately in a better position to 'choose' than those who lack such advantages (see, for example, Smith and Noble 1995). 'Parental choice' of schools is a good example of the way in which social policies interact with families' social and economic position, and consequently can have unequal effects.

The influence of the white nuclear family as a model of family life is not only evident in government policy, it is also evident in professional decision making. For example, some checklists of risk factors relating to child protection have included parental status as a significant factor and suggest that children living in stepfamilies may be at greater risk of abuse (for example, Greenland 1987). This approach and others like it are not only based on a mis-understanding of research evidence, but apparently also on the view that non-nuclear families are more likely to be 'dysfunctional' (Brodie & Berridge 1996a). Similarly, professionals do not always take account of the needs of minority ethnic families; the idea that black families and communities are close knit and will therefore provide the necessary support for families experiencing difficulties can mitigate against effective service provision (Barn *et al.* 1997).

A flawed ideology?

Criticism of the ideology surrounding the nuclear family has frequently centred on the fact that this model fails to take account of the inequalities in power which exist within families. There is now much greater acceptance of the feminist position that these inadequacies relate to gender, and that the family is an institution based on patriarchy, that is, the exercise of male power (Gittings 1993). It is only by recognising the existence of these relationships that action can be taken in cases where that power is abused, for example in the area of domestic violence.

Social policy has failed to take account of changes in gender relationships within families in a number of ways. Inequalities in the economy mean that women tend to be concentrated in part-time or temporary jobs and are more likely to experience low pay. A high proportion of mothers in paid employment also work 'unsocial' hours in the evenings or at weekends (Ferri & Smith 1996). This situation is especially serious for lone parent families, which tend to be headed by women and are over-represented among the poor. Lone mothers are more likely to be unemployed and less likely to have access to part-time work than married women, and this differential has increased over time (Office for National Statistics 1996). The lack of affordable, good quality child care also means that they are disadvantaged as single parents, as in two parent households fathers are able to share responsibility for child care (Kumar 1993). Most women continue to rely heavily on family and friends to look after their children, with only a tiny minority having

access to child care provided by their employers (OPCS 1993; Ferri & Smith 1996). This has become a matter of considerable controversy under the Labour government, which in late 1997 confirmed that lone parent benefit would be cut as part of an initiative to encourage lone parents into work (*The Times*, 20 November 1997). Without the availability of appro-priate child care, this is not a realistic option for many lone mothers and this policy may potentially further impoverish some families.

At the same time that 'the family' has been held up as desirable, evidence suggests that other areas of policy have combined to erode the quality of family life. Utting (1995) states that there has been 'a policy drift under successive governments away from recognising the costs and demands of parenthood' and links this to growing inequality in society more generally. Bradshaw (1997) argues that families with children have been particularly adversely affected. Kumar (1993) has shown that child poverty has increased dramatically since 1979, and specifically that the number of children living in poverty has increased from 10% to over 30% of the total UK population. Children from minority ethnic groups are particularly affected. Families who are poor are more likely to live in inadequate housing and to experience poor health. Such information suggests that there is often a gap between political rhetoric and the day-to-day realities and practices of family life.

1.5 FAMILIES AND CHILDREN IN NEED

The provision of services to families who are experiencing difficulties is an important part of social policy and the Children Act 1989 is particularly sig-nificant in providing a framework for this. The Act was introduced in the wake of a series of crises con-cerning the care and protection of children during the 1970s and 1980s, involving cases of serious physical and sexual abuse. A substantial body of research had also demonstrated shortcomings in state care for children (Department for Health and Social Security 1985). Importantly, the Act differs in important ways from other social care legislation introduced during the same period, most notably that relating to com-munity care and criminal justice (Packman & Jordan

1991) and in several respects can be argued to present a very different model of family relationships.

The main purpose of the legislation is described as promoting and safeguarding the welfare of children, and it introduces a number of new ideas and concepts. One of the most important changes made by the Children Act 1989 relates to its definition of 'children in need'. Section 17 (10) of the Act defines 'children in need' as follows:

'. . . a child shall be taken to be in need if:

(a)   he is unlikely to achieve or maintain, or to have the opportunity of achieving or maintaining, a reasonable standard of health or development without the provision for him of services by a local authority under this Part;

(b)   his health or development is likely to be significantly impaired, or further impaired, without the provision of such services; or

(c)   he is disabled.' (HMSO 1989)

The total number of children in need is estimated to be in the region of 350,000 children at any one time, but this group is by no means static and children and families will move in and out of this category. Emphasis has increasingly been given to the development of inter-agency responses to families experiencing difficulties, and this approach is embedded within the Children Act 1989 and other legislation relating to children. Local authorities are also required to produce comprehensive 'Children's Service Plans' which are intended to produce more integrated policy and practice.

Partnership with parents

In regard to the relationships between parents and their children and the state, the Act is based on the concept of partnership. It recognises that children are best looked after within their families, and that 'unwarranted intervention' in family life should be avoided. Even when family breakdown occurs, parents retain 'parental responsibility', which is the 'collection of duties, rights and authority which a parent has in respect of his child' (DoH, 1989). The idea that the state does not simply take over these responsibilities is reflected in the language; children are no longer 'taken into care' but are 'looked after' by the local authority. However, partnership with parents is a concept which is not always easy to

implement. It has been argued that services continue to be focused on 'crisis intervention', specifically in the area of child protection, and that insufficient emphasis is given to prevention and support for parents experiencing difficulties (DoH 1995). Problems of partnerships may be particularly acute in cases where children have been abused or where parents appear to reject children. In one study of children living apart from their parents it was found that, while the importance of partnership was recognised by professionals, judgements about the quality of parenting meant that in some cases little or no work was undertaken to maintain parental involvement, especially that of fathers (Masson *et al.* 1997). Chapter 6 considers in more detail the complex issues surrounding children at risk.

Culture and ethnicity

The Children Act 1989 places a new duty on local authorities to 'give due consideration' to children's 'religious persuasion, racial origin and cultural and linguistic background' when making decisions about them (section 22 (5) (*c*)). This has been viewed as an important step forward in taking account of ethnic diversity. However, a number of difficulties remain, not least that families from some minority ethnic groups are often amongst the poorest in British society. Racism continues to pervade many areas of social life and research has found, for example, that children from minority ethnic groups experience considerable racist abuse at school (Troyna & Hatcher 1992). Some children, most notably African-Caribbean boys, are at much greater risk of exclusion from school (Brodie & Berridge 1996b; Gillborn & Gipps 1996).

There are also difficulties relating to the delivery of services to minority ethnic groups. There has frequently been a failure to distinguish between the needs of different ethnic groups, and it has been argued that policy is too generalised in this respect (Barn *et al.* 1977). Good practice can be fragmentary, and professionals can easily flounder through a lack of information. In some areas of social care, individuals from ethnic communities have been unable to access services, and this has sometimes been perceived as an indication of lack of need or self-sufficiency.

Fitches (1995), discussing the provision of health services to Asian families, emphasises that professionals must take account of – and where possible adapt – existing cultural practices. For example, in Bangladeshi families, concepts of mental and physical disability are often very different. If families from different ethnic groups are to be given appropriate support in such circumstances, it is essential that information is available to professionals and that good practice is shared. There is also a need for more and better research.

Children living away from home

There is a long tradition of the removal of children from their families. The distinction between good and bad families has meant that when the state has intervened in family life it has removed children elsewhere. Thus the history of child welfare is largely that of the removal of children to a wide range of institutions for correction and care (Frost & Stein 1989). The Children Act 1989, however, emphasises the prevention of family breakdown and professional work to maintain families, but still a small proportion of children will at some point live apart from their parents in foster or residential care. This number has greatly reduced since the introduction of the Act and in 1995–96 some 50,000 children were looked after; the majority (30,000) by foster carers, a further 8000 were living in residential accommodation, and the remainder were looked after while remaining within their own families.

Research evidence suggests that children looked after include some of the most disadvantaged children living in Britain today. Their families are more likely to be dependent on state benefits, to be headed by a single parent and to be living in poor housing (Bebbington & Miles 1989). Many of those children who are looked after in foster and residential care have been abused and some will present extremely challenging behaviour (Berridge 1997; Berridge & Brodie 1997). Most children who are looked after spend only a short time apart from their parents and will return home within a few weeks. It is therefore essential that sufficient support services are available to families when young people return, and that agencies work together effectively to facilitate this.

Children in trouble

The link between childhood and innocence makes the development of policy relating to children who commit criminal offences or who are more generally perceived to be 'troublesome' especially problematic. For example, in the run up to the 1997 general election the hitherto almost traditional difference between the response of the political Left and Right to young people who commit crimes appeared to collapse altogether. The mood was one of 'listen less and punish more', with an emphasis on the need for more responsible parenting. However, in an era of changing concepts of families the definition of what a more responsible parent might be remains problematic.

The moral problem of troublesome youth is also increasingly complex (see Kroll & Barrett 1995, for fuller discussion) and the political point scoring over who is toughest on crime be it Left or Right does little to help. Already the 'bad' versus 'sad' and 'just deserts' versus 'welfare' debates produce both contradictory images and responses towards young offenders (Cavadino & Dignon 1992). Moral outrage in itself has not so far proved constructive (Stevenson 1993).

In particular, recognition of the troubled backgrounds of many young offenders is not easily obscured. Research has shown that 'the tangled roots of delinquency' are to be found in a complex interrelationship between poor economic circumstances and living environment, educational and behavioural difficulties, relationship problems and care-related factors, such as poor parental supervision (Utting et al. 1993).

In policy terms, the pendulum appears to have been stuck for some time at John Major's maxim of 'understand less and condemn more'. More creative responses are required but these would involve considerable political risk-taking; as no Minister wishes to be labelled 'soft on crime' so the cycle is perpetuated. New conceptual models such as mentoring and multi-disciplinary responses may not be the panacea once thought, but they are, at least, introducing alternative approaches to what has been an increasingly gloomy scenario concerning young offenders. In view of the increasing responsibilities and duties placed on young offenders and their families by the Criminal Justice Acts of the early 1990s, it should be remembered that young offenders themselves have rights, as enshrined particularly in the Children Act 1989.

1.6 CONCLUSION

This chapter has attempted to provide some insight into the complex workings of contemporary families in Britain and their relationships with the state. Whilst in a short discussion it is impossible to do full justice to the rich diversity of family life which exists in Britain at the end of the twentieth century, it is clear that, in terms of the policies which have helped structure family life, there are many tensions and contradictions. Many of these result from the fact that, while the white nuclear family continues to exercise considerable social and political influence, the nature of family life is very much more complex. Crucially, families must be considered not only in terms of a particular cultural milieu, but also taking account of the relationships which are constituted by age and gender.

The governments of Margaret Thatcher and John Major radically changed the face of social policy relating to families. The Labour government proposes a new set of changes which will no doubt have an impact on the shape of family life and present new challenges for professionals responsible for providing support to parents and their children. In the light of this it is essential that professionals, irrespective of their role, keep up to date with both social and professional developments in order to facilitate best practice in the fields of health and social care.

REFERENCES

Aries, P. (1996) *Centuries of Childhood.* Pimlico, London.

Barn, R., Sinclair, R. & Ferdinand, D. (1997) *Acting on Principle.* BAAF/Commission for Racial Equality, London.

Bebbington, A. & Miles, J. (1989) The background of children who enter local authority care. *British Journal of Social Work,* **19** (5), 349–69.

Berridge, D. (1997) *Foster Care: A Research Review.* The Stationery Office, London.

Berridge, D. & Brodie, I. (1998) *Children's Homes Revisited.* Jessica Kingsley, London.

Bradshaw, J. (1997) Poverty and deprivation in the United Kingdom. *Research, Policy and Planning,* **14** (1), 4–14.

Brodie, I. & Berridge, D. (1996a) *Child Abuse and Step-families. Fact File 4.* National Stepfamily Association, London.

Brodie, I. & Berridge, D. (1996b) *Exclusion from School: Research Themes and Issues.* University of Luton Press.

Butt, J. & Mirza, K. (1996) *Social Care and Black Communities.* HMSO, London.

Cavadino, M. & Dignon, J. (1992) From System Disaster to Systems Management. In: *The Penal System: An Introduction* (eds M. Cavadino & J. Dignon), Sage, London.

Cockett, C. & Tripp, J. (1994) *Family Breakdown and its Impact on Children.* Family Policy Studies Unit, London.

Dean, H. (ed.) (1995) *Parents' Duties, Children's Debts.* Arena, Aldershot.

Dench, G. (1996) *Exploring variations in men's family roles,* Joseph Rowntree Findings 99. Joseph Rowntree Foundation, York.

Dennis, N. & Erdos, G. (1993) *Families without Fatherhood.* ILEA Health and Welfare Unit, London.

Department of Health and Social Security (1985) *Social Work Decisions in Child Care.* HMSO, London.

Department of Health (1989) *An introduction to the Children Act 1989.* HMSO, London.

Department of Health (1995) *Child Protection: Messages from Research.* HMSO, London.

Ferri, E. & Smith, K. (1996) *Parenting in the 1990s.* Family Policy Studies Centre Joseph Rowntree Foundation.

Fitches, R. (1995) Ethnicity, culture and parenthood. In: *Parents' Duties, Children's Debts* (ed. H. Dean). Arena, Aldershot.

Frost, N. & Stein, M. (1989) *The Politics of Child Welfare.* Harvester Wheatsheaf, Hemel Hempstead.

Gillborn, D. & Gipps, C. (1996) *Recent Research on the Achievements of Ethnic Minority Pupils.* HMSO, London.

Gittings, D. (1993) *The Family in Question.* Macmillan, London.

Greenland, C. (1987) Child protection: the law and dangerousness. In: *Child Abuse* (ed. S. Stevenson). Harvester Wheatsheaf, Hemel Hempstead.

Halsey, A. (1993) Changes in the family. *Children and Society,* **7** (2), 125–36.

Haskey, J. (1991) Estimated numbers and demographic characteristics of one-parent families in Great Britain. *Population Trends,* **65**, HMSO, London, pp. 35–43.

Haskey, J. (1993) Trends in the numbers of one-parent families in Great Britain. *Population Trends,* **71**, HMSO, London.

Haskey, J. (1994) Stepfamilies and stepchildren in Great Britain. *Population Trends,* No. 81, Autumn, OPCS.

HMSO (1989) *Children Act.* HMSO, London.

James, A. & Jenks, C. (1996) Public perceptions of childhood criminality. *British Journal of Sociology,* **47** (2), 315–31.

Jenks, C. (1996) *The Sociology of Childhood.* Batsford, London.

Kroll, B. & Barrett, D. (1995) Troublesome children: failure and moral liability. In: *Parents' Duties, Children's Debts* (ed. H. Dean). Arena, Aldershot.

Kumar, U. (1993) *Poverty and Inequality in the UK: The effects on children.* National Children's Bureau, London.

Lindsay, M. (1992) *An Introduction to Children's Rights. Highlight 113.* National Children's Bureau, London.

Masson, J., Harrison, C. & Pavlovic, A. (1997) *Working with children and 'lost' parents: putting partnership into practice.* Joseph Rowntree Foundation, York.

Murray, C. (1996) *Charles Murray and the Underclass: The Developing Debate.* IEA Health and Welfare Unit, London.

Office for National Statistics (1996) *Living in Britain: Results from the 1995 General Household Survey.* HMSO, London.

OPCS (1993) *General Household Survey 1991.* HMSO, London.

OPCS (1995) *Population Trends.* **82**, Winter, HMSO, London.

Packman, J. & Jordan, B. (1991) The Children's Act: looking forward, looking back, *British Journal of Social Work*, **21**, 315–27.

Pinchbeck, I. & Hewitt, M. (1973) *Children in English Society.* Routledge and Kegan Paul, London.

Smith, T. & Noble, M. (1995) *Education Divides.* Child Poverty Action Group, London.

Stevenson, O. (1993) Foreword. In: *Beyond Blame: Child Abuse Tragedies Revisited* (eds P. Reder, S. Duncan and M. Gray). Routledge, London.

The Times, 20 November 1997.

Troyna, B. & Hatcher, R. (1982) *Racism in Children's Lives.* Routledge and Kegan Paul in association with the National Children's Bureau, London.

Utting, D. (1995) *Family and Parenthood: Supporting Families, Preventing Breakdown.* Social Policy Summary 4, Joseph Rowntree Foundation, February, 1995.

Utting, D., Bright, J. & Henricson, C. (1993) *Crime and the Family.* Occasional Paper 16, Family Policy Studies Centre, London.

FURTHER READING

James, A. & Prout, A. (eds) (1996) *Constructing and Reconstructing Childhood.* Falmer, London.

Thompson, D. (1995) Constructing the 'private' carer: Daughters of reform? In: *Parents' Duties, Children's Debts* (ed. H. Dean). Arena, Aldershot.

2

The Developing Child
Kate Cernik

Most societies see children as an investment in the future. Good quality education and children's health care services are frequently viewed as a high priority and are often the subject of political debate. From conception onwards, child health is promoted by the state through the provision of maternity, health visiting and school nursing services, dedicated to ensure that all children reach their maximum potential. This chapter is concerned with some of the recent debates and evidence concerning child health policy in the UK. It outlines the milestones in the development of normal children and considers the promotion of health and development.

2.2 THE DEVELOPMENT OF CHILD HEALTH PROMOTION SERVICES

As the NHS has changed over the last decade in response to health care reforms, so has the way in which child health services are delivered. An understanding of the policies that are currently shaping services is important for those involved in the delivery of services. A thorough analysis and overhaul of services in the UK was undertaken by a joint working party under the chairmanship of Professor David Hall (Hall 1989).

This review into the delivery of child health surveillance (CHS) was indicated for the following reasons:

(1) There was a growing recognition that all health care activities need to be reviewed in the light of productivity and cost effectiveness. Child health surveillance was traditionally carried out by district health authorities using a mixture of systems, some formal, some informal, some serviced by general practitioners, others by clinical medical officers and some by health visitors. Most existing services have been organised along the lines originally suggested by the Court Report 1976.

(2) New methods of evaluating community medicine and epidemiology have developed, resulting in a more rigorous approach to the evaluation of screening tests. The value of screening tests will be described further on in more detail.

(3) Research has shown that sometimes screening can do more harm than good in that the tests may be poor and inaccurate. This causes congestion of referral systems, and sometimes unnecessary procedures.

(4) Consumer sensitivity has changed: parents now expect to be consulted about decisions that affect their children, and may be prepared to challenge professional expertise.

(5) The Education Act (1981), which came about as a result of the Warnock Report, has led away from a labelling or diagnostic approach to children with special needs, towards the provision of descriptive analyses of a child's strengths and weaknesses (statements). This puts a different emphasis on the detection of developmental abnormalities.

(6) The WHO has postulated that too much emphasis has been placed on the detection of defects and not enough on preventive and educational activities (WHO 1978).

Child health services

The current organisation of child health services places prime responsibility for the delivery of the Child Health Promotion Programme (CHP) with the primary care services – health visitors and GPs in particular. Health care reforms in the UK have given GPs a pivotal role in the delivery of health promotion services. General practitioners have been given financial incentives for achieving high levels of immunisation and delivering child health surveillance. This has led to a reduction in the volume of services offered by NHS Trust staff. In addition the services offered by Trusts are moving away from the routine work of child health clinics towards specialist work in other areas, such as audiology or child protection, that is secondary care. Health visitors have become more closely integrated in primary health care teams, and are increasingly the key workers in child health promotion within the team. Many health visitors are now organising such clinics in GP practice premises and immunising infants. Hall (1996) recognises the importance of these developments and recommends that the programme needs to be delivered according to the following key fundamental principles:

- the programme should be based on the principles of primary prevention;
- partnership with parents is essential;
- collaboration with other agencies needs to be developed and maintained;
- any screening procedures used should be rigorous. Pathways for referral should be clear and well audited;
- the programme should be appropriately targeted on those in greatest need;
- there should be a change in emphasis. This should move away from screening and to surveillance;
- all screening or assessment should carry with it an educational value rather than a medical or fault-finding value;
- parent-held records should be used.

The screening debate

The classic definition of screening, by the American Commission on chronic illness, dates back to 1957 and is still helpful today.

> 'The presumptive identification of unrecognised disease or defect by the application of tests, examinations and other procedures, which can be applied rapidly. Screening tests sort out apparently well persons who may have a disease from those who probably do not. A screening test is not intended to be diagnostic.' (Hall 1996)

However, there still remains an important debate as to whether or not the currently used screening tests in child health programmes meet the requirements of modern screening programmes. The Wilson-Jungner principles of screening are now widely accepted as a guide for assessing the value of screening programmes (Figure 2.1).

Hall (1996) concludes that very few of the current screening activities fulfil these criteria and questions the benefits of universal screening. He suggests that health reviews should be viewed as an opportunity for parents to:

- receive reassurance about their child's progress;
- receive information that will help them to promote health, that is anticipatory guidance;
- be given an opportunity to seek expert advice and guidance on problems that the parents perceive as causing difficulties.

Thus health reviews are an opportunity for health professionals to:

- promote health education messages such as immunisation and accident prevention;
- maintain a body of knowledge in the community among parents and professionals, about child health and development.

2.3 WORKING WITH CHILDREN – ISSUES IN ASSESSMENT

For health professionals working in the promotion of child health, a sound knowledge of normal child development is essential in order that they can:

- The condition should be an important one.
- There should be acceptable treatment available for the condition.
- Facilities for diagnosis/treatment should be available.
- The condition should have a latent or early symptomatic stage.
- There should be a suitable test or examination available.
- The test should be acceptable to the population that is to be screened.
- The natural history of the disease should be adequately understood.
- There should be an agreed policy on who to treat as patients.
- The cost of case-finding should be economically worthwhile.
- Case-finding should be a continuous project.

Haggard (1990) adds four further caveats:
- The incidental harm done by screening, and by the information that it gives, should be small in comparison to the total benefits from the screening-assessment-treatment system.
- There should be agreed guidelines on whom to divulge the provisional and final results and on when and how this is best done; there should be transitional counselling support where necessary.
- All screening arrangements should be reviewed from time to time in the light of changes in demography, culture, health services, technologies, and the epidemiology of the target conditions.
- Because cases are not homogeneous, the balance of costs, benefits and risks from screening, assessments and treatments has to be worked out on a stratified basis, and the definition of the target group has to be revised so that this balance is favourable for all strata within it.

Figure 2.1 The principles of screening, (Wilson-Jungner 1968 and Haggard 1990, with acknowledgement to Archives of Disease in Childhood BMA Publications).

- Identify normal development in the children they see, so that deviations from the norm can be managed or appropriately referred. For example, a child who is not saying any words at 18 months may have a hearing problem or a serious developmental delay.
- Use their knowledge to inform and educate parents and give anticipatory guidance where appropriate. For example, babies develop the ability to roll over at around 5–6 months, after this age it is unsafe to leave them unsupervised on a bed or changing table.
- Encourage parents to provide appropriate play and stimulation for their children. For example, very young babies enjoy watching brightly coloured moving objects such as mobiles.
- Prepare parents to help their children become part of the social world, for example help parents choose appropriate pre-school experiences for the children such as playschools or nurseries.
- Help the parents of children with special needs to understand the scope and limitations of their children's abilities.

Most of the child health promotion programme is

delivered by health visitors working in the home and at clinics. Clinics are increasingly located in GP practice premises, although many are still found in Health Care Trust buildings where medical support is provided by community medical officers (CMOs) who are employed by Trusts. Trusts also supply a range of support services for children, including:

- dental care
- speech therapy
- orthoptic services
- chiropody
- services for children with special needs
- continence promotion services
- audiology services
- school nursing
- child protection advice and support.

Trusts may also offer other services such as family therapists, child and adolescent psychiatry, and most of these services are provided through a network of clinics. Parents can attend clinics where their children can have weight checks, developmental checks and parents can have access to advice from health visitors and doctors. In general, parents are satisfied with the services offered in these clinics (Sharpe & Lowenthal 1992).

The main criticisms identified in various recent postal surveys of clinic users are: lack of access because of location or times, lack of privacy, dirty clinics, long waiting times, inattentiveness of staff, the clinic is too busy, rushed or crowded (Sharpe & Lowenthal 1992; Sefi & Grice 1994; Sutton *et al.* 1995). The authors of these reports suggest a number of improvements, which would enhance uptake of services and increase client satisfaction including:

- more privacy in consultations with the health visitor;
- provision of refreshments;
- play area/crèche facilities;
- more convenient times;
- appointments system;
- improved information about service provision.

Assessing development

There are many approaches used to measure children's developmental progress. One of the simplest was developed by Mary Sheridan (1983) and is the basis of much current practice. The emphasis is on identifying normality and making appropriate referrals if there are deviations from the norm. The scheme is based on a description of how the average child develops physical skills and behaviours whereby development is divided into four categories that are described in the order of chronological age:

- gross motor – the ability to walk
- fine motor and vision – hand–eye co–ordination
- speech and language – the ability to communicate
- socialisation – the ability to interact with others.

Developmental milestones

Milestones are events that mark progress in the child's development. Whilst development is a continuous process, most parents will recall key events such as a first smile, the emergence of the first tooth or the first faltering steps that their child makes. Children develop at different paces, so milestones will be achieved at a variety of chronological ages but they do occur in a certain order and within a particular age range. A child that does not achieve key milestones at key ages may be neurologically delayed. Another important char-

acteristic of development is that once skills are developed they are not easily lost, so a child whose development regresses will need further assessment and possible referral. Table 2.1 draws on the work of Sheridan (1983) and Illingworth (1987) in describing important milestones. Important checks recommended by Hall (1996) are shown alongside each stage.

2.4 PREMATURE AND LOW BIRTH WEIGHT BABIES

'Low birth weight' or 'small for dates' babies are usually defined as babies who weigh less than 2500 g when born at 40 weeks gestation. Such babies may have subsequent problems. Middle *et al.* (1996) report that low birth weight children are at higher risk of developmental and educational delay than other children, and that the degree of difficulty is higher in very low weight babies, that is those less than 1500 g at birth.

Pre-term babies may also share these characteristics, but these babies generally 'catch up' with their peers within a year or two. Illingworth (1987) notes the following features of pre-term babies:

- The pre-term baby is likely to sleep far more of the time than does a full term baby.
- The pre-term baby cries less, and the cry may be feeble and short.
- They may move differently – in a less co-ordinated fashion.
- They are reluctant feeders with a poorly developed sucking reflex.
- They have poorer muscle tone.
- In the prone position, the pre-term baby lies flat with the pelvis low and the knees to the side of the abdomen. A full term baby lies with the pelvis high and knees up under the abdomen.
- The pre-term baby's head can be rotated more than that of the full term baby.
- The reflexes are altered and may be more difficult to obtain.

Health professionals need to take account of prematurity when assessing development, but no hard and fast rules can determine how long the effects of prematurity will be manifested. They need to be

Table 2.1 Developmental milestones, child surveillance and health promotion.

Age	Developmental milestones[1]	Screening tests and assessments[2]	Health promotion[3]
Birth	Neonatal reflexes present Muscle tone appropriate When prone with legs pulled under abdomen – pelvis high. In ventral suspension – elbows flex, hips partly extended.	Weight and head circumference Check hips Check testicular descent Physical examinations including heart Check eyes – red reflex Consider audiometry if high risk Phenylketonuria and thyroid test	Cot death/sleep positions Feeding and nutrition Sibling management Safety equipment Hygiene/skin care
2–4 weeks	Can raise head from prone Neonatal reflexes still present Complete head lag on pull to sit Hands closed – grasp reflex present	Physical exam Check for jaundice Check hips Check testicular descent	Immunisation Feeding and nutrition Colic, crying and comfort Sleep management Adult smoking Managing minor ailments
6–8 weeks	Begins to hold head in mid-line Pelvis flat in prone position Hands start to open Follows object with eyes Smiles – begins to vocalise	Begin course of primary immunisation Weighing at parent's request	Feeding and nutrition Weaning Avoid prop feeding Play and stimulation
6–9 months	Begins to bear weight Creeps along floor may stand with support Sits with support Rolls over Holds objects and transfers from hand to hand and uses pincer grasp Puts objects in mouth Babbles, imitates, says Dada/Mama Curious to explore surroundings	Distraction test of hearing Examine eyes for squint Check immunisation status	Safety in the home Choking Nutrition: establishing a healthy diet Dental care Avoiding sunburn Play and stimulation Establishing sleep patterns
13 months	Crawls on hands and feet May walk holding one hand Throws objects to the ground (casting) Understands simple phrases Uses a few words with meaning	MMR vaccination	

Age	Developmental milestones	Checks	Health topics

18–24 months	Walking – may be able to run
	Walks up stairs – holding a hand
	Throws ball or toy without falling
	No longer casts or mouths objects
	Can use a spoon without rotation
	Builds a tower of 3 or 4 bricks
	Takes off gloves/socks
	Holds pencil and scribbles
	Knows up to 20 words – points to parts of the body – jargon and intelligible words – joins words
	Mimics parents
	Becoming dry in the day
		Check walking and gait
		Measure height
		Explain why comprehension is more important than expressed language
		Discuss hearing or vision concerns
		Discuss potential iron deficiency
			Accident prevention
			  – falls
			  – drowning
			  – poisoning
			  – road safety
			  – parental smoking
			Stimulation and play
			Social contact with others
			Management of behaviour – tantrums, sleep, negativity
			Toilet training
			Diet and nutrition
			Footwear

39–42 months	Jumps off step. Stands on one foot
	Rides tricycle
	Can build tower of 9–10 cubes
	Dresses/undresses – may manage buttons
	Draws a man – can copy circle and cross
	May count to 10
	Recites nursery rhymes
	Asks questions – all the time!
	Plays with others – may have imaginary friend
	Dry at night – usually!
		Check all immunisations complete
		Discuss vision hearing and language acquisition – refer if necessary
		Discuss education – any problems which may result in special educational needs
		Measure height – weigh if necessary – plot
		Check testicular descent
		Physical examination if required
			Accidents prevention
			  – fires
			  – drowning
			  – road safety
			Nutrition
			Dental care
			Preparation for school
			Play with other children
			Dealing with minor illness

54–66 months (school entry)	Skips with both feet – hops proficiently May be able to write name – can copy triangle Knows colours, knows own age – may know days of week – repeats 4 digits May tie shoelaces Understands complex speech Speech clear Copes with toileting independently	Discuss parental and teacher concerns Review pre-school records Measure height and plot Test vision using Snellen chart Check hearing with Sweep test	Nutrition and food choices Road safety School routines and sleep Dental health Enuresis (if appropriate)

1 Sheridan 1983; Illingworth 1987.
2 Based on Hall 1996.
3 Based on Hall 1996.

aware of the increased vulnerability of such children and refer appropriately.

Primary prevention

In the main, health professionals need to address the area of improved ante-natal care and the primary prevention of the risk factors associated with pre-term delivery and low birth weight. These risk factors are often associated with socio-economic disadvantage and include: poor maternal nutrition, smoking, mental ill health, poor housing, alcohol and drug misuse. Other factors are early or late motherhood, multiple pregnancy, maternal illness or obstetric difficulties (Illingworth 1987). Many of these are theoretically preventable, although the extent to which individual health workers can have any impact on problems which are more to do with the structure of society is debatable.

2.5 GROWTH

Steady gain in weight and height tells parents that their children are healthy and developing normally and monitoring growth through regular weighing has been a traditional service offered in child health clinics. But how valuable is regular weighing? There is no doubt that failure to thrive or weight loss in babies can indicate serious disease, particularly so if a baby who has been steadily gaining weight suddenly stops growing or loses weight. On the other hand, regular weighing can produce parental anxiety, and may in some circumstances undermine parental self-confidence.

Weight gain is normally plotted on a standard centile chart. These charts are compiled from huge numbers of measurements taken from a range of normal children, and are likely to change from time to time as nutritional standards improve. Hall (1996) recommends the use of the 1990 nine-centile chart (Child Growth Foundation 1990) (see Appendix 2.1). Centile charts offer an opportunity to measure weight, height and head circumference.

Reasons why normal infants may not follow centiles are as follows:

■ feeding techniques – breast fed babies may put on weight at a different rate from infants fed on for-

mula milks (Chapters 8 and 9 consider infant feeding in some detail);
■ minor illness such as colds;
■ adaptation to genetically determined size which may be different at birth;
■ normal ebb and flow in growth rate.

Occasionally growth monitoring may reveal more serious problems: for instance cardiovascular or other disease may be detected by lack of growth. Failure to thrive for reasons of neglect or abuse may be revealed by weighing, either when a child presents at clinic or if a child who is deemed 'at risk' is being monitored. Skuse *et al.* (1995) suggest that failure to thrive is a risk factor for neglect, however previous research has overstated its importance. There is an association between slow weight gain and sudden infant death syndrome. However, the differences are unlikely to be useful for predictive purposes (Williams *et al.* 1990).

The plotting and interpretation of centile charts requires skill and experience. Parental, social, nutritional and other factors may affect growth. Hall (1996) suggests that health professionals should avoid putting undue emphasis on routine weighing – indeed he suggests that there is no reason why parents should not weigh babies and plot the values on centile charts themselves if they wish.

Primary prevention

Primary prevention of failure to thrive through inadequate weight gain is achieved mainly through the promotion of healthy nutrition throughout childhood. Helping parents make healthy food choices for their young children is a role for health visitors. The promotion of breast feeding, advice about formula milk feeding and weaning are important to infants. In the case of older children the school health and educational services have a role to play.

2.6 WALKING

Parents often attach great importance to the development of the ability to walk. The age range at which babies start to walk is wide; from nine months to two years. Ainsworth (1967) suggests that early walking is brought about by a close mother/baby relationship and by cultural and social factors. On the other hand, delayed motor development may be due to familial factors, an unsuitable environment, lack of opportunity, lack of confidence, personality, learning difficulties, physical disability, visual or hearing defects or abnormal modes of locomotion such as bottom shuffling (Illingworth 1987).

By the age of 18 months 97% of children can walk (Neligan & Pridham 1969). In a survey of 410 late walking children; Johnson *et al.* (1990) found that 56% had an associated abnormality diagnosed before the age of three, and, of these, a third had cerebral palsy. Almost half, 46%, were pre-term babies. Another factor which may contribute to a delay in walking may be the use of baby walkers (Crouchman 1986); no long-term delay was associated with their use, however, interference with normal experiences such as floor play and pulling to stand could affect the course of development. These effects were only apparent in infants who spent long periods of time in baby walkers.

Any deviations from the norm cause great anxiety on the part of parents. A common deviation from the crawl-stand-walk sequence is the bottom shuffle. Bottom shuffling babies move around by sitting upright and jerking themselves forwards or backwards with a series of bumps. As the hands are free and the field of vision is increased there is little incentive for the child to move on to the walking stage. Illingworth (1987) suggests that most babies who devise alternative methods of locomotion such as shuffling or rolling will be delayed walkers and that parents can be reassured that if a child can bottom shuffle he or she will eventually walk.

Primary prevention

Children will acquire motor skills at their own pace. The role of the health professional is to encourage parents to allow their infants to learn to move around and explore their environment in safety by:

- putting mats on the floor for babies from an early age so that they can practise kicking, rolling around;
- limiting the use of baby walkers;
- providing suitable toys, such as trolleys or sit-ons;
- encouraging babies to weight bear by playing with them on their knees;

- providing safety equipment, such as stair gates and fire guards;
- removing hazardous objects as babies start exploring – this can be done by asking parents to crawl the same routes that their infants are likely to take and danger spot!

This kind of advice giving can be given in a variety of situations including the home, in clinics, in hospitals – especially Accident and Emergency units, and within parent groups – for example mother and baby groups, play groups and so on.

2.7 SCREENING FOR VISUAL DEFECTS

The development of visual function depends to a large extent on normal anatomical and physiological development. A full term infant has relatively well developed eyes in so much as all ocular tissues are differentiated, but the axial length is less than that of the adult eye. The retina is fully developed except for the fovea. The fovea develops rapidly with an increase in the density of the cones and the speed of development contributes to the rapid increase in visual acuity from birth to six months of age. At birth, visual acuity is thought to be approximately 6/240, increasing to 6/180 at one month, 6/18 to 6/6 at age three years. (See Appendix 2.2 for an explanation of visual acuity levels.) Stereopsis, the ability to perceive depth, is known to develop at around five months, having an abrupt onset (Birch *et al.* 1985).

Visual defects vary from those resulting from refractive errors such as hypermetropia, caused by insufficient axial development of the eye, and myopia, strabismus and colour blindness to somewhat more serious problems such as cataract and retinopathy or even infection such as toxicariasis. The mere existence of refractive errors increases the chance of developing strabismus and amblyopia, a term referring to the persistence of a visual deficit after refractive correction.

Hall (1996: p. 9) states that: 'The surveillance and monitoring of child health and development is regarded as good practice'. It has been widely assumed that the value of such programmes is self-evident; the earlier the problem is detected, the sooner our moral duty to provide treatment and to provide the optimum chance of recovery can be initiated. With respect to visual screening for amblyopia, strabismus and refractive error, an established scientific basis does not exist. There are wide variations in the pattern of visual screening within the UK, which may be partly attributed to the varying socio-economic conditions of different geographical areas (Woodruff *et al.* 1994). Although pre-school visual screening is routine in almost all health districts of England and Wales, at present there is no nationally adopted policy regarding the existence, content or timing of visual screening programmes, or indeed guidelines as to who should perform the testing (Bolger *et al.* 1991; Edwards *et al.* 1993).

This uncertain picture underlies the statement from 'Effective Health Care' (April 1998) that:

> 'Research is needed to establish whether pre-school screening is of benefit. Pending further research, and the recommendations of the National Screening Committee, it would seem inappropriate to initiate new programmes, or extend or dismantle existing ones.'

A further difficulty is that the prevalence of amblyopia is difficult to assess. Estimates vary depending upon the sample of population screened and the tests and criteria used, but it is most commonly quoted as between 2 and 2.5% of the general population and up to 5% of the pre-school population (Taylor 1987; Thompson *et al.* 1991; Von Noorden 1996).

Current practice

Most current orthoptic screening programmes use six tests to assess visual acuity and the presence of a strabismus or abnormal eye movements (Beardsell 1989; Edwards *et al.* 1993; Carney & Norton 1994; Vardy *et al.* 1995). The usual tests are uniocular visual acuity testing using the Single Sheridan Gardiner test at 6 metres, the cover test, ocular movements, convergence and checking for binocular vision by using a prism and stereotest. It is accepted that the measurement of visual acuity at the age of three and a half years is difficult and if screening were to be performed at a younger age than this, there would likely be an unacceptably high recall rate (Beardsell 1989). However, a test needs to be chosen which is simple to perform and sufficiently reliable to detect all cases of

amblyopia. Much discussion has taken place over the use of the Single Sheridan Gardiner test and a linear version of the test comprising letters of the same size (Hall 1996). The linear test requires greater scrutiny and identification of letters is significantly more difficult because of a crowding effect which is characteristic of amblyopia (Stuart & Burian 1961). If a linear test is not used, cases of amblyopia will be missed (Elston 1995). However, it can also be said that if genuine low vision is found using a single Sheridan Gardiner test, then linear acuity will almost always be worse (Carney & Norton 1994). The linear test is not feasible as a screening test merely because it requires a greater degree of understanding and motivation than most three and a half year olds possess. Other tests have been considered as an alternative to the linear test as a way of introducing a crowding phenomenon. The Cambridge Crowding Cards create the desired effect by having a central letter surrounded by four different letters of the same size (Atkinson *et al.* 1987), but a pronounced crowding effect was produced suggesting that the test is difficult to comprehend rather than due to amblyopia (Atkinson *et al.* 1988). The accepted level of acuity for referral is considered to be 6/12 or worse (Hall 1996), but many orthoptists would express concern over this level and would, undoubtedly, refer at 6/9.

Much discussion has taken place over the timing of screening. In Nottingham, screening programmes undertaken by school nurses on children of five years of age concluded that, although the system was effective at detecting defects, problems resulted in the lack of follow-up (Hardman-Lea & Haworth 1989). They argued that many cases of amblyopia were discovered prior to school age probably because the defect was more obvious to the parents. The Hall report (1996) concludes that, 'Universal screening of pre-school children could not be recommended in the absence of any evidence that this produces a better outcome in terms of visual acuity.'

De Vries (1985) strongly believes that, with reference to amblyopia caused by different refractive errors between the two eyes, the effect of age on the success rate of treatment is important and therefore that screening for amblyogenic factors should be aimed at as young an age group as is possible to test. Late referral has been found to have an adverse effect on outcome (Edwards *et al.* 1993; Collins & Hannah 1996). One of the most compelling reasons for early diagnosis is quite simply that parents want it (Hall

1996). Parents believe that they have a right to know of any concerns about their child's development at the earliest possible stage, and early diagnosis, if accompanied by adequate explanation of the condition and its treatment, facilitates adaptation to any difficulties the child may be experiencing as well as compliance with the treatment regime.

A debate also exists as to who is best able to perform visual screening. It is a question that is bound up with issues of time, cost and reliability of the personnel involved, be they general practitioners, health visitors, community medical officers or orthoptists. Health visitors make a large number of false positive referrals (Edwards *et al.* 1989), but it must be recorded that these personnel only received half a day's training in visual assessment. Beardsell (1989) believes that orthoptists have the advantage of being able to base referral on the interpretation of the combined results of the other tests, thus making them more effective screeners. This same opinion has been expressed by others (Bolger *et al.* 1991; Fathy & Elton 1993). Collins and Hannah (1996) support this view, but also reiterate that early testing with a high degree of accuracy can only be achieved if orthoptists perform the tests.

It is paramount that any screening programme needs to be cost-effective. Hall (1996) states that a detailed review of the potential savings of community visual screening is required and it is very difficult to assess the full financial impact that an efficient screening programme may have. Colour vision defects occur in 8% of boys and 0.5% of girls (Illingworth 1987) and the routine testing of children for colour vision may be included in many screening programmes (Ehrlich *et al.* 1983). Hall (1996) recommends the use of colour vision screening by either the Ishihara or City test at the beginning of secondary school for educational or career planning reasons.

Primary prevention

The other cause of visual problems may be accidental injury. To this end, health professionals need to be aware of hazards which could endanger the eyes. They should encourage parents to:
- seek prompt medical help for eye injuries or infection;
- remove or pad furniture with sharp corners;
- ensure that toys are safe;
- ensure that glass doors are made of safety glass;

- put hazardous chemicals/drugs out of reach of small children;
- take fire safety precautions and install a smoke detector;
- regularly worm pets and maintain good standards of hygiene including hand washing;
- lobby local councils to ensure that play areas and equipment are well maintained and kept dog-free.

Appendix 2.2 at the end of this chapter explains technical terms used in visual screening.

2.8 SCREENING FOR HEARING DEFECTS

Young babies respond to noises by showing the Moro or 'startle' reflex when exposed to a loud, sudden noise. They also respond to the human voice more than other noises. Schneider *et al.* (1980) found that babies are able to distinguish between high and low pitched sounds and Clifton *et al.* (1981) found that quite young babies can locate the source of sound. Salt (1960) found that babies are soothed by rhythmic, heartbeat like sounds, a fact which has been exploited by some mothers using tape recordings of heartbeat sounds. Whilst the ability to hear is essential for the normal development of speech and language, communication and the ability to interact with others, significant congenital hearing loss affects approximately 840 children per year in the UK (Effective Health Care 1998).

If a child has a loss of hearing, urgent referral, assessment and intervention is required to ensure that the impact of deafness on a child's developmental progress is minimised. Hearing problems can either be *conductive* or *sensorineural*. Sensorineural hearing loss is usually congenital, or arises from subsequent infections such as meningitis, whereas conductive hearing loss is usually the result of middle ear problems such as otitis media and can be acute or chronic.

Conductive loss

Where hearing loss is conductive, the cause is fluid or sticky secretions in the middle ear interfering with the transmission of sound to the cochlea. Chronic ear infections and otitis media are more common in children whose parents smoke and in children with congenital abnormalities such as cleft palate, Down's syndrome and other facial malformation syndromes (Hall 1996). Conductive loss is common, with up to half of all schoolchildren experiencing loss at some stage. Hall suggests that transient loss is unlikely to affect normal development but persistent or severe loss may result in delayed language acquisition. Surgical treatment may be helpful, but a wait-and-see attitude is generally applied as conservative management of the problem may be as effective as surgery (Hogan *et al.* 1997). This subject is again considered in Chapter 13.

Sensorineural Loss

Sensorineural loss occurs when there is a lesion of the cochlea or auditory nerves. There are a number of risk factors associated with sensorineural loss including: low birth weight, prolonged neo-natal ventilation, prolonged jaundice, ototoxic drugs, hypoxia, neonatal meningitis, congenital infections such as rubella, or a family history of a close relative needing a hearing aid under the age of five years. Sensorineural loss is permanent. Few babies are, however, completely deaf and even small babies can be fitted with hearing aids to ensure that they can make optimum use of any residual hearing.

Early detection of hearing loss

Hall (1996) advocates screening of all children for hearing defects in the first year. This normally takes place at around eight months of age and is undertaken by the health visitor. Parental education and vigilance are also important in the early detection of hearing problems, but cannot be relied upon because hearing impaired children are seldom deaf to all frequencies. In addition, they become skilled at picking up visual or olfactory cues, so hearing problems may not be apparent.

For high risk infants the identification of hearing problems should take place earlier. Assessment of risk of hearing problems depends on good history taking, which can be done at birth or within the first six weeks. For infants whose history suggests high risk, there should be an immediate referral for specialist audiometric assessment. The potential of universal screening of very young infants using sophisticated

technology such as 'evoked otoacoustic emissions' (EOAE) has been assessed in some areas of the UK and there is good evidence to suggest that it is both effective and cost-efficient (Effective Health Care 1998). The use of parent questionnaires such as McCormick's (1983) is also proving useful in helping parents determine if their child is not hearing normally.

Current practice: the distraction test

For most low risk infants, the distraction test of hearing is still widely used. It is used in about 80% of health districts and a achieves a coverage of about 90% of all infants. Two people are required to perform the distraction test which is suitable for babies aged 7–10 months; one person acts as a distracter and the other as the tester. The parent is asked to sit on the chair holding the baby comfortably on his or her knee. The baby should not be wearing a hat or constrictive clothing which could prevent turning around. The baby should ideally be well, free from colds and not tired or irritable. The distracter's job is to keep the child looking in front whilst the tester makes noises behind the child to see if he or she responds to specific sounds. The tester moves around so that the baby cannot anticipate the 'game'. The sounds include a high frequency rattle, a high 'ssss', a low frequency mumble and a low frequency warbler if available. All the sounds made should be checked with a sound meter to ensure that they are below 30 dB. The tester should avoid wearing perfume, making shadows or wearing eye-catching clothing. Babies are deemed to have passed the test if they turn and locate the sounds. The test is in no way diagnostic. Babies who do not respond to the sounds should be referred for further assessment.

Morgan (1996) provides a useful review on the value of the distraction test. The current consensus is that it fails to detect a significant number of hearing problems and that universal neo-natal hearing screening is more effective and cost-effective than the health visitor distraction test at detecting significant hearing loss. Table 2.2 is a summary of screening tests available for hearing loss in infants (Effective Health Care 1998).

For older children, taking a careful history including incidence of illnesses such as measles or meningitis, and speech and language development, will identify children who need testing. The most

Table 2.2 A summary of screening tests for hearing loss (from *Effective Health Care*, 1998).

Tests	Comments
(1) Infant distraction test (IDT)	
(1)a Traditional health visitor distraction test (HVDT) – universal in most districts	Test carried out at 6–9 months, usually in protected time. Cost about £25 per test including follow-up[1]
(1)b Targeted IDT	Proposed in tandem with universal neo-natal screning on equity grounds
(1)c BeST test	New one person IDT, with calibrated sound source
(2) Transient evoked otoacoustic emissions (TEOAE)	Quick test carried out within days of birth. Measures acoustic energy generated by the healthy cochlea in response to wide band clicks using a lightweight ear canal probe. Cost £14 per test. Presently most used for well babies. Need agreed criteria for pass/refer
(3) Maximum length sequence stimuli (MLS TEOAE)	New very quick version of TEOAE that may have advantages in noisy situations
(4) Distortion product otoacoustic emissions (DPOAE)	Many implementations, need to monitor literature as to outcome
(5) Auditory brainstorm response (ABR)	Test carried out within days of birth. Wide band clicks are presented to one ear and the resulting electrical potentials of the early auditory pathways are measured using surface electrodes. Some ABR machines make pass or refer decisions, others need trained operators. High recurrent costs or long test times on some implementations. Presently most used in NICU/SCBU children
(6) Portable auditory response cradle (PARC)	Automated, quick, behavioural test which presents a 70–80 dB SPL high pass noise to one or both of the baby's ears via an earphone or probe. The baby's response is measured by a cradle and associated computer software which compares head turns and body movements in periods with the sound on and off. An automated decision algorithm is used to pass or refer. Probably good for severe and profound impairments

1 The full cost of health visitor (HV) time does not allow for the fact that HVs may be visiting the home anyway. However, if done in conjunction with several other activities its accuracy and therefore its value is likely to be reduced. (Reproduced with kind permission of NHS Centre for Reviews and Dissemination, University of York)

commonly used tests are speech discrimination tests such as the McCormick toy test, or the use of an audiometer. The usefulness of these tests is limited by the reliance on the child's co-operation, which may be limited if the child has special needs or language problems.

Primary prevention

Health professionals have a role in the prevention of hearing loss by:

- helping parents to change their smoking behaviour;

- encouraging the uptake of the Hib vaccine which protects against haemophilus meningitis;
- promoting pre-conceptual care – especially rubella screening,
- ensuring that acute ear infections are appropriately treated – remind parents to complete antibiotic treatment if prescribed.

2.9 COMMUNICATION SKILLS

Early communication between mothers and their babies has been the subject of a great deal of research.

Crying is an important form of early communication. In a classic work Brazelton (1974) studied the quality of mother-infant interaction and found that early interaction influences attachment of mother and baby. He described seven phrases of reciprocal interaction:

(1) **Initiation**	The baby looks at his mother.
(2) **Orientation**	The infant's face brightens as he looks at his mother.
(3) **Site of attention**	If the mother has responded to the first two phases the infant sends out cues with facial expressions and movements.
(4) **Acceleration**	Body activities intensify and the infant may smile if the mother smiles.
(5) **Peak of excitement**	Jerky and intense movements highlight the peak of interaction, he may suck his fingers and move his arms and legs.
(6) **Deceleration**	Gradual slowing down of movements, and dulling of facial expression.
(7) **Withdrawal**	The infant plays an active role in ending the interaction of turning away and quieting down.

Brazelton's study demonstrates how the baby takes an active part in social development, and how important the ability to see and hear is to the development of the normal, social child.

Language development can be divided into the pre-linguistic and the linguistic phases. The pre-linguistic phase is characterised by sounds such as differentiated crying, cooing, babbling and so forth, with the first words being used with meaning at the end of the first 12 months. During this time the baby will be developing the ability to understand the meaning of speech, known as receptive language. Expressive language develops in the child's second and third years. When speech begins to develop at 15 months, single words are used with meaning and sing-song 'jargoning' accompanies most activities. During the second year of life the vocabulary increases to about 300 words (Bee 1989).

Children should have a good understanding of most receptive speech, that is what is said to them, by three to four years old. Most three year olds can produce complex sentences although there may be problems of articulation and grammar, for example they may call all fruits apples. This is known as **over-generalisation**. Children may adapt the rules of grammar in, for instance, the use of plurals and by saying 'sheeps' or in the use of tenses by saying 'dided'. Most of these irregularities will have disappeared by the fourth birthday. The pre-schooler likes to practise newly acquired language skills incessantly, often to the exasperation of those around!

Detecting language problems

Obviously children with hearing difficulties or other serious disorders are likely to have delayed speech development. For other children, however, the rate of speech and language development varies greatly from child to child (Bates *et al.* 1993). The lack of a definition of 'language delay' coupled with difficulties in gaining a child's co-operation make screening unrealistic (Hall 1989). Difficulties also arise where English is a second language.

Delayed language acquisition may result in educational or behavioural difficulties and are often the source of anxiety for parents. Hall (1996) suggests that children who have difficulty understanding language may have more problems than those who have problems with expressing themselves. The impact of speech therapy in the long term has not been evaluated, but may help in the short term and provide parents with valuable support. In the absence of clear guidelines on the detection and treatment of language problems, how can health professionals help parents who are worrying about their children's language?

Checking hearing is an obvious beginning. Deciding with the parents whether the child understands language is the next step. If understanding is clearly absent, referral may be necessary to rule out serious disorders such as autism or associated communication disorders which require specialist management. For other children who understand what is being said to them, but who have difficulty articulating words or forming sentences, most will develop normal speech by the time they are in school. Nevertheless such children should be encouraged to join playgroups and nurseries and make the most of opportunities to learn through play. Assessment and intervention by a speech therapist can be helpful, although it is not currently clear which children would fail to progress without such interventions (Effective Health Care 1998).

Primary prevention

Parents naturally talk to children in a way which enhances their ability to learn speech. As long ago as 1977 Snow and Ferguson identified the way in which mothers speak to children and the way in which it enhances language development calling it 'motherese'. The richness of language spoken in the home will enhance the vocabulary of its children. Early intervention programmes such as the 'Child Development Programme', which uses structured health visiting to enhance maternal skills, is an example of primary prevention in this area (Barker 1992).

Health professionals can promote language development by:

- encouraging parents to play with and stimulate their babies and young children;
- providing and promoting support groups for young parents, for example the Cope Street project (Rowe & Miles 1991);
- advising parents about suitable play materials such as books.

2.10 CONCLUSION

The role of health professionals in promoting child health is undergoing a process of change. Whilst the traditional role of the child health services has been to detect disability and delay and to promote health education, the emphasis now is on working in partnership with parents to promote child health in the widest possible terms. Health visitors, in particular, have an opportunity to deliver a child health promotion programme geared to the needs of children and their parents. Their unique position as home visitors located within the primary health care team should help them to deliver such a service. Whilst this chapter has not given a detailed account of public health approaches, the importance of delivering a service based on the philosophy of 'Health for All'

(WHO 1978) should not be underestimated. This states that health care services should be: primary care led, accessible, equitable, collaborative and responsive. The shift in emphasis away from biomedical approaches to care, and towards social models of care, is something that everyone involved in the delivery of the service should promote.

ACKNOWLEDGEMENTS

The section on screening for visual defects was contributed by Helen Orton, Lecturer in Orthoptics at the University of Liverpool. We gratefully acknowledge her contribution.

REFERENCES

Ainsworth, M. (1967) *Infancy in Wuganda*. Baltimore, Johns Hopkins Press.

Atkinson, J., Anker, S., Evans, C., Hall, R. & Pimm-Smith, E. (1988) Visual acuity testing of young children with the Cambridge Crowding Cards at three and six years. *Acta Ophthalmology*, **66**, 505–8.

Atkinson, J., Anker, S., Evans, C. & McIntyre, A. (1987) The Cambridge Crowding Cards for pre-school visual acuity testing. *Transcript VIth International Orthoptics Congress*, Harrogate, 482–6.

Barker, W. (1992) *The Bristol Child Development Programme*. Early child development unit, University of Bristol.

Bates, E., Dale, P.S. & Thal, D. (1993) Individual differences and their implications for theories of language development. In: *Handbook of child language* (ed. P. Fletcher & B. MacWhinney). Blackwell, Oxford.

Brazelton, T.B. (1980) Behavioural competence of the new born infant. In: *Parent–infant relationship* (ed. Paul Taylor). Grune & Stratton, New York.

Beardsell, R. (1989) Orthoptic visual screening at three and a half years by Huntingdon Health Authority. *British Orthoptic Journal*, **46**, 7–13.

Bee, H. (1989) *The developing child*, 5th edn. Harper & Row, New York.

Birch, E.E., Shimojo, S. & Held, R. (1985) Preferential looking assessment of fusion and steriopsis in infants aged one to six months. *Invt. Ophthalmol. Vis. Sci.*, **26**, 366–70.

Bolger, P.G., Stewart-Brown, S.L., Newcombe, E. and Starbuck, A. (1991) Visual screening in pre-school children: comparison of orthoptists and clinical medical officers as primary screeners. *British Medical Journal*, 303, 1291–4.

Brazelton, T.B., Koslowski, B. & Main, M. (1974) *The Origins of Reciprocity: The Early Mother–Infant Interaction.*

Carney, P.S. & Norton, P. (1994) A study of children with minor visual defects referred for primary school screening. *British Orthoptics Journal*, 51, 6–9.

Child Growth Foundation (1993) *Nine-centile growth chart.* Child Growth Foundation, available from: 2 Mayfield Avenue, London W4 1PW.

Clifton, R.K., Morrongiello, B.A., Kulig, J. & Dowd, J.M. (1981) New borns' orientation towards sound: possible implications for cortical development. *Child Development*, 52, 833–8.

Collins, A. & Hannah, J. (1996) Anisometropia: orthoptists and early diagnosis make the difference. *British Orthoptic Journal*, 53, 31–5.

Crouchman, M. (1986) The effects of babywalkers on early locomotor ability. *Developmental Medicine and Child Neurology*, 28, 757–61.

Edwards, R.S., Whitelaw, A.J. & Abbott, A.G. (1989) Orthoptists as pre-school screeners: a two and a half year study. *British Orthoptic Journal*, 46, 14–19.

Edwards, R.S., Whitelaw, A.J. & Abbott, A.G. (1993) The outcome of pre-school visual screening, *British Orthoptic Journal*, 50, 2–6.

Effective Health Care (1998) Pre-school hearing, speech, language and vision screening. NHS Centre for Reviews and Dissemination, 4 (2), University of York.

Elston, J. (1995) Pre-school visual screening (Editorial). *British Journal of Ophthalmology*, 79, 1063–5.

Ehrlich, M., Reinechke, R. & Simons, K. (1983) Pre-school vision screening for amblyopia, strabismus. Programmes, methods, guidelines. *Survey of Ophthalomology*, 28, 145–63.

Fathy, V.C., Elton, P.J. (1993) Orthoptic screening for three and four year olds. *Public Health*, 107, 19–23.

Hall, D.M.B. (1996) *Health for all Children*, 3rd edn. Oxford University Press, Oxford.

Hall, D. (ed.) (1989) *Health for all children – a programme of child surveillance.* Oxford Medical Press, Oxford.

Hall, D., Hill, P. & Ellemen, D. (1990) *The Child Surveillance Handbook.* Radcliffe Medical Press, Oxford.

Hardman-Lea, S.J. & Haworth, S.M. (1989) An assessment of the present system for visual screening of school children in Nottingham. *British Orthoptic Journal*, 46, 20–25.

Hogan, S.C., Stratford, K.J. & Moore, D.R. (1997) Duration and reassurance of otitis media with effusion. *British Medical Journal*, 314, 350–3.

Illingworth, R. (1983) *The Normal Child*, 8th edn. Churchill Livingstone, Edinburgh.

Illingworth, R. (1987) *The Development of the Infant and Young Child*, 9th edn. Churchill Livingstone, Edinburgh.

Johnson, A., Goddard, O. & Ashurst, A. (1990) Is late walking a marker of morbidity? *Archives of Disease in Childhood*, 65, 486–8.

McCormick, B. (1983) Hearing screening by health visitors: a critical appraisal of the distraction test. *Health Visitor*, 56 (12), 449–51.

Middle, C., Johnson, A., Aderdice, F., Petty, T. & MacFarlane, A. *et al.* (1996) Birth weight and health and development at the age of seven years. *Child Health Care and Development*, 22, 55–71.

Morgan, S. (1996) The value of the health visitor distraction test. *Health Visitor*, 69 (10), 417–18.

Neligan, G. & Pridham, D. (1969) Norms for standard developmental milestones by sex, social class and place in the family. *Developmental Medicine Child Neurology*, 11, 413–22.

Rowe, A. & Miles, M. (1994) Coping strategy. *Nursing Times*, 90, 32–4.

Salk, L. (1960) The effects of the normal heartbeat on the behaviour of the normal infant; implications for mental health. *World Mental Health*, 12, 168–75.

Schneider, B. *et al.* (1980) High frequency sensitivity in infants. *Science*, 207(4434), 1003–4.

Sefi, S. & Grice, D. (1994) Parents' views of clinics. *Health Visitors*, 67 (2), 62.

Sharpe, H. & Lowenthal, D. (1992) Reasons for attending GP or Health Authority clinics. *Health Visitor*, 65 (10), 149–51.

Sheridan, M. (1983) *From Birth to Five*. NFER Nelson, Windsor.

Skuse, D.G., Gill, D., Reilly, S., Wolke, D. & Lynch, M.A. (1995) Failure to thrive and the risk of child abuse: a prospective population survey. *Journal of Medical Screening*, 2 (3), 145–9.

Snow, C.E. & Ferguson, C.A. (eds) (1977) *Talking to Children*. Cambridge University Press, Cambridge.

Stuart, J.A., Burian, H.M. (1961) A study of separation difficulty: its relationship to visual acuity in normal and amblyopic eyes. *American Journal of Opthalmology*, 53, 471–7.

Sutton, J.C., Jagger, C. & Smith, L.K. (1995) Parents' views of health surveillance. *Archives of Diseases in Childhood*, 73, 57–61.

Taylor, D. (1987) Screening for squint and poor vision. *Archives of Diseases in Childhood*, 62, 982–3.

Thompson, J.R., Woodruff, G., Hiscox, F., Strong, N. & Minshull, C. (1991) The incidence and prevalence of amblyopia detected in childhood. *Public Health*, 105, 455–63.

Williams, S.M., Taylor B.J., Ford, R.P. & Nelson, E.A.

(1990) Growth velocity before sudden infant death. *Archives of Diseases in Childhood*, **65** (12), 1315–18.

Woodruff, G., Hiscox, F., Thompson, J.R. & Smith, L.K. (1994) Factors affecting the outcome of children treated for amblyopia. *Eye*, **8**, 627–31.

World Health Authority (1978) *Health for All – Alma Ater Declaration*. WHO, Geneva.

Vardy, J.M., Brailsford, S.A., Anderson, J.D. & Milne, C. (1995) Is 6/9 visual acuity acceptable? Are our screening standards too high? *British Orthoptic Journal*, **52**, 41–52.

Von Noorden, G.K. (1996) *Binocular vision and ocular motility: Theory and management of Strabismus*, 5th edn. Mosby, St Louis.

FURTHER READING

Ainsworth, M.D.S. (1973) The development of infant–mother attachment. In: Review of Child Development Research, Vol. 3 (eds B.M. Caldwell & H.N. Ricciuti). Academic Press, New York.

Department of Education and Science (1978) *Warnock Report on Special Educational Needs*. HMSO, London.

De Vries, J. (1985) Anisometropia in children: analysis of a hospital based population. *Ophthalmology*, **69**, 504–507.

DHSS (1988) *Causes of Blindness and Partial Sight among Children aged under 16*. Statistical Bulletin No. 3/9/88. HMSO, London.

Haggard, M.P. (1990) Hearing screening in children – state of the art(s). *Archives of Diseases in Childhood*, **65**, 1193–8.

Mein, J. & Trimble, R. (1991) *Diagnosis and Management of Ocular Motility Disorders*, 2nd edn. Blackwell Scientific Publications, Oxford.

Nottingham, H.A. (1991) *45 Cope Street*. Nottingham Health Authority.

Snyder, L. (1978) Communicative and cognitive abilities and disabilities in the sensorimotor period. *Merrill-Palmer Quarterly*, **24**, 161–86.

Wilson, J.M.G. & Jungner, G. (1968) *Principles and Practice of Screening for Disease*. WHO, Geneva.

APPENDIX 2.1: THE 1996 NINE-CENTILE GROWTH CHART BOYS BIRTH–1 YEAR

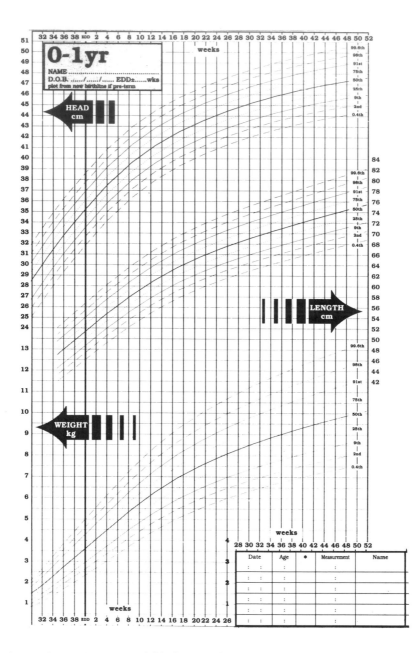

© Child Growth Foundation. Copies available from Harlow Printing, Maxwell Street, South Shields NE33 4PU.

APPENDIX 2.2: TECHNICAL TERMS USED IN VISUAL SCREENING

Strabismus: a condition in which one or other of the visual axis is not directed towards the object of fixation. **It may be:**

esotropia – when one or other eye deviates nasally (inwards)

exotropia – when one or other eye deviates temporally (outwards)

hypotropia – when one eye is rotated downwards

hypertropia – when one eye is rotated upwards

Amblyopia: defective visual acuity in one or both eyes which persists after correction of the refractive error and removal of any pathological obstacle to vision.

Hypermetropia: parallel rays of light come to focus behind the retina (alternatively referred to as long-sight). It may be corrected by the use of a convex (plus) lens which refracts the light rays so they come to a focus on the retina (Figure 2.3).

Myopia: parallel rays of light come to focus in front of the retina (alternatively referred to as short-sight). It may be corrected by the use of a concave (minus) lens so that the light rays come to a focus on the retina (Figure 2.4).

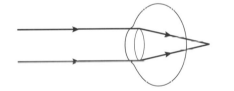
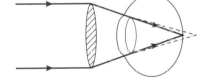

Figure 2.3   Hypermetropia.

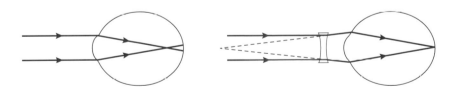

Figure 2.4   Myopia.

Explanation of visual acuity (VA) levels

6/6 VA	means that a patient is able to see a letter on the vision chart which is designed to be seen at 6 metres and is therefore said to have normal visual acuity
6/18 VA	the 6 represents the distance to testing; the 18 represents the distance at which that particular sized letter should be seen by the normal eye – thus 6/18 VA represents reduced VA as that sized letter is being seen by the patient when it should be seen at a distance of 18 metres, but they are only seeing it at 6 metres
6/4 VA	represents above average vision – therefore a patient is able to see a particular sized letter, designed to be seen at 4 metres by the normal eye, at 6 metres

Fovea: area within the retina which is responsible for the maximum visual acuity. Also has the highest density of cones, which are responsible for colour vision.

3

Promoting Psychological Health: A Focus on Children Within Families

Sam Warner

3.1 INTRODUCTION

What constitutes an ideal family environment in which to bring up children has been the subject of great debate in recent years. Changing patterns of family structure have given rise to anxieties regarding the supposed erosion of traditional family values, and at the same time concern about the deleterious effect of this on the nation's children. In society generally, views of family structures, such as single-parent families and, in particular, those headed by women, have become enmeshed in moralistic arguments that preclude serious evaluation of those factors which contribute to a healthy psychological environment.

The aim of this chapter is to examine psychological evidence concerning the best way to provide psychological health. This is to enable health professionals to identify some of the factors that are important in contributing to an emotionally healthy family environment, a place in which children's needs can be identified and met. It is also necessary to highlight those parenting behaviours which contribute to poor psychological development and behavioural disturbance. Minimum standards of parenting are laid out in the Children Act 1989 (DoH 1990) and operationalised in documents, such as 'Working Together' (HMSO 1991). When these minimum standards have been contravened poor parenting becomes abusive and the focus of much concern. As Puckering *et al.* (1994: 299) have noted, 'parenting is a complex, demanding and vital job for

which there are no qualifications, no training, little support and maximum discredit when it goes wrong.' It is important, therefore, to identify what works, as much as what does not. Additionally, this chapter will identify when children's behaviour indicates a serious level of concern, and when and how to access further help.

3.2 CREATING A WARM FAMILY ATMOSPHERE

Positive parenting and psychological health

A warm family atmosphere is developed through interactions between three main factors:

(1) aspects associated with parenting styles;
(2) factors associated with children themselves;
(3) the specific cultural and local contexts in which family life takes place.

Attachment theory, which is based on the work of Bowlby (1969; 1973) and Ainsworth (1967), and developed by Rutter (1972), attempts to theorise the precise impact of the child's early relationships with parental figures on later emotional development and the ability to sustain loving and close relationships with others. Bowlby (1969) argued that the primary relationship with the parental figure is internalised as a model for future encounters and acts as a template for determining the individual's capacity for emotional proximity and ability to receive, seek and to give care. From this perspective the parent has considerable impact on the emotional growth and development of the child and if we, as a community, are to provide a psychologically healthy environment in which to raise children, we must care for the parents.

Through the provision of consistent and appropriate care a child develops a sense of trust and security and becomes positively attached to significant others. The speed and intensity of response to the child's physical and psychological needs impacts on this sense of trust and the sensitivity with which care is delivered is of paramount importance. The parent must be sensitive to the child's cues and respond appropriately within the context of a warm and loving relationship. Hence, secure and positive attachments are enabled by the provision of a family environment which includes a primary and specific caretaker, who offers consistent care, safety and security (Rutter 1972). There should be adequate stimulation and encouragement for growth, grounded in reasonable expectations and support in times of stress. Experience in expressing and identifying emotions will be encouraged through having needs recognised and met.

When the parent's ability to offer consistent care and support is compromised evidence exists to suggest that children's abilities and mental health will be impaired later in life. Thus, factors which affect the quality and consistency of the parent–child relationship are significant. For example, children of parents who have been diagnosed as having mental illnesses have been shown to be at increased risk of developing psychiatric disorders themselves (Rutter & Quinton 1984). Mothers who suffer from postnatal depression have been shown to be negatively associated with their child's psychological development (Murray 1992).

Because of the type of evidence which links quality of parenting with subsequent development, a great deal of effort has been made to explore the specific dimensions of care that contribute to a child's sense of wellbeing. A large number of attempts have been made to identify those parenting styles which are associated with increased psychological health in children, and a number of measures have been developed to establish what these are.

Evaluating parenting styles and defining positive parent—child relationships

The nature of parent–child interactions, the factors which impinge on them and the effect of these on the child's development and adjustment constitute a significant proportion of all research in psychopathology and developmental psychology (Rey *et al.* 1993). Building on the work of Bowlby, Ainsworth and Rutter, Parker *et al.* (1979) aimed to define and measure the principal dimensions of bonding and in this to examine the parental contribution to the child–parent relationship. Using a factor analytic design, Parker *et al.* isolated two factors which were found to be significant in defining the quality of the parental bond: those of care and of over-protection, which were theoretically anticipated in the attachment and bonding literature.

Out of this work Parker *et al.* developed the 'parental bonding instrument', or PBI, specifically to measure these factors. They defined care as a continuum ranging from affection, emotional warmth, empathy and closeness to emotional coldness, indifference and neglect. Excessive control was characterised as including over-protection, intrusion, excessive contact, infantilisation and the prevention of independent behaviour.

In Parker *et al.*'s (1979) original study over-protection was found to be associated with lack of care. Parents who scored low on the care dimension but were given high protection scores were defined as being in the 'affectionless control' quadrant. Thomasgard and Metz (1993) made a distinction between 'affectionless control' which represents overprotection and 'affectionate constraint,' which, they argued, more closely represents an indulgent form of parent–child interaction. 'Affectionless control', it is argued, is specifically implicated as the most harmful parenting style. In their review of the research literature relating to parenting styles, Thomasgard and Metz (1993) concluded that 'a lack of care contributed to low self-esteem in the child, and excessive parental control interfered with the development of the child's social competence and autonomy'.

However, it must be noted that, not all studies involving the PBI supported these findings. MacKinnon *et al.* (1989) found that whilst scores on the PBI scales were unaffected by negative life events, such as bereavement, illness, accident or injury, they, unlike other researchers, failed to find a greater number of people with affective symptoms who scored their parents as high affectionless controllers. In a later study however, MacKinnon *et al.* (1993) did find that lack of care was a primary risk factor in individuals with a history of depression compared with controls. Over-protection was not found to be a significant risk factor. Similar results were obtained by Rodriguez Vega *et al.* (1993), who found that there was a significant increase in depression of women who scored their mothers as less caring, and one or both parents as extremely cold on the PBI, although again the effects of over-control were equivocal. However, Fonagy *et al.* (1996) more generally found that psychiatric patients' accounts of their childhoods are significantly different from non-psychiatric controls.

The PBI has been used primarily with adult populations. Although some investigations with younger participants have been carried out, the results have been contradictory. For example, Rey *et al.* (1993) found that emotional disorder in adolescents was not associated with perceived parental affectionless control. MacKinnon *et al.* (1989) suggest that adults' memories of childhood are selective, rather than a uniform recollection, and are more likely to represent more recent experiences associated with later childhood. It may be, therefore, that what is remembered as an adult, differs significantly from what is described by those still in childhood. Although, as MacKinnon *et al.* (1993) argue, in terms of adult pathology, what is recalled in adulthood may be more important than detailed exploration of actual childhood events.

Given some of these difficulties associated with retrospective studies, other methods have been used to investigate parenting behaviour. Alternative methods of evaluation include concurrent studies and the use of direct observation, and more open-ended measures such as semi-structured interview (for example, the Adult Attachment Interview, Main & Goldwyn 1990; and the Narrative Completion Task for children, Buchsbaum *et al.* 1992). These measures tend to support the view that, in a general sense, less positive interactions were associated with greater increases of negative behaviour in children (Browne & Saqi 1988).

3.3 MEDIATING FACTORS AND CRITICAL APPRAISAL

Methodological criticisms

Despite the wealth of research linking early parenting experiences with later psychological adjustment, causal relationships have proved difficult to establish. Burman (1994) argues that this is not least because of methodological and theoretical flaws, such as an over-reliance on prospective and retrospective studies of deviant populations, and a lack of clarity in defining central concepts, such as attachment and bonding. Additionally, statistical association does not establish the direction of effect, or define the etiologic relationship.

Burman (1994) questions the utility of instruments such as the PBI, when ultimately all that is established is that quality of care is (unsurprisingly) central to positive parenting. Thomasgard and Metz (1993) further criticise the use of the PBI, for failing to clarify the dimension of parental over-protection. They note that, whilst both indulgent and controlling behaviours in parents have been used to indicate over-protection, they may be associated with different earlier events and consequences. They argue that what constitutes over-protection cannot be understood outside of the particular socio-cultural circumstance and in relation to the needs of the individual child. As such, the notion of a global measure of over-protection is untenable. Rather, dimensions of care and control need to be evaluated in relation to specific mediating factors, some of which will be discussed below.

Socio-cultural factors

The relative value of different parenting styles will be mediated by the specific relationship the child and carer have with their environment, both in terms of the immediate family and the larger social context. With regard to the immediate family context, criticism has been made of the fact that the focus of interest regarding positive parenting has been largely in terms of maternal behaviour and characteristics of fathers have too often been left untheorised or assumed as the same. Little attention has been paid to whether this is the case or, indeed, whether alternative theoretical models are required to understand fathering. There has been an over-reliance on dominant notions of women as the primary care-taker and men as the primary breadwinner. Burman (1994) argues that practical as well as ideological factors are relevant here. She notes that as mothers are more likely to be available during the day, they make more convenient research 'subjects', hence the mother-focused orientation of much investigation and discussion. Ultimately, the nuclear unit represents the 'norm' against which all other family arrangements are rendered invisible and/or defined as deviant (terms such as 'reconstituted' (stepfamilies) and 'pretended' ('parents' are gay/lesbian) proliferate).

Additionally, most studies assume that two-parent households are always heterosexual. Where alternative child care arrangements, such as day care, and alternative family structures are investigated these are invariably researched within a damage limitation model (Burman 1994). Slater & Power (1987) note that whilst there is evidence to suggest that children within single-parent families or where there is divorce or marital distress are at greater risk of psychopathology than those from relatively stable intact two-parent families, negative conclusions are too readily assumed. It is argued (Slater & Power 1987) that it is the transition from two-parent to one-parent households and the stress of divorce that mediate distress for both the child and carer, and thus detract from parenting behaviour, rather than the simple fact of number of carers. According to their study parenting attitudes and behaviours were much greater predictors of children's adjustment than family structure. Furthermore, they found that this was particularly the case in single-parent families, who, they argue, might be more at risk from the distress associated with transition and temporal stressors. They additionally concluded that what is adaptive in one-parent families may not be adaptive for two-parent families, and hence, specific parenting skills appear to be needed for specific outcomes in specific family structures.

Thus, how a family functions will vary over time with families showing more unhelpful ways of functioning at times of stress. Mediating factors will include other unhappy life events, such as deaths and unemployment. The interactional effect of life events on parenting styles may thus be more evident when these are investigated at the time of occurrence, rather than retrospectively as in MacKinnon et al.'s (1989) study.

In relation to family structure attachment issues between siblings should be considered (Bretherton 1992). Additionally, whilst much research concentrates on child–carer dyads, that is just two members in the relationship, many families consist of more than one child, and so relationships are far from 'dyadic'. The effects of non-traditional family structures, where primary relationships may include, for example, those between grandparent and child, remain largely unexplored. Further exploration of the effects of differences in parenting behaviours within families is also required.

The impact of wider cultural and ethnic issues has received too little consideration of what constitutes adequate care and protection, despite the fact that cultural prescriptions have profound influences on what is defined as acceptable parenting behaviour. For example, orthodox religious groups will place more restrictions on the behaviour of children than more liberal groupings. This has led Burman (1994) to conclude that there has been a failure to understand the child in the context, not only of his or her immediate family surroundings, but also in relation to the impact of social-historical influences on the construction of the family unit itself. As such, issues relating to how particular families adapt and are resilient to specific social and cultural stresses are not considered. The result of this is yet more condemnation for what may be more properly understood as adaptive behaviour. Thomasgard and Metz (1993) note, for example, that 'over-protection' may be desirable in lower socio-economic homes where inner city life presents very real dangers to development. It is inappropriate, therefore, for people to evaluate parenting styles without reference to the socio-cultural context and Herbert (1996a: 19) has concluded that, 'parents who do what they, and the community to which they belong believe is right for the child are the most effective parents.'

Factors associated with children

Different children will respond in different ways to the same events. For example, children may respond to inconsistent parenting by becoming either over-anxious or aggressive and defiant. In their study of adolescents, Rey et al. (1993) note that PBI scores were not stable across gender and age. One explanation for this is that developmental considerations are important in elucidating appropriate expectations regarding children's behaviour, and some parents may have difficulty adapting to the changing needs of their children. Rey *et al.* argue, parenting behaviour is as likely to be attenuated by the child's conduct as the child's behaviour is influenced by parenting style. They note that increased behavioural disinhibition on the part of the child may evoke more controlling parenting behaviours. A one-way relationship between a parent's action and a child's behaviour cannot therefore be assumed, and the picture may be complex and interactive.

Children may be unresponsive or act antisocially for a variety of reasons including personality variables as well as factors associated with particular physical conditions, which means children have specific disabilities or biological vulnerabilities which affect their ability to communicate. In a study of mothers who had premature babies, Bradley *et al.* (1995) found that children's adaptive social behaviour was related to parental responsivity, acceptance of the child and avoidance of restriction and punishment. As premature babies may be less responsive to normal social cues it is argued that this makes them especially vulnerable to parenting inadequacies. Creating a warm family environment is dependent therefore not only on the actions of parents and the socio-cultural context, but the specific personality, developmental needs and abilities of the child itself.

A multifactorial model

Given the fact that creating a warm family atmosphere is affected by more than simply the behaviour of parents, numerous authors have proposed a multi-factorial model of parenting (Slater & Power 1987; Thomasgard & Metz 1993; Bradley *et al.* 1995).

Clearly the quality and quantity of monitoring, supervision, stimulation and interaction within the home is important, but so too is the socio-cultural context. This has led theorists such as Burman (1994) to argue that relationships should form the basic unit of analysis rather than individuals, be they carer or child. She notes that a focus on pre-constituted individuals can have the dual effect of removing attention from more social issues and contribute to a climate of accausality and blame. Building on a more relational understanding of parenting, Bretherton (1992) suggests that concepts formed about parenting would benefit from 'dialogic' or narrative approaches derived from social construction theory whereby multiple realities can be evaluated and conceived.

Such approaches go some way to grappling with the complexity that characterises human relations. A multifactorial model which does not pre-privilege any one aspect of the basic triadic relationship enables a more social developmental psychology, and provides a non-judgemental context in which to encourage and enable the evolution of psychologically healthy family environments.

3.4 HELPING CARERS CARE FOR THEIR CHILDREN

Positive parenting may be encouraged by helping parents to explore all those factors which impinge on psychological health. When parents are unresponsive to the particular needs of the child and environment, they can be helped to increase their sensitivity and empathy towards their children by being encouraged to model and attend to explicit and consistent communication. Additionally, empathy, warmth and enjoyment can be encouraged by helping adults (re-)learn how to play with their children and to reframe negative behaviour in terms of positive understandings. The use of play and the availability of toys goes some way to creating a stimulating atmosphere. Encouraging parents to use their own feelings to make sense of what their child is feeling can also increase empathy. If parents, for example can be helped to understand that their feelings of uselessness and rejection may mirror their child's, they are less likely to act out their feelings of rejection on the child, and are more likely to treat their child with understanding.

Some evidence exists to support the notion that, when parents are encouraged to develop these skills, the parent–child relationship can be improved. Parent training and support programmes have demonstrated some success. Lieberman *et al.* (1991), for example, found that maternal empathy and interaction with the child can be increased by therapy input, although the effects of such interventions have not always been found to be effective or long-lasting (Puckering *et al.* 1994).

Where intervention has been demonstrated as being particularly effective a facilitative approach which enhances carers' self-esteem has been identified as being of central significance. For example, Machen (1996) found general satisfaction for first time mothers regarding health visiting services where such an approach was adopted. Rowe & Miles (1994) evaluated positively a comprehensive community service comprising focused groups, a drop-in service and volunteer visitors whose philsophy for intervention was based on enhancing mothers' abilities to make choices and thus raise their self-esteem. This was achieved by the mothers themselves setting the agenda for intervention and via adopting a non-blaming approach to information-giving practices. This study replicates other findings which suggest that clients view their own experiences of health visiting positively when intervention is relationship-centred rather than problem-focused (Appleton 1994). Barker in 1992 reported his large-scale study which demonstrated that health visitor intervention was associated with positive change in home environment and child development variables. The most significant contribution to changes in the children was associated with changes in mother's self-esteem. As such, early and comprehensive interventions, such as the Child Development Programme (Barker 1992) can be effective.

Given that the ways parents deal with their own children will, in part, be a function of their own parenting experiences, it is important, when assessing the quality of parental care and family environment, to include a detailed exploration of both parents' family histories, as this should give some indication of both negative and positive expectations of family life. Assessment should also involve a complete history of the child and current concerns and behaviours from the perspective of all concerned, framed within an understanding of the specific cultural and social contexts. This history taking should be supplemented by direct observation.

Where pre-school children are concerned, health visitors have a key role in identifying and monitoring vulnerable families who may require increased support. This is particularly important as vulnerable familes are perhaps the least likely to seek help themselves (Appleton 1994; 1996). Hence, assessment of need for intervention is of critical importance. Whilst the approach outlined above requires a considerable commitment in terms of time, skills and resources there appears to be little evidence that this process can be condensed.

Appleton (1994) and Browne (1995) reviewed the literature regarding the role of health visitiors in identifying and working with vulnerable families and concluded that screening tests, checklists and scoring systems have not been demonstrated to be valid or effective. Rather, there is a need for observation and participatory practice, which seeks to support rather than to blame. For example, Browne (1995) suggests that health visitors should be trained in the assessment of parent–child interactions, as targeting relationship interactions for intervention rather than focusing on parent psychopathology has more chance of raising self-esteem. Problems with defining 'vulnerability' notwithstanding, a related issue concerns the difficulty of providing for families once identified. Adequate resources and services are not always available (Appleton 1996), or the offered support not taken up (Oakley 1994).

However, identification of specific concerns and issues will facilitate change, as any problems can be addressed individually, in contrast to parents' and children feeling overwhelmed by global and immutable concerns. From this perspective, these problems are largely viewed as symptomatic of relationship difficulties, rather than residing in individuals who are 'to blame'. This approach, however, should not deny the very real differences in power that exist between children and adults. Common negative behaviours in children, such as tantrums, aggression and excessive anxiety can also benefit from being understood in the context of relationship exchanges and will be explored below.

3.5 NEGATIVE BEHAVIOURS

Tantrums and aggression

Tantrums and aggressive or antisocial behaviour can be understood as maladaptive ways of dealing with the environment, and may be learned responses to inconsistent and harsh parenting. Patterson (1982) has found that antisocial children have parents who lack the skills to manage common child-rearing difficulties, and are more likely to issue negative and vague directives than controls. He argues that antisocial children learn to exert control over their parents' behaviour by developing equally coercive strategies. Children and carers act in increasingly aversive ways which become mutually reinforcing. The child gets what he or she wants by acting aggressively and hence learns this is an effective method of communication. The carer meantime gains peace at the price of capitulation and the child stops shouting/hitting. Whilst it may be difficult to identify cause and effect, the result is that the mutual reinforcement of poor parenting and aggressive behaviour in children means that these negative interactions can become well established and resistant to change (see Herbert 1996b).

Some evidence exists which suggests that abusive parents are more consistent in their negative inter-actions with children than in their positive ones. Cerezo and D'Ocon (1995) found that abusive mothers were more indiscriminate in giving attention to their children following prosocial behaviour, but much more consistent in their attention following antisocial behaviour. Given the importance of con-sistency for children's emotional wellbeing, aggressive and negative behaviour on the part of children can be understood as a functional adaptation that increases certainty. Negative behaviour may give rise to nega-tive attention, but at least it is predictable. Again, a mutually reinforcing relationship is established. In the case of Cerezo and D'Ocon's mothers, they note that abusive mothers tend to be depressed, feel incompe-tent, financially stressed and are isolated. They sug-gest that these mothers may be helped by helping them discriminate between stress and their children's behaviour. Additionally, intervention which raises mothers' self-esteem and directly addresses the effects of poverty can go some way to enabling a return to more positive and consistent interactions.

When to be worried about tantrums and aggression

All children must explore the limits of their world and, in this sense, it would be worrying if children did not at times act aggressively and antisocially. Con-cerns regarding children's behaviour should be understood in terms of how realistic carers' expecta-tions are. What is acceptable behaviour in a younger child may be inappropriate in an older one, and issues relating to cognitive maturity and the distinction between action and intention needs to be considered (Herbert 1991). Additionally, an aggressive two year old does not cause the same amount of damage or harm as an aggressive twelve year old, and the effects

of behaviour will be implicated in deciding on the need for intervention. If behaviour persists and remains unacceptably severe in terms of the developmental age of the child and the demands of his or her environment, further action should be taken. Investigation should aim to find out whether a child's behaviour is a learned response to the environment and/or a communication of underlying distress.

How to evaluate and alter aggressive and antisocial behaviour

Numerous scales have been developed to evaluate aspects of parent–child interaction (Herbert 1991 for review). However, as suggested earlier there is no short cut to taking a detailed history and having first-hand knowledge of the child and family. It is crucial to have a clear understanding of the developmental level of the child regarding all relevant indices, including the emotional, physical, sexual, cognitive and linguistic.

There are some useful psychological tools that can be used to explore negative reinforcement cycles and learned behaviour in order to encourage parents to initiate positive interactions. Parents can be asked to record the antecedents, behaviours and consequences (ABC) of undesirable behaviour. Such recordings provide the means for analysing direct causal influ-ences that are close in time to the behaviour and, thus, may be considered to be functionally related to them. Causal influences may implicate specific persons, places, times and circumstances. Thus, the recording of ABCs can be used to analyse and moderate the setting conditions that give rise to aggression, and mediate the reinforcing consequences by enabling specification and localisation of the problem. Another useful mnemonic is FIND which refers to the frequency, intensity, number and duration of behaviours. Recording this information can offer a baseline for what is acceptable behaviour and what is not. Undesirable behaviour should be ignored or time out taken to cool down, whilst positive and prosocial behaviour should be praised and rewarded. A focus on, and over-criticism of, negative behaviours should be kept to a minimum because of their association with negative interaction cycles.

Childhood anxieties

Again as demonstrated earlier, negative and insecure attachments deriving from inconsistent and harsh parenting can result in increased anxiety in children as well as other antisocial behaviour. As the world for such children is an erratic place, they have limited scope for developing logical thinking or of identifying and labelling emotions accurately. As a result of this children may feel insecure and mistrustful, and lack the discrimination to cope with normal stress and anxiety. Because of this they may be unable to develop strategies for handling novel and stressful situations.

Inconsistent parenting, as suggested earlier, is often associated with unreasonable expectations, and this can contribute to enmeshing child and parent in a negatively reinforcing cycle. For example, a child who feels insecure in his or her attachments to his or her carer may deal with this by becoming more clingy. The carer may feel overwhelmed by the child and believe that the child is too old to be behaving in this manner, and, hence, attempts to withdraw further. This has the effect of exacerbating anxiety in the child and so on.

When to be worried about childhood anxieties

Some level of anxiety is adaptive. It is necessary to have fears about the world, without these children would be unable to develop a sense of danger. Common childhood anxieties include phobias, avoidant behaviours, such as school refusal, and separation anxiety. Anxiety at separation and change manifests in different ways at different ages and in different cultures. It is normal for children who have been cared for primarily by one carer to exhibit anxiety at being with strangers at about 12 months, but would be of concern if the child was ten years old. However, situational variables should also be considered. A ten-year-old child may exhibit more clingy behaviour in response to being ill. Anxiety only becomes problematic when it interferes with a child's ability to engage fully with the world, is beyond normal expectations and is of long duration.

Again it is important to consider what the surface communication of anxiety tells us about the underlying issue or fear. Recording ABCs and FINDs can be helpful in establishing the nature of the anxiety and whether there is a cause for concern. Specific and direct communication, facilitated by the aforementioned mnemonics, is useful in understanding the nature of the fear, and can be used to help the child to make sense of his or her worries. In this way, it is

possible to tease out specific anxieties from generalised problems associated with family situation and/or cultural setting.

Evaluating and altering behaviour

Children who experience extreme anxiety will show behavioural, emotional and physiological symptoms, all of which will need addressing and will benefit from being recorded. Similar interventions, involving parents and/or children, to those described for altering aggressive behaviour can be utilised. Additionally, as physiological symptoms can in themselves be frightening, children can be helped by learning about how their body works and given additional training to label and understand their feelings.

3.6 FURTHER HELP

When to access further help

As indicated in previous sections there are a number of scales and measures which can be used to indicate when behaviour becomes serious enough to require professional intervention. However, general screening tools used by health visitors to identify vulnerable families have largely proved to be invalid and ineffective (Appleton 1994). Other than this, helping parents to develop positive ways of caring can begin with validating their concerns and worries and enhancing self-esteem. If parents express concerns regarding their children they should be listened to. When immediate discussion seems unable to make sense of concerns or alleviate worries, parents should be encouraged to seek out other professionals who have specialist knowledge.

How to access further help and where to go

Where younger children are concerned, the first line of contact will normally be the health visitor whose main role is to offer help and advice regarding recognition and assessment of feeding and parenting. If the health visitor and/or the parents still have concerns, the second source of support and advice is via the general practitioner. Some GP practices now offer on-site support in the form of community nurses and counsellors. The GP may also operate as the 'gate-keeper' to other, more specialist, services such as child psychology, psychiatry, psychiatric nursing, social work and so on. The former services aim to explore underlying interactions and interpret behaviour with the aim of seeking strategies and solutions. Most child mental health services operate within a multi-disciplinary framework and offer a range of services, including individual support, advice and therapy for children and their carers. Some services offer specific input in the form of parenting groups. Groups may provide education, counselling and/or advice-giving and may be crisis and/or problem-focused. Additionally, most localities will have community projects that are aimed at offering advice, support and respite for isolated and struggling carers and self-referrals may be accepted. Some localities may offer community-based services that are specifically targeted at particular ethnic and cultural groups. Social services are normally a good source of information regarding such projects as well as providing their own family centres, family aids and nurseries. They also have lead responsibility for statutory child care and protection. For parents who are reluctant to join groups or make use of services a number of books and resources can be found in book shops and local libraries. For example, the British Psychological Society has recently published a series of books regarding common childhood problems under the series title *Parents, Adolescents and Child Training Skills*.

3.7 CONCLUSION

A warm family environment which promotes psychological health in children is best understood as a function of a number of factors including the parent(s), child(ren), extended family, socio-cultural context and the family's and individual's capacity for resilience and adaptability. As any evaluation of the appropriate level of care and control is multifactorial, global and static measures have limited utility. Different families will require different strategies of care, and roles and needs will change over time. As such, the quality and consistency of care is more important than who or how many people offer it. Any assessment of family functioning should address all the above factors and involve a detailed history of all concerned. The preferred focus of interest should be in the relationships themselves, rather than in attempting to blame individuals. Help should be offered in terms of partnership and support for all those affected.

REFERENCES

Ainsworth, M.D.S. (1967) *Infancy in Uganda: Infant Care and the Growth of Love*. Johns Hopkins University Press, Baltimore.

Appleton, J.V. (1994) The role of the health visitor in identifying and working with vulnerable families in relation to child protection: A review of the literature. *Journal of Advanced Nursing*, **20**, 167–75.

Appleton, J.V. (1996) Working with vulnerable families: a health visiting perspective. *Journal of Advanced Nursing*, **23**, 912–18.

Barker, W. (1992) Health visiting: action research in a controlled environment. *International Journal of Nursing Studies*, **29** (3), 251–9.

Bowlby, J. (1969) *Attachment and Loss, Vol. 1: Attachment*. Basic Books, New York.

Bowlby, J. (1973) *Attachment and Loss, Vol. 2: Separation*. Basic Books, New York.

Bradley, R.H., Whiteside, L., Mundfrom, D.J., Blevins-Knabe, B., Casey, P.H., Caldwell, B.M., Kelleher, K.H., Pope, S. & Barrett, K. (1995) Home environment and adaptive social behaviour among premature, low birth weight children: alternative models of environmental action. *Journal of Pediatric Psychology*, **20** (3), 347–62.

Bretherton, I. (1992) The origins of attachment theory: John Bowlby and Mary Ainsworth. *Developmental Psychology*, **28** (5), 759–75.

Browne, K. (1995) Preventing child maltreatment through community nursing. *Journal of Advanced Nursing*, **24**, 57–63.

Browne, K. & Saqi, S. (1988) Mother–Infant interaction and attachment in physical abusing families. *Journal of Reproductive and Infant Psychology*, **6**, 163–82.

Buchsbaum, H.K., Toth, S.L., Clyman, R.B., Cichetti, D. & Emde, R.N. (1992) The use of a narrative story stem technique with maltreated children: implications for theory and practice. *Development and Psychopathology*, **4**, 603–25.

Burman, E. (1994) *Deconstructing Developmental Psychology*. Routledge, London.

Cerezo, M.A. & D'Ocon, A. (1995) Maternal inconsistent socialization: an interactional pattern with maltreated children. *Child Abuse Review*, **4**, 14–31.

Department of Health (1990) *An introduction to the Children Act 1989*. HMSO, London.

Fonagy, P., Leigh, T., Steele, M., Steele, H., Kennedy, R., Mattoon, G., Target, M. & Gerber, A. (1996) The relationship of attachment status, psychiatric classification, and response to psychotherapy. *Journal of Consulting and Clinical Psychology*, **64** (1), 22–31.

Herbert, M. (1991) *Clinical Child Psychology: Social Learning, Development and Behaviour*. John Wiley & Sons, Chichester.

Herbert, M. (1996a) *Assessing Children in Need and their Parents*. BPS Books, Leicester.

Herbert, M. (1996b) *Feuding and Fighting: A Guide to the Management of Aggression and Quarrelling in Children*. BPS Books, Leicester.

HMSO (1991) *Working together under the Children Act 1989: A guide to arrangements for inter-agency co-operation for the protection of children from abuse*. HMSO, London.

Lieberman, A.F., Weston, D.R. & Pawl, J.H. (1991) Preventative intervention and outcome with anxiously attached dyads. *Child Development*, **62**, 199–209.

Machen, I. (1996) The relevance of health visiting policy to contemporary mothers. *Journal of Advanced Nursing*, **24**, 350–6.

MacKinnon, A.J., Henderson, A.S., Scott, R. & Duncan-Jones, P. (1989) The parental bonding instrument (PBI): an epidemiological study in a general population sample. *Psychological Medicine*, **19**, 1023–34.

MacKinnon, A.J., Henderson, A.S. & Andrews, G. (1993) Prenatal 'affectionless control' as an antecedent to adult depression: a risk factor refined. *Psychological Medicine*, **23**, 135–41.

Main, M. & Goldwyn, R. (1990) Adult attachment rating and classification system. In: *A Topology of Human Attachment Organisation Assessed in Discourse, Drawings and Interviews* (ed. M. Main). Cambridge University Press, New York.

Murray, L. (1992) The impact of postnatal depression on infant development. *Journal of Child Psychology and Psychiatry*, **33**, 543–61.

Oakley, A., Manther, M., Rajan, L. & Turner, H. (1994) Supporting vulnerable families: an evaluation of NEW-PIN. *Health Visitor*, **68** (5), 188–9.

Parker, G., Tupling, H. & Brown, L.B. (1979) A parental bonding instrument. *British Journal of Medical Psychology*, **52**, 1–10.

Patterson, G.R. (1982) *Coersive Family Process*. Castalia, Oregon.

Puckering, C., Mills, M., Cox, A.D. & Mattson-Graff, M. (1994) Process and evaluation of a group intervention for mothers with parenting difficulties. *Child Abuse Review*, **3**, 299–310.

Rey, J.M., Bird, K.D., Kopec-Schrader, E., & Richards, R.N. (1993) Effects of gender, age and diagnosis on perceived parental care and protection in adolescents. *Acta Psychiatrica Scandinavia*, **88**, 440–46.

Rodriguez Vega, B., Bayon, C., Franco, B., Canas, F., Graell, M. & Salvador, M. (1993) Parental rearing and intimate relations in women's depression. *Acta Psychiatrica Scandinavia*, **88**, 193–7.

Rowe, A., Miles, M. (1994) Coping strategy. *Nursing Times*, **90** (10), 32–4.

Rutter, M. (1972) *Maternal Deprivation Reassessed*. Penguin, Harmondsworth.

Rutter, M. & Quinton, D. (1984) Parental psychiatric disorder: effects on children. *Psychological Medicine*, **14**, 835–80.

Slater, M.A. & Power, T.G. (1987) Multidimentional assessment of parenting in single-parent families. *Family Intervention, Assessment and Theory*, **4**, 197–228.

Thomasgard, M. & Metz, W.P. (1993) Parental over-protection revisited. *Child Psychiatry and Human Development*, **24** (2), 67–80.

4

Caring Within Families
Kate Cernik

4.1 INTRODUCTION

On the whole in Britain today children are cared for by families. This means that the promotion of child health care largely falls within the responsibility of the family in general and mothers in particular. Despite this in Britain today many families make arrangements for their children to be cared for outside the home and/or by people other than family members. This chapter will consider evidence relating to these current trends in care in four key areas: caring for children; influencing the care children receive; positive parenting; and preventing accidents.

4.2 CARING FOR CHILDREN

For the most part it is mothers who provide the care a child needs. Graham (1984) identified that health care is largely women's work in the home. Women manage household resources to provide food, warmth and clothing – often at the expense of their own health. They also act directly to promote health and prevent illness by ensuring home safety, managing childhood illness and arranging their children's lives. Graham also found that mothers are in closest contact with the child health services and are more likely to take their children to the clinic for immunisations or health checks. They also decide when to seek medical care for their children. In Berry Mayall's (1986) study of how 135 London mothers cared for their children's

health, she found that mothers had a high level of awareness of health issues, such as diet and safety, but that constraints – especially lack of money – often led them to make considerable compromises (see also Pearson *et al.* 1993).

Working mothers

One of the most significant changes in child care in the UK over the last 10 years has been the increase in the number of women in the workplace, so that in 1994 69% of mothers with children under 15 were working. This trend towards women working (OPCS 1995) is, however, influenced by a number of factors. For instance the availability of child care is likely to be pivotal, women with very young children are less likely to work, as are women with two or more children. Such factors also affect whether a women works full or part time. The following reasons underlie this current trend:

- there are more part-time jobs available;
- women who are lone parents need to work to support their families;
- high male job insecurity has meant that a second income has become increasingly important to increase economic security for families;
- professional women have higher expectations and aspirations than their mothers and see employment as a means of gaining self-fulfilment (see for instance, *Guardian*, 26 May 1997, on successful women in their careers and life styles).

As more women with young children keep their jobs after having children, a new industry of child care has emerged. The main providers of child care are:

- friends and family
- childminders
- day nurseries
- nannies or au pairs.

Childminders are usually mothers with young children who provide child care for other children in their own homes for a moderate fee – usually paid at an hourly rate. They normally provide meals and offer children a 'home from home'. Childminders have to be registered by social services departments and to do this they must satisfy a social services inspector that their home provides a safe environment for children. In addition, they undergo a police check. Childminders are then told how many places they may offer depending on the size of their home and the number and ages of their own families.

Day nurseries may be run by social services departments or as private businesses. Nurseries run by social services provide places for vulnerable children and are not usually available to working mothers except in special circumstances. Private day nurseries

must be registered. The charges normally depend on local market forces. Staff who work in day nurseries are likely to hold a recognised child care qualification such as the Nursery Nurses Examination Board (NNEB).

The number of private day nurseries has increased as has the number of registered childminders. In addition the availability of places for the under four's in primary school or nursery class continues to increase; in 1977 57% of three and four year olds were attending school, often part-time (OPCS 1997).

The choice of child care is often dependent on income. Nannies and au pairs are the choices open to women with considerable financial resources. The costs of child care for low paid mothers may be prohibitive, so family and friends will be the only option. For most mothers if family and friends are unavailable the choice is between day nurseries and childminders, if the cost is affordable. Table 4.1 outlines the relative advantages and disadvantages of these options.

Community nurses and health visitors have a role in helping parents make informed choices about child

Table 4.1   Relative advantages and disadvantages of choosing day nurseries and childminders for day care.

Day nurseries		Childminders	
Advantages	**Disadvantages**	**Advantages**	**Disadvantages**
Reliable form of child care	May be expensive	A family environment	May be problems with family illness
Trained staff	Increased risk of infections	Probably close to home	Few checks on standards of care
Opportunity for child to mix with other children	Lack of continuity of care	Potential for flexibility about hours	Mother and care giver may have differing attitudes to child care, e.g. discipline
May be educational element	Hours may be inconvenient for shift workers	May be able to attend playgroup in preparation for school	Informal contract which may break down
More than one care giver	The child must fit in with the nursery routine	The child can have likes and dislikes catered for	May be problems if holidays do not coincide
Formal contract for care	Will be excluded if unwell	Small numbers of children	May have additional 'unofficial' children to mind May have different attitudes to pets, hygiene, etc.

care. Parents should be encouraged to look critically at the child care choices available to them. Perhaps the most important criterion of all is trust and this cannot be measured objectively. Parents need to know that they can trust the individuals who are caring for their children. Parents should be encouraged to explore all the options open to them and to visit childminders and day nurseries and take their time in making their choice.

Scarr and Dunn (1987) provide a checklist of questions for parents to consider when choosing child care:

- Do the babies or children appear happy and involved in play?
- Do the children get timely and pleasant meals and snacks?
- Do the children get adequate rest and naps?
- Are the children reasonably clean?
- Are there enough books, toys, games and opportunities for varied play?
- Does the space available to the children allow for both harmonious play with the other children, and individual choices of how to spend time?
- Is the place attractively decorated and arranged from the child's point of view?
- Does the minder or nursery staff know enough about children to provide good care?
- Are the babies and children supervised closely but not intrusively?
- Is there careful supervision of the babies in potentially dangerous spaces, and the children with potentially dangerous material?
- Is every opportunity to talk with babies and children used? Are there regular times of the day for reading, music, painting and outdoor play, for free play and play alone?
- Are there times when the children are alone and times when they are doing things together with other children?
- How does the minder or staff communicate with parents about their children's activities, development, problems and special talents? Is the transition from home to childminder or nursery and back again eased by those in charge?

Whichever way the family is assisted with child care, parents themselves have the most important influence on their children. What makes a good parent? People will answer this question in a variety of ways. The answer will be influenced by a number of factors such as age, social class, level of education, ethnic origin and, very importantly, personal experience of childhood. Styles of parenting have been demonstrated to have profound effects on the child, as discussed in Chapter 3.

4.3 INFLUENCING THE CARE CHILDREN RECEIVE

Promoting child health means promoting family health. The arrival of a child in the family results in a major change in life style for parents, siblings, and others. For health promoters these changes offer an opportunity for interventions which will have a beneficial effect on the health of the nation as a whole. Some interventions are child-orientated such as immunisation, the promotion of breastfeeding and so on, but there is also an opportunity to influence other family members about issues such as diet and smoking.

Health promotion has been traditionally offered by health visitors visiting the families with children under five in their homes. As health visiting services have become more stretched, alternative approaches may be more appropriate. Targeting of services towards families in greatest need has been widely advocated (Hall 1996; National Health Service Management Executive 1996). The argument against targeting health care interventions such as health visiting is that it is likely to lead to the stigmatisation of families and the ultimate rejection of the service by those in greatest need. An alternative approach to targeting is based on community diagnosis. Tools for identifying vulnerable families using checklists have usually been found to be of limited value. Families do not always conform to stereotypes, for example the single teenage mother may well be able to provide an excellent environment for the growth and development of children, whilst an affluent professional parent may live a chaotic life which fails to provide the security that children need.

A more successful approach to the targeting of resources is to examine the needs of specific communities or population groups, (e.g. Orr 1992). Interest in developing equitable distribution of resources has led to the development of a number of approaches to assessing the health needs of communities and the families that live in them. Figure 4.1 is a summary of the most commonly used community assessment tools.

The information gleaned from such approaches shown in Figure 4.1 can be used by a number of individuals and organisations including:

- individual health care practitioners – to identify work priorities;
- primary health care teams to identify health promotion priorities;
- nurse managers for workforce planning;
- purchasers of health care for resource allocation and forward planning.

Many of the factors which influence parents' ability to parent are not under the control of health professionals. For many parents resources rather than health education are needed to bring children up in an optimal environment. For instance many studies (Graham 1984; Mayall 1986; Pearson *et al.* 1993) have found that poverty has a huge impact on the way in which families are able to provide a healthy environment for their children. This problem affects many children; in 1993–1995 two in five people in the bottom fifth of the national income tables came from families with dependent children (OPCS 1997). The adverse effects of poverty on health have been well known for many years (Townsend *et al.* 1988) and community nurses are aware that many families they are working with live in poverty. Whilst some poor families often struggle with very limited resources to provide optimum child care, nurses often perceive that their clients lack the knowledge and ability to cope with their children. (Edwards & Popay 1994). In particular, diet and income are discussed in Chapter 9.

Families and mothers in particular are the custodians of children's health and therefore supporting and working with families is a valuable way of improving the health of the population. The projects described here are community based and have attempted to improve children's health by targeting vulnerable families using an empowerment model to increase the self-esteem of mothers.

4.4 POSITIVE PARENTING

Concepts such as **positive parenting** and **good enough parenting** are now influencing the provision of services. These concepts rest on the premise that by educating mothers and raising their confidence and self-esteem, improved parenting and child health will follow. The traditional approaches to helping parents, based on a traditional educational approach, that is 'teaching' of parents by community nurses, have often been seen to undermine mothers by 'professionalising' parenting. Health education messages about parenting are often at odds with parents' real experiences (Mayall & Foster 1989). The image of the 'perfect' parent has been reinforced by child care manuals, psychologists and governments

Jarman index Jarman (1983)	A measure of need derived from a study of the demands made on GP practices
Townsend deprivation score Townsend *et al.* (1988)	A scoring system identifying poverty based on Census data
Poverty profiling Blackburn (1991; 1992)	Focuses on identifying local patterns of poverty
Rapid appraisal Annett & Riflan (1990)	Developed from developing world approaches using community networks to develop health needs assessments
Caseload/practice/community profiles Billings (1996)	Identifying needs within specified areas

Figure 4.1 Common tools for assessing the health needs of communities and families that live within them.

(Richardson 1993). Three examples of projects using 'positive parenting' approaches are described below.

The Child Development Programme

The Child Development Programme uses many of the concepts of 'good enough' care. The programme was developed by Walter Barker at the University of Bristol and became widely used in the 1980s and early 1990s (Barker 1991; 1992). It is a structured programme of education designed for first time parents using health visitors to work in partnership with mothers to improve children's environments. A selection of material from the Child Development Programme appears in Appendix 6, pp. 220–43 in Luker & Orr (1992).

Cope Street

Similarly, the Cope Street Project was based in a socially deprived part of Nottingham with poor housing, high unemployment and a high level of single parenthood. Based in a terraced house in the heart of the area, a multiprofessional team consisting of health visitors, midwives, nursery nurses and adult education workers offered young women a radical health promotion service. The stated aim of the project was 'to work in partnership with parents and improve child and family health in those families who have contact'. Young women were referred or attended through word of mouth and advertising. As well as advice, child care and informal support, the women were encouraged to participate in group work (Billingham 1989).

The groups varied from non-thematic groups with an open agenda to structured groups with specific themes. The emphasis on group work came from perspectives on adult education. The evaluation has concentrated on the views of the service users. This process approach to evaluation has informed the development of the project. The evaluation showed that the project was greatly valued by its users who had gained knowledge and confidence about themselves and their parenting skills (Rowe 1993).

NEWPIN

NEWPIN – the New Parent Infant Network – was established in 1980. There are now several centres in England. The aim of NEWPIN is to offer support for vulnerable families and prevent family breakdown.

Supported by the voluntary sector, and much appreciated by health visitors, the centres provide drop-in services and crèches. Parents who may be experiencing difficulties such as depression or social isolation are encouraged to participate in training programmes which will help them to develop their parenting skills and enhance their self-esteem. Parents may self-refer, but are usually referred to NEWPIN by health visitors or social workers or other professionals. Evaluation of NEWPIN has been somewhat mixed (Oakley *et al.* 1994), but it offers a useful alternative to traditional individualised approaches to helping parents. Whilst group-based approaches offer an innovative and exciting way of working with families, many of the concepts which underpin these approaches can be incorporated into more traditional health care approaches.

Parent-held records

Parent-held child health records have been developed over the last decade and have been strongly advocated by Hall (1996). The development in parent-held records reflects changing attitudes to parents by health professionals. They have the potential to provide a tool for working in partnership with parents. Parents can now see everything that is recorded about their child. This has forced health professionals to give greater consideration to what they write in records and has also changed the way in which they communicate. The records are given to parents shortly after their baby's birth and contain:

- information about the baby's birth;
- information and centile charts on growth and development;
- a record of development checks and progress;
- a record of immunisations;
- a record of childhood illnesses;
- health education material.

Parents and health professionals may write in the records which are kept by the parents. Parents are asked to bring them to any appointments with health visitors, GPs, clinic or hospital staff. Evaluations of the use of parent-held records have been favourable from both the parents' and health professionals' points of view. (Macfarlane & Saffin 1990; Charles 1994). One of the most important benefits of the records is the way it encourages health professionals to communicate with families in a more open and participative way. A dislike of 'people writing things down about them' was recorded in a study of mothers and health visitors (Mayall & Foster 1989). Handing back responsibility for records to parents can be seen as working more in partnership – one of the key concepts of positive parenting approaches.

4.5 PREVENTING ACCIDENTS

More pre-school children die from accidents than from any other reason. Many are seriously injured and disabled. Accidents in the home cause 37% of all deaths in the one to five age group, after age five most accidental deaths are due to road traffic accidents (DoH 1993). Two million children attend accident and emergency departments every year, 125,000 of them are admitted to hospital, and this accounts for approximately one-fifth of all paediatric hospital admissions (Child Accident Prevention Trust 1989). From these statistics it can be seen that in economic and social terms, accidents are an enormous problem, to say nothing of the pain and grief caused to individuals and their families. Childhood accidents are targeted as an area of priority in the 'Health of the Nation' initiative. The aim is to reduce the death rate from accidents among children under 14 by at least 33% by the year 2005, (DoH 1992). Strategies for achieving this end are discussed in Smith (1991).

Factors which affect accidents in childhood include:

- gender – more boys have accidents than girls;
- social class and deprivation – accidents are more prevalent in socio-economically deprived families;
- personal factors – such as curiosity, clumsiness, age level of daring and so on;
- level of parental supervision – families that are under pressure because of divorce or a 'chaotic' life style may have lower parental supervision (Child Accident Prevention Trust 1989).

The reasons for childhood accidents are largely environmental. Socio-economically deprived children are less likely to live in homes with gardens, more likely to live near dangerous streets and are less likely to be supervised at play. Promoting child safety has traditionally been approached using traditional health promotion approaches directed towards the behaviour of individuals. This ignores the factors which are largely responsible for creating unsafe environments such as increased traffic close to housing, a lack of park land in inner cities and a lack of suitable play areas.

What role do community nurses have in the prevention of childhood accidents? Health visitors in particular have a key role in preventing accidents in the home because of the extent of their work with families with children under five and their unique function of home visiting. Nelson and Dines' (1995) review of the literature of accident prevention offers guidelines drawn from various studies of accident prevention and health visiting and offers a comprehensive checklist of mainly individual approaches (Figure 4.2). Individual families can be targeted for accident prevention, using such strategies as these. The Department of Health (1993) examines the role that health professionals could play in changing the environments in which accidents occur. The main suggestions are for community nurses to participate in developing local alliances with other agencies such as the police, local schools, environmental health departments and so forth, and to take part in specific projects such as the DUMP (disposal of unwanted medicines) campaign.

Other potential areas for health workers to become involved include:

- local 'play it safe' campaigns;
- lobbying to improve road safety;
- safety equipment loan schemes;
- solvent abuse campaigns;
- fire prevention (especially the promotion of smoke detecting devices).

In terms of evidence for effectiveness the summary shown in Figure 4.3 is from Effective Health Care (1996).

4.6 CONCLUSIONS

This chapter has looked at various approaches to helping and supporting families to promote the health

- Advice given should focus on single actions that will have a lasting effect.
- Advice given should be about hazards present at the time in each home.
- The amount of advice should be limited and not combined with a variety of other advice about childcare.
- The purpose of the visit should be clear and an appointment made.
- Detailed information regarding the availability of safety devices and any financial help available should be given (Colver *et al.* 1982).
- Health visitor intervention should follow an assessment of the client and the environment.
- Education should be tailored to the child's developmental needs.
- The method of presentation used by health visitors should be improved by actively involving the client and ensuring that methods are appropriate for the client.
- Practical and theoretical training for health visitors should be improved.
- Accident and emergency notification systems should be improved. Laidman (1989).
- The basis for all safety advice should be a good relationship between the health visitor and family.
- Post accident support visits should be improved. Health visitors should communicate openly about referral routes for accident and emergency contacts.
- Many of the safety needs of parents could be met through group work, using structured participative activities.
- Parents' knowledge of the local area should be used to contribute to decisions about priorities for local campaign work.
- Coombes' (1991) study also demonstrated that many parents wanted increased knowledge about first aid.

Figure 4.2 Checklist for accident prevention. (Adapted from Nelson & Dines 1995. Reproduced with the kind permission of *Health Visitor.*)

- There is good evidence that the use of cycle helmets and child care seat restraints can reduce serious injury to children involved in road traffic accidents.
- Urban road safety measures such as the provision of crossing patrollers, measures to redistribute traffic and improve the safety of individual roads can reduce the rate and severity of childhood accidents.
- The use of safety devices in the home such as smoke detectors, child resistant containers and thermostatic control for tap water can reduce the risks of home injuries. Targeting of households at higher risk combined with home visits, education and the free distribution of devices is likely to make the most impact.
- Educational programmes by themselves appear to have little effect. However, a number of community programmes which involve local participation and use a broad range of interventions have been effective at reducing childhood injuries from a wide variety of causes. These need to be based on accurate data derived from surveillance systems.

Figure 4.3 Evidence of effectiveness of strategies/programmes designed for accident prevention. (Effective Health Care 1996. Reproduced with the kind permission of NHS Centre for Reviews and Dissemination, University of York.)

of children. Community nurses who promote the health of children are likely in the future to be delivering more targeted approaches to those in greatest need. Intersectoral approaches to family health care will also continue to develop, especially in the pre-

vention of childhood accidents. It is very likely that such nurses will increasingly also work in partnership with parents through individual home visiting and through group work.

REFERENCES

Annett, H. & Riflan, S. (1990) *Improving Urban Health*. World Health Organisation. Geneva.

Barker, W. (1991) *Empowering Parents: the Evolution, Evaluation and Expansion of a Programme. Network for Developmental Intiatives in the Community*. University of Bristol, Bristol.

Barker, W. (1992) Health visiting: action research is a controlled environment. *International Journal of Nursing Studies*, **29** (3), 251–9.

Billingham, K. (1989) 45 Cope Street: working in partnership with parents. *Health Visitor*, **62** (5), 156–7.

Billings, J. (1996) *Profiling for Health: the Process and Practice*. Health Visitors Association, London.

Blackburn, C. (1991) *Poverty and Health: Working with Families*. Open University, Milton Keynes.

Blackburn, C. (1992) *Poverty Profiling: A Guide for Community Nurses*. Health Visitors Association, London.

Charles, R.P. (1994) An evaluation of parent held records. *Health Visitor*, **67** (8), 270–72.

Child Accident Prevention Trust (1989) *Basic Principles of Accident Prevention. A Guide to Action*. Child Accident Prevention Trust, London.

Coombes, G. (1991) *You Can't Watch them 24 Hours a Day*. Child Accident Prevention Trust, London.

Colver, A.F., Hutchingson, P.J. & Judson, E.C. (1982) Promoting children's home safety. *BMJ*, **285**, 1177–80.

Department of Health (1992) *The Health of the Nation: a Strategy for Health in England*. HMSO, London.

Department of Health (1993) *The Health of the Nation. Key Area Handbook: Accidents*. HMSO, London.

Edwards, J. & Popay, J. (1994) Contradictions of support and self-help: views from providers of community health and social services to families with young children. *Health & Social Care in the Community*, **2** (1), 31–40.

Effective Health Care (1996) Preventing unintentional injuries in children and young adolescents. Effective Health Care, Universities of Leeds & York, **2** (5), 1.

Graham, H. (1984) *Women, Health and the Family*. Wheatsheaf Books, Brighton.

Guardian (1997) Smashing the glass ceiling. 26 May 1997, G2, 2–4.

Hall, D. (ed.) (1996) *Health for all Children – a Programme of Child Surveillance*, 3rd edn. Oxford Medical Press, Oxford.

Jarman, B. (1983) Identification of underprivileged areas. *BMJ*, **285**, 1705–9.

Luker, K.A. & Orr, J. (1992) *Health Visiting: Towards Community Health Nursing*. Blackwell Scientific Publications, Oxford.

Macfarlane, J.A. & Saffin (1990) Do general practitioners and health visitors like parent held child health records? *British Journal of General Practice*, **40**, 106–8.

Mayall, B. (1986) *Keeping Children Healthy*. Allen and Unwin, London.

Mayall, B. & Foster, M. (1989) *Child Health Care: Living with Children, Working for Children*. Heinemann, Oxford.

National Health Services Management Executive (1996) *Child Health in the Community: a Guide to Good Practice*. HMSO, London.

Nelson, E. & Dines, A. (1995) The health visitor and accident prevention. *Health Visitor*, **68** (7), 280–83.

Oakley, A., Mauther, M., Rajan, L. & Turner, H. (1994) Supporting vulnerable families: an evaluation of NEWPIN. *Health Visitor*, **68** (5), 188–91.

Oppenheim, C. (1990) *Poverty: the Facts*. Child poverty action group, London OPCS (1995) Social Trends, HMSO, London.

OPCS (1995) *Social Trends 25*. HMSO, London.

OPCS (1997) *Social Trends 27*. HMSO, London.

Orr, J. (1992) Chapter 3, Health visiting and the community. In: *Health Visiting: Towards Community Health Nursing*, (eds K.A. Luker & J. Orr). Blackwell Scientific Publications, Oxford, pp. 73–106.

Pearson, M., Dawson, C., Moore, H. & Spencer, S. (1993) Health on Borrowed Time? Priorities and meeting needs in low income households. *Health and Social Care in the Community*, **1** (1), 45–54.

Richardson, D. (1993) *Women, Motherhood and Childrearing*. Macmillan Basingstoke.

Rowe, A. (1993) Cope Street revisited. *Health Visitor*, **66** (10), 358–9.

Scarr, S. & Dunn, J. (1987) *Mothercare/Othercare*. Penguin, Middlesex.

Smith, R. (1991) *The Health of the Nation, The BMJ View*. British Medical Journal, London.

Townsend, P., Davidson, N. & Whitehead, M. (1988) *Inequalities in Health*. Penguin, London.

FURTHER READING

Dowler, E. & Calvert, C. (1995) *Nutrition and Diet in Lone Parent Families in London*. Family Policy Studies Centre, London.

Laidman, P. (1987) Health visiting and preventing accidents to children. Research Report 12. Child Accident Prevention Trust, London.

5

Post-natal Depression: Minimising the Impact

Catherine Gaskell

5.1 INTRODUCTION

Post-natal depression (PND) is an illness that can occur at any time during the year after birth, and the greatest risk of onset is in the first month after delivery. It is the most common complication of the post-natal period. The illness can have a devastating effect on the mother's relationship with her child, partner and extended family and friends, and can leave her clinically depressed with a range of distressing symptoms.

Primary health care workers such as health visitors, GPs, midwives and practice nurses are in key positions to recognise the symptoms, and are therefore ideally placed to advise on commencing treatment. In the 1990s this consists of both professional and personal help, involving medication, counselling, hospitalisation in extreme cases, family support, rest, adequate nutrition and contact with other mothers. Appendix 5.1 at the end of this chapter gives a list of self-help agencies which are useful contacts for the practitioner to refer to.

5.2 PREVALENCE

Three separate states of mood disturbance post-partum are commonly cited (Brown 1979). These are: post-partum blues, post-partum depression, and post-partum psychosis.

Post-partum blues

More commonly known as 'baby blues', this condition may commonly occur in the post-natal ward, and last from a few hours to a few days, or, occasionally weeks. Between 50–70% of post-partum women suffer from this experience, symptoms of which include tearfulness, excitement, extreme tiredness and an overall emotional fragility. Some people believe it coincides with the start of lactation, and others that being in hospital contributes to it. It is not an illness or disorder because of the mild and transient nature of the mood changes, and their very common prevalence. In some cases, the blues may progress into depression, or may coincide with the onset of psychosis.

Post-partum depression

This is a more serious and long-term condition with prevalence rates around 14% (O'Hara & Swain 1996). Symptoms are more severe (see Figure 5.1 for a list of 11 major symptoms of post-natal depression). The peak time of incidence is in the first month (Cox *et al.* 1993), and the nature and severity of depression is similar to depression in other settings. The range and severity affects treatment options and management. Very severe illness may require psychiatric outpatient or inpatient treatment. This treatment usually occurs in acute psychiatric wards, which may have a limited number of mother and baby beds, or the mother may be admitted separately. More rarely, women may be admitted into specialist mother and baby units, which specialise in joint admissions and intensive treatment

Despondency	The mother may feel nothing she does is any good; life is not worth living. The mother may express hopeless/helpless feelings.
Feeling a failure	The mother may voice negative feelings on her ability to perform tasks. She tends to withdraw socially.
Feeling guilty	Due to feeling a failure, unable to cope. Feelings of not loving the baby enough. Feelings of not wanting the baby. Feeling not the same as other mothers.
Feeling irritable/restless	Some women experience PMT-like symptoms. Feelings of anger and hostility towards baby, self or partner.
Loss of appetite	Combined with rapid weight loss.
Loss of sex drive	Avoidance or fear of intimacy. This is nearly universal after childbirth, but is much more severe and persistent in women who are depressed.
Tearfulness	Crying excessively, the mother feeling that she cries without a reason.
Severe fatigue	Feeling permanently exhausted. Waking feeling tired and unrefreshed.
Poor concentration	Reading may not now be enjoyable or even watching TV.
Sleep disturbance	Difficulty in getting to sleep, waking early and not returning to sleep.
Thoughts of death	Ending it all and escape.

Figure 5.1 Eleven major symptoms of post-natal depression.

involving the family. Most cases are, however, managed in the primary health care setting.

Post-partum psychosis

This condition is also referred to as puerperal psychosis. The incidence rate is usually found to be 1 in 1000 deliveries (Paffenberger 1964; Kendell *et al.* 1987). This is an extremely serious state where the mother is psychotic, and may be hallucinating and unable to care for herself or baby. Other symptoms include insomnia, exhaustion and elated mood. Rapid hospitalisation is usual due to the risks of harm to mother and baby through loss of contact with reality.

In this chapter we concentrate on post-partum depression, its effects and treatment.

5.3 THEORIES

Since the time of Louis Marcé, 1858, theories of the origin of post-natal illness have been expounded, promoted and then discounted. They have ranged from hormonal – deficiencies of progesterone (Dalton 1980) through to social causes (Brown & Harris 1978; Oakley 1980). Elliot *et al.* (1985) suggested that post-natal depression could be a natural response to stressors associated with, or coinciding with, motherhood.

Evidence from research has contributed more understanding, and has begun to test previously held beliefs. Investigations for causes of onset fall broadly into two overlapping categories, psychosocial, and neuro-endocrine. The general consensus is that non-psychotic depression after childbirth is predominantly provoked by factors such as deprived early experience of parenting, poor social support, life stress and difficulties in the marital relationship (Kumar 1982; Beck 1996; Sheppard 1997). Another major influence is a history of a depressive disorder (O'Hara & Zekoski 1988; Beck 1996).

Neuro-endocrine links are still under investigation, but many researchers and clinicians in the field are tending to hold with the view put forward by Kumar *et al.* (1995), that 'psychosocial and environmental factors appear to be the main contributors to the occurrence of non-psychotic post-natal depression.' This view is supported by the meta-analysis of 44 studies reported by Beck (1996). In this analysis, significant effects were associated with eight predictor variables: pre-natal depression, child care stress, life stress, social support, pre-natal anxiety, maternity blues, marital dissatisfaction and a history of previous depression.

5.4 SIGNS AND SYMPTOMS

Focusing on signs and symptoms will give the health care practitioner some diagnostic information, but will not explain fully how the woman feels, nor the effect on her child or partner/family. Symptoms can develop at any time from one week to one year after birth. (See Figure 5.1 for symptoms.) A women does not need to experience all of these symptoms to be suffering from PND. They may occur to a lesser degree, and can be seen as variants or extremes of normal changes and fears experienced after birth, for example severe fatigue.

Dr Diane Semprevivo (1966) in her classic book, *The Lived Experience of Post-Partum Mental Illness*, described in detail several sets of distressing symptoms expressed by post-natally depressed women. She identified them as:

Resentment – where the mothering role turns into a resentment of the infant. A mother may question her decision to have had the child.

Inadequacy – The feelings of being unable to cope with the baby and the daily requirements, also carrying out other activities, such as self-care and managing the household.

Lack of or reduction in maternal feelings – Many women express distress regarding their lack of attachment or feelings for their baby. Robson and Kumar (1980) found that immediate post-natal reactions of detachment to the newborn baby did not appear to have prolonged emotional complications, however mothers who were depressed three months after the birth were more likely to express feelings of dislike or detachment in relation to their babies.

A combination of symptoms namely sleep disturbance, feeling a failure and despondency and any mother voicing thoughts of death or harm to her baby, would need immediate further investigation. Mead, Bower

and Gask (1997) explore the considerable potential for nurses in primary care to make an impact in terms of the prevention and management of emotional problems, and Thompson (1997) shows how important it is to take account of cultural and linguistic differences when detecting difficulties. One area where there has been considerable interest is the screening of women for depression after childbirth. For instance Broadhead (1996, pers. comm.), recommends that women should be screened for depression at the sixth week post-natal check. Although not a replacement for clinical judgement, screening tools have been developed, and in particular the Edinburgh Post-natal Depression Scale (EPDS) is widely used.

History of EPDS

Cox, Holden & Sagovsky (1987) developed a scale with 10 items, referred to as the EPDS, which registers the quality of mood, and it is now recognised as a useful measure to help practitioners identify postnatal depression. It is completed by the woman, (ideally when she is alone), takes approximately five minutes, and can be easily scored with the maximum score being 30. A score of over 12 suggests that clinical depression may not be present. Item 10 on the scale can alert health professionals to assess the risk of deliberate self-harm or suicide (see Appendix 5.2).

5.5 MANAGEMENT

Primary care

A common criticism by parents (Holden *et al.* 1989) was that ante-natal preparation had concentrated on the practical aspects of pregnancy, delivery and basic infant care, and that insufficient attention is devoted to the possibility of low mood and change in roles and status. As long ago as 1960 Gordon and Gordon reported that women who were encouraged during pregnancy to confide in their husbands, and enlist their practical help, not only got more help, but were less likely to become depressed.

Primary care may also involve prevention, with appropriate interventions directed at women and their families during pregnancy. Prevention can begin in the pre-birth classes, as well as through contacts in health centre settings. Nurses working in primary care are ideally placed to put women in touch with others in a similar setting. Educational leaflets can be available in waiting rooms. Advice on facilities which are available to offer support in their area should be provided for both partners.

Midwives are also in a position to gain a history of past mental illness when clerking pregnant patients, and to inform other health services that a vulnerable patient is in the system and to provide extra support pre-and post-birth. Kumar (1990) points out that there can be few better opportunities for preventative care than in the obstetric setting, given mothers' repeated contacts with medical and paramedical staff. Clement (1995) explores the potential preventive value of ante-natal visiting targeted at women with low emotional wellbeing. In addition some health authorities have community psychiatric nurses with special interest in post-natal mental health, who are assigned to care for women either after they have been in hospital, or who are deemed vulnerable due to a prior history of mental illness. According to Oates (1988), predictive vulnerability factors can be detected readily, during pregnancy and the first six weeks after childbirth, by family doctors and other members of the primary care team, and suitable follow-up care provided. A newly reported checklist (Beck 1998) may be of value in helping health professionals to identify women at risk.

Health visitors have a key role in providing information, advice and counselling post-birth to new mothers, encouraging the mother to talk through the tremendous changes that are occurring, both in role and status, for both herself and her partner. A health visitor can provide reassurance and support on the physical effects of labour, and in caring for a demanding baby – tiredness, weight loss or gain and irritability. Encouraging mothers to talk through expectations, difficulties and dilemmas that occur in the early weeks post-birth, may all help in reducing anxiety and the concerns that often accompany parenthood. If these interventions are not effective and symptoms of PND become apparent, then further treatments and involvement of the wider multi-disciplinary team occur.

Medication

About 25% of women with post-natal depression, will require medication, outpatient referral and/or help from a specialist mental health team. If post-natal depression is persistent and associated with biological features (i.e., lack of sleep, sex drive, and appetite), women are generally prescribed antidepressant medication. Women who require admission will usually have been on antidepressants but, if not, antidepressants will usually be commenced and advice on side effects given. Women will be closely monitored, and sleep routines will be enhanced by staff supporting them during night feeds and baby's restless times.

Recommended antidepressants are tricyclic drugs and serotonin selective re-uptake inhibitors (SSRIs). Tricyclic drugs may cause some drowsiness and may be given at night. They have some anticholinergic side effects such as dry mouth, blurred vision and possible urinary retention, which could manifest itself in the baby if breast feeding. However, it is generally considered safe to breast feed whilst on antidepressants, providing the baby is healthy. Yoshida and Kumar (1996) have shown that the baby's cognitive development is not significantly impaired. The benefit of breast feeding may outweigh possible undesirable effects if the mother is taking tricyclic antidepressants. This is thought to be the case when using tricyclic drugs – much less is known about SSRI medication.

Alternative therapies

Some women have reported beneficial effects from massage and aromatherapy in milder cases of PND. This may be due to a number of reasons, not the least, that it is time for themselves away from the baby. Any relaxing and calming treatment such as yoga, relaxation tapes, reflexology are useful as an adjunct to traditional treatment and in the preventative phases.

Support groups

Some women benefit from meeting other women in similar situations, others find this too depressing. Consider the range of support groups available locally or nationally (see Appendix 5.1 which lists self-help agencies). Making links with mother-and-baby groups, play sessions or any other baby/child related activity can be a way of getting a mother to mix. Groups may be advertised at a GP's surgery via the health visitor. Babies also benefit from the social stimulation and activity and can learn and develop through imitation.

Tips for mothers – how to help yourself

■ Take advantage of offers of help that you feel comfortable with. You may have been in control, organised, efficient, confident; the one who helped others, pre-birth. It is now your turn to accept help and it does not mean you are a failure.

■ Avoid making major decisions – stress exacerbates a range of other symptoms. Try not to plan a house move, career change, or trip overseas whilst the baby is small and you are not on top form.

■ Exercise. It probably feels like the last thing you want to do. It may feel as though you have no spare energy to contemplate it. It will, however, boost your reserves. It can be pushing the pram around the park or going to the shops but exercise daily, aiming for 20 minutes.

■ Sleep – try to get unbroken sleep. Hand over night care to partner or friends. Nap during the day. Go to bed early. Use the weekends. Build up energy reserves by sleeping when and where you can.

■ Nutrition – especially when breast feeding, eat healthily and, if you cannot cook and feel too ill to prepare food, take supplements and vitamins. Think of the care you took in choosing food when pregnant; think of yourself now.

■ Talk to people and tell your health visitor or GP about how you feel. Express your feelings, showing them can make you feel unburdened, but also release tension and frustration. Choose a sympathetic audience. Expressing feelings of despondency at some mother and baby groups may not get the required sympathetic non-judgemental response. Link up with PND groups or support groups via your health visitor. Share your feelings.

■ Consider drug treatment if offered. It will not usually be for a prolonged period, and antidepressants are not addictive. It may help relieve the symptoms enough to help you take advantage of counselling or time apart from your baby. It may also lessen or reduce the impact of your illness on your baby and enable you to recover quickly.

Management in the community

Broadhead (1996, pers. comm.) comments that, if a woman is thought to have PND, she should be offered listening visits from a member of the Primary Care Team. He has outlined seven steps that primary practitioners can take in their management of a post-natally ill woman:

(1) Ask questions.
(2) Listen and talk.
(3) Ask about suicide and thoughts of harming the baby.
(4) Give information.
(5) Look at the options for networking.
(6) Talk about the use of antidepressants.
(7) Plan follow-up.

The view that an early intervention involving talking and information-giving is useful is confirmed by a paper by Gerrard *et al.* (1993). Health visitors were trained in the use of EPDS and in screening, intervention and preventative strategies, in a research study in Edinburgh, Lewisham and North Staffordshire. The findings from the health visitors were that it had been a positive experience and that structured listening was a positive intervention for the mothers to whom it was offered.

Assessing risk

If a mother becomes extremely unwell in the community, and unable to meet her own, or the baby's physical/emotional needs, or through unpredictability of mental state, has lost contact with reality or lapsed into psychosis, there may be a considerable risk to the infant's wellbeing, Cassin (1996) writes that three dimensions should be considered when assessing possible risk to an infant from its mother in the home environment. She stresses the need for communication among health professionals as health visitors in particular have a child protection remit. The dimensions are:

Mother's mental state

■ Preoccupation with certain activities.
■ Levels of concentration – is the mother completing tasks or distracted?
■ Anger towards baby, self or others.
■ Voicing of strange beliefs or thoughts – particularly involving baby.
■ Presence of auditory hallucinations (hearing voices).

Family members' feedback

- Is the mother acting differently?
- Is she responding normally to them?
- Does she relate to the baby as per normal?

Professionals' observations of baby (health visitor/midwives)

- Weight gain/loss.
- Developmental milestones normal.
- Signs of neglect/abuse.

Tertiary management

There is a limited range of treatment options for the severely post-natally depressed woman. Severely depressed mothers who are unable to care for themselves or their babies may need to be admitted to an inpatient mother and baby unit. There are few dedicated mother and baby units, many are regional and require travelling some distance and are frequently over-subscribed. Some NHS Trusts admit into acute units causing a separation of mother and child.

5.6 WIDER EFFECTS

Effects on the family

The family and close friends can be seen as a source of important support or can be perceived as interfering. A depressed mother will be sensitive to perceived criticisms, and can experience feeling taken over or overwhelmed by offers of help. The nurse can encourage the mother's empowerment by allowing her to choose what activities she wants help with, delegating practical activities, such as housework and ironing, rather than having baby care removed by well meaning relatives.

Using a supportive network of family and friends can be useful in talking through mixed and painful emotions, and for the mother to allow herself to be supported. Partners may be able to help in this process if they can maintain a non-judgemental approach, and avoid telling the woman to 'pull herself together'. Changes in role for both partners often arise at this

time. The mother may perceive herself as having previously been in control, a competent and self-reliant person. The flexibility demanded by a baby and initial lack of routine is an enormous change to adapt to. Encouraging the mother to ask for help to delegate housework and lower standards for herself will involve her in relinquishing control and she will require support. Partners will also need to consider role change in and out of the home. Fathers may need to take extra leave, reduce hours away from the home, support their partner and provide consistency for the baby. Within the home, fathers may need to examine and change previously held beliefs on traditional roles, learn practical baby care and take on night feeds and so on so that the mother is provided with maximum rest.

Nurses clearly have an important role in education, support and modelling for both parents and relatives.

Effects on the partner

There is clear evidence that the lack of marital support or a disharmonious marital relationship are important factors in predicting a recurrence of post-partum episodes of mental illness (Kendell *et al.* 1987). What can the health practitioner do to help support this relationship, which may be central to the recovery of the patient? One approach is working with the partner/family to allow them to recognise that the illness affects everyone, and that the process of recovery will require adjustment for the family as a whole. This could involve the health practitioner in:

- providing health education via literature on PND;
- allowing the partner to ventilate his fears and anxieties concerning his partner's distress;
- encouraging the partner/family to speak to their GP for further assistance;
- meeting other partners in similar situations.

Fathers/partners need to try to be supportive and caring, but also to realise their limitations and maintain some detachment. It is exhausting caring for someone with post-natal depression for long periods of time; so the health professionals can encourage the development of other support systems. There is strong evidence for the efficiency of couple therapy, both in terms of improving the quality of the relationship (Jacobson & Addis 1993), and in helping to address psychiatric symptoms in one of the partners (Hulson 1992). Several studies have shown the value of couple therapy in depression (e.g., Jacobson *et al.* 1993).

The health practitioner can also work as an advisor and educator on the symptoms of PND which also overlap with normal concomitants of motherhood and, although distressing, usually pass with support.

Reduced libido

Most women lose the desire for sex for up to 4–6 weeks after childbirth and some for much longer. The reasons may include tiredness and complications or consequences of the delivery, particularly if an episiotomy or stitches were involved, fear of pain post delivery, or fear of pregnancy so soon after birth.

Exhaustion

The stress of baby care, plus a depression, usually drains a new mother's physical and emotional reserves of energy. Support and absence of pressure are advised and the opportunity to talk through what is happening for both partners, can reduce tension and expectations.

Broken sleep

Night feeds, and coping with the demands of other children, can cause a broken sleep pattern and increase general exhaustion. Involving the partner in making and giving feeds of formula, or expressing breast milk or sharing feeds is helpful in reducing this.

Fathers can also experience loss of libido and the other symptoms due to the experience of birth or their partner's pain. The role of the health practitioner again would be that of health promotion, providing advice, reassurance and normalising the situation.

Effects on the baby

Murray (1992) reported that depressed mothers related differently to sons and daughters. A number of researchers have suggested that boys are generally more vulnerable to psychosocial risk factors such as divorce or marital discord (Grych & Finsham 1990). In a paper written by Sharp *et al.* (1995) 'maternal depression in the first year post-partum was asso-

ciated with lower scores on tests of intellectual attainment as children approached their fourth birthdays'. This raises concerns that, as community nurses, we have a role to play in prevention and management of mental illness/depression associated with childbirth, if we hope to reduce the impact for children in later life.

Babies are primarily dependent on their mothers for nurturing and stimulation. If this is lacking, or is not sensitive (i.e., in tune) then there may be adverse consequences for the baby's psychological development. Mothers feel miserable enough when they are depressed, and many find the added guilt that they may be harming their baby's development to be unbearable. Ignoring the problem is not going to solve it. What is needed is early detection of depression, and work with the mother to find strategies which empower her to relate happily and successfully with her baby (e.g., in short bursts), and to ask for help in between.

5.7 CONCLUSION

Post-natal depression can be devastating. It affects not only the mother in her ability to care and bond with her baby, but all her close and intimate relationships. It can, if untreated, have long-term consequences for the whole family. The role of any health practitioner working with women and families experiencing these difficulties will be broad and encompasses several aspects:

■ Support and reassurance of the mother and family once symptoms occur and advising on reducing symptoms.
■ Careful monitoring and aftercare planning. Liaison with a wide range of health care professionals and ensuring continued community support.
■ Referral on to voluntary support groups/community mental health teams.
■ Health promotion for both mother and child.

The overall aims are that the illness of post-natal depression and the distress it causes can be dealt with as sensitively, safely and quickly as possible.

REFERENCES

Appleby, L., Gregoire, A., Platz, C., Prince, M. & Kumar, R. (1994) Screening women for high risk of post-natal depression. *Journal of Psychosomatic Research*, **38**, 539–45.

Beck, C.T. (1996) A meta-analysis of predictors of post-partum depression. *Nursing Research*, **45** (5), 297–303.

Beck, C.T. (1998) A checklist to identify women at risk for developing postpartum depression. *Journal of Obstetric, Gynaecological and Neonatal Nursing*, **27** (1), 39–46.

Brown, G. & Harris, T. (1978) *Social Origins of Depression*. Tavistock Publications, London.

Brown, W.A. (1979) *Psychological Care During Pregnancy and Post-Partum Period*. Rowen Press, New York.

Cassin, A.L. (1996) Acute maternal mental illness – infants at risk. *Psychiatric Care*, **2**, 202–5.

Clement, S. (1995) 'Listening Visits' in pregnancy: a strategy for preventing postnatal depression. *Midwifery*, **11** (2), 75–80.

Cox, J.L., Murray, D. & Chapman, D.A. (1993) A controlled study of onset, duration and prevalence of post-natal depression. *British Journal of Psychiatry*, **163**, 27–31.

Dalton, K. (1980) *Depression after Childbirth*. Oxford University Press, Oxford.

Elliot, S.A., Watson, J.P. & Brough, D.I. (1985) Transition to parenthood by British couples. *Journal of Reproductive & Infant Psychology*, **3**, 28–39.

Gerrard, J., Holden, J.M., Elliot, S.H. *et al.* (1993) A trainer's perspective of an innovative training programme to teach health visitor's about the detection, treatment and prevention of postnatal depression. *Journal of Advanced Nursing*, **18**, 1822–32.

Gordon, R.E. & Gordon, K.K. (1960) Social factors in prevention of post-partum emotional adjustment. *Obstetrics & Gynaecology*, **15**, 433–8.

Grych, J.H. & Fincham, F.D. (1990) Marital conflict & children's adjustment; A contextual framework. *Psychological Bulletin*, **108**, 267–90.

Holden, J.M., Sagovsky, R. & Cox, J.L. (1989) Counselling in the general practice setting; a controlled study of health visitors' intervention in the treatment of post-natal depression. *British Medical Journal*, **289**, 223–6.

Hulson, B. (1992) Relationship problems and mental illness; indications for couple therapy. *Sexual & Marital Therapy*, **7**, 173–87.

Jacobson, N.S. & Addis, M.E. (1993) Research on couples and couple therapy; What do we know? Where are we going? *Journal of Consulting & Clinical Psychology*, **61**, 93–5.

Jacobson, N.S., Fruzzetti, A.E. & Dobson, E. (1993) Couple therapy as a treatment for depression II. The effects of relationship quality and therapy on depressive relapse. *Journal of Consulting Clinical Psychology*, **61**, 516–19.

Kendell, R.E., Chalmers, L. & Platz, C. (1987) Epidemiology of a puerperal psychosis. *British Journal of Psychiatry*, **150**, 662–73.

Kumar, R. (1982) Neurotic disorders in childbearing women. In: *Motherhood & Mental Illness* (eds I.F. Brockington & R. Kumar). Academic Press, London, pp. 71–118.

Kumar, R. (1990) An overview of post-partum psychiatric disorders. *NAACOGS. Clinical Issues in Perinatal & Women's Health Nursing*, **3**, 351–8.

Kumar, R. & Robson, K.M. (1984) A prospective study of emotional disorders in childbearing women. *British Journal of Psychiatry*, **144**, 35–7.

Kumar, R., Marks, M., Platz, C. & Yoshida, K. (1995) Clinical survey of a psychiatric mother and baby unit with characteristics of 100 consequent admissions. *Journal of Affective Disorders*, **33**, 11–22.

Mead, N., Bower, P. & Gask, L. (1997) Emotional problems in primary care: what is the potential for increasing the role of nurses? *Journal of Advanced Nursing*, **26** (5), 879–90.

Murray, L. (1992) The impact of postnatal depression on infant development. *Journal of Child Psychology & Psychiatry*, **33** (3) 543–61.

Oakley, A. (1980) *'Women Confined' Towards a Sociology of Childbirth*. Martin Robertson, Oxford.

Oates, M.R. (1988) *The Development of An Integrated Community Orientated Service for Severe Postnatal Illness*, Vol. 2, Cause & Consequences (eds R. Kumar & I.F. Brockington). John Wright, London.

Oates, M.R. (1994) Post-natal mental illness: organisation & function of a psychiatric service. In: *Aspects of Perinatal Psychiatry. Use and misuse of EPDS* (eds J. Cox & J. Holden). Gaskell Press, London.

O'Hara, M.W. & Zekoski, E.M. (1988) Post-partum depression: a comprehensive review. In: *Motherhood & Mental Illness*. Vol. 2, *Causes and Consequences* (eds R. Kumar & I.F. Brockington). Wright, London, pp. 17–63.

O'Hara, M.W. & Swain, A.M. (1996) Rats of risk of post-partum depression meta-analysis. *International Review of Psychiatry*, 1996, **8**, 37–54.

Paffenbarger, R.S. (1964) Epidemiological aspects of para-partum mental illness. *British Journal of Preventative & Social Medicine*, **18**, 189–95.

Robson, K.M. & Kumar, R. (1980) Delayed onset of maternal affection after childbirth. *British Journal of Psychiatry*, **36**, 347–53.

Semprevivo, D. (1966) The lived experience of a post-partum mental illness. Rush University. Submitted in partial fulfilment of the requirements for the degree of Doctor of Nursing Science, Illinois.

Sharp, D., Hay, D., Powlby, S., Schmucher, G., Allen, H. & Kumar, R. (1995) The impact of post-natal depression on boys' intellectual development. *Journal of Child Psychology & Psychiatry*, **36**, 1315–37.

Sheppard, M. (1997) Depression in female health visitor consulters: social and demographic facets. *Journal of Advanced Nursing*, **26** (5), 921–9.

Thompson, K. (1997) Detecting postnatal depression in Asian women. *Health Visitor*, **70** (6), 226-8.

Yoshida, K. & Kumar, R. (1996) Breastfeeding & Psychotropic drugs. *International Review of Psychiatry*, **8** (1), March 1996, Carfax, Oxfordshire.

FURTHER READING

Cox, J.L. (1986) *Post-Natal Depression – A Guide for Health Professionals*. Churchill Livingstone, Edinburgh.

Cox, J.L., Holden, J.M. & Sagovsky, R. (1987) Detection of post-natal depression; development of a 10 item Edinburgh Post-natal Depression Scale. *British Journal of Psychiatry*, **150**, 782–6.

Holden, J.M., Sagovsky, R. & Cox, J.L. (1989) Counselling in general practice setting: a controlled study of health visitor intervention in the treatment of postnatal depression. *British Medical Journal*, **298**, 223–6.

Lovestone, S. & Kumar, C. (1993) Postnatal psychiatric illness: the impact on partners. *British Journal of Psychiatry*, **163**, 210–16.

APPENDIX 5.1: SELF HELP AND SUPPORTIVE AGENCIES

MAMA (Meet a Mum Association)

14 Willis Road, South Croydon, Surrey (0181 665 0357). Offers support and friendship to new mothers, particularly with PND. Can link depressed mums with recovering mums. Also prints leaflets about PND.

The Association for Postnatal Illness

25 Jerdan Place, London SW6 1BE (0171 386 0868). Helps women suffering from PND and has links with MAMA.

The National Childbirth Trust

Alexandra House, Oldham Terrace, London W3 6NH (0181 992 8637). A national organisation which may have groups or supporters in local areas for depressed women.

National NEWPIN

Sutherland House, 35 Sutherland Square, London SE17 3EE (0171 703 6326). Provides peer support, group work and counselling, particularly for women whose children are on the 'at risk' register. Good support for isolated women/families.

Cry-sis

BM Cry-sis, London WC1N 3XX (0171 404 5011). A self-help support group run by parents who have experienced the problems of crying or sleepless babies/young children. Volunteers take telephone calls and advise or reassure parents on practical issues concerning their baby; or simply listen. They do not provide medical advice.

Homestart

Voluntary home-visiting scheme, offering friendship and practical support to families/carers where there are children under five; 140 schemes are currently running in the UK.

Parent Link

The Parent Network, 44–46 Caversham Road, London NW5 2DS (0171 735 1214). A group where parents with a trained group leader can learn new parenting skills to help deal with their children.

Relate

Formerly the National Marriage Guidance Council. See your local directory for the nearest branch, or contact headquarters.

Institute of Family Therapy

24–32 New Stephenson Way, London NW1 2HX (0171 391 9150). Voluntary organisation which works with families, couples and individuals on their inter-personal relationships.

Useful books for parents

Sapstead, A. (1990) *Banish Post-baby Blues*, Thorsons.
Marshall, F. (1993) *Coping with Postnatal Depression*, Sheldon Press.
Dix, C. (1985) *The New Mother Syndrome*, Unwin.

APPENDIX 5.2: EDINBURGH POST-NATAL DEPRESSION SCALE[1]

In the past seven days

(1) *I have been able to laugh and see the funny side of things:*

- [ ] As much as I always could
- [ ] Not quite so much now
- [ ] Definitely not so much now
- [ ] Not at all.

(2) *I have looked forward with enjoyment to things:*

- [ ] As much as I ever did
- [ ] Rather less than I used to
- [ ] Definitely less than I used to
- [ ] Hardly at all.

(3) **I have blamed myself unnecessarily whn things went wrong:*

- [ ] Yes, most of the time
- [ ] Yes, some of the time
- [ ] Not very often
- [ ] No, never.

(4) *I have felt worried and anxious for no very good reason:*

- [ ] No, not at all
- [ ] Hardly ever
- [ ] Yes, sometimes
- [ ] Yes, very often.

(5) **I have felt scared or panicky for no very good reason:*

- [ ] Yes, quite a lot
- [ ] Yes, sometimes
- [ ] No, not much
- [ ] No, not at all.

(6) **Things have been getting on top of me:*

- [ ] Yes, most of the time I haven't been able to cope at all
- [ ] Yes, sometimes I haven't been coping as well as usual
- [ ] No, most of the time I have coped quite well
- [ ] No, I have been coping as well as ever.

(7) **I have been so unhappy that I have had difficulty sleeping:*

- [ ] Yes, most of the time
- [ ] Yes, sometimes
- [ ] Not very often
- [ ] No, not at all.

(8) **I have felt sad and miserable:*

- [ ] Yes, most of the time
- [ ] Yes, quite often
- [ ] Not very often
- [ ] No, not at all.

(9) **I have been so unhappy that I have been crying:*

- [ ] Yes, most of the time
- [ ] Yes, quite often
- [ ] Only occasionally
- [ ] No, never.

(10) **The thought of harming myself has occurred to me:*

- [ ] Yes, quite often
- [ ] Sometimes
- [ ] Hardly ever
- [ ] Never.

---

[1] Questions with asterisks * 3, 5, 6, 7, 8, 9, 10 are scored by 3,2,1,0.
　Questions without asterisks are scored by 0, 1, 2, 3.
Reproduced by kind permission of Professor J. Cox and Gaskell Press, London.

6

The Child at Risk: Working with Families and the Child Protection System

Brian Corby

State concern about the abuse of children within their own families, while by no means a new phenomenon (Corby 1993), was re-established and reframed in Britain in the late 1960s. Then the paediatric profession, following on from the work of Kempe in the USA, began to develop an interest in the physical mistreatment of babies and young children (Parton 1985, pp. 48–68). This resulted in a major shift in thinking about parental ill-treatment of children. Previously, the main focus of state intervention had been on neglect, which occasionally incorporated cruelty and, even more rarely, incest. Such forms of ill-treatment were seen largely as products of poverty, ignorance and stress. Baby battering, later termed non-accidental injury to children, was seen to result more from individual pathology than from general deprivation. Greater emphasis was placed on the need for more active direct intervention in families to protect children in these circumstances.

This shift in focus was reflected in the Maria Colwell inquiry report published in 1974 (DHSS 1974). Maria, aged seven, had been killed by her step-father after being returned from care to live with him and her natural mother. Much emphasis was placed in the report on the fact that Maria was highly resistant to such a return, and that her wishes were seen by social workers as secondary to those of her birth mother. There was also considerable concern that, after her return, different health and welfare professionals, who all had some knowledge of Maria's deterioration, failed to communicate and share this information. As a result of these findings by the inquiry, two significant changes followed. Firstly, there was the establishment of a formal inter-agency system for dealing with child abuse. The system in England and Wales was characterised by three features:

- Area Review Committees which were inter-disciplinary forums for middle and higher managers of police, health, welfare and education departments. (The main functions of this body were to enhance interprofessional co-ordination and co-operation, to ensure that central government guidelines were incorporated into local practice and to monitor and review problematic cases.)
- Interdisciplinary Case Conferences – these were held on each new case considered to be serious enough to warrant formal consultation.
- Non-accidental injury registers which were used to record the names of children deemed to have been abused or at risk of abuse.

This system has in essence persisted to the present time with various modifications and updatings. Area Review Committees are now termed Area Child Protection Committees, and non-accidental injury registers are now called Child Protection Registers.

The second significant change was in terms of legislation (the 1975 Children Act) which placed greater emphasis on the child's needs for protection against her or his parents.

Against this background this chapter will discuss

policy and evidence concerning the child protection system, community nursing and child protection, and investigating children at risk.

6.2 THE CHILD PROTECTION SYSTEM

The development of the system

Between the mid-1970s and the late 1980s the child protection system expanded dramatically. Initially, the medical profession (mainly through the work of paediatricians) and, in some parts of the country, the National Society for the Prevention of Cruelty to Children (NSPCC), took lead roles in the system. Gradually, however, the main responsibility for all aspects of child protection work was taken over by social services departments. The rate and nature of the growth of the child protection system merits closer inspection. There were 37 public inquiries into the deaths of children as a result of ill-treatment by their carers between 1973 and 1989 (DHSS 1982; DoH 1991a). These inquiries nearly all pointed to two main concerns: Firstly, failures on the part of individual professionals (usually social workers) to focus on the child's best interests as distinct from those of the family, and secondly, failures in communication between professionals.

The net outcome of these messages was to concentrate professional attention more and more on abuse incidents, and on ensuring that interprofessional procedures were strictly adhered to. The main effects of this were twofold: firstly, the number of children on child protection registers in England rose exponentially from 11,800 in 1978 to 45,300 in 1991. This stretched professional resources to their limits resulting in a large proportion of the community child care resources in social services departments being diverted into child protection work. The second effect was that social services department social workers, who had the lead role in this work, moved away from a family-oriented approach to such an extent that they came to be seen by parents as child-snatchers. This term is not justified by children in care statistics at the time, but is probably a fair perception of the style of intervention if not the effect.

Another key development in the 1980s was the broadening of concerns about risks to children. Whereas physical abuse and neglect had been almost the sole causes of concern throughout the 1970s, from the early 1980s onwards there was an increasing awareness of more complex and challenging forms of abuse, that is sexual abuse and (to a lesser extent) emotional abuse. This awareness is reflected in the number of registrations in these categories. In 1984 the numbers of children registered for sexual and emotional abuse in England were 1088 and 200 respectively. By 1991 registrations in these categories had risen to 5600 and 2600.

The current context and a change of direction

There were signs of disquiet about the impact of these developments in the late 1980s. Events at Cleveland brought matters to a head. Here, in the first six months of 1987, 121 children were taken into care on the grounds of sexual abuse, a rate of case confirmation which far exceeded that of other areas at this time, and that of Cleveland itself prior to this period. The resulting inquiry report (Butler-Sloss 1988) raised concerns about the lack of co-operation between social workers and police, and between paediatricians and police surgeons. It was particularly critical of the lack of open communication with parents by professionals as to the causes of their concerns and of the processes whereby children were in many cases subjected to repeated interviews and medical examinations. As a consequence of these events, the 1989 Children Act, implemented in 1991, placed greater requirements on social workers to justify and explain the purposes of statutory intervention. It required them to pay more attention to children's rights and parental responsibilities. Child protection guidelines issued in 1991 (DoH 1991b) also emphasised these issues. An important offshoot of this shift was that parents and children were, in normal circumstances, to be invited to attend child protection conferences throughout. They were to be much more closely involved in the process of child abuse work than before.

The 1990s have seen further developments away from the approaches that were encouraged throughout the 1970s and 1980s. Public inquiries such as those at the Orkneys (Clyde 1992) and Rochdale (Lyon & de Cruz 1993) have strengthened the notion of overzealous intervention particularly by social workers. There have also been reductions in the numbers of children on child protection registers in England. In 1995 there were 34,954 children and young people on registers, a decrease of approximately 10,000 since 1991. However, these figures need to be treated with some care. Numbers have been reduced partly because of the disuse of the category of 'grave concern', and also because the system of deregistration has become far more efficient. The number of additions to the register in 1995 was 30,444, roughly the same as in 1991.

Messages from research

In 1995 the Department of Health published a series of reports on research projects which it had initiated in the early 1990s (DoH 1995). The main message of much of this research was that the child protection system, while serving to protect children to some degree, had major dysfunctional effects which needed attention. The first of these was that opportunities were being missed to work with parents to reduce risks to their children. The system was being operated in a way that was perceived as too punitive by parents. More work was needed to involve them in the process and to engage them more fully in efforts to improve their child care practices.

The second was that the child protection system because of a blinkered focus on incidents of abuse was missing out on opportunities to help and support families with more general child care problems and difficulties. This latter dysfunction was particularly identified in the research project carried out by Gibbons *et al.* (1995) which followed the progress of 1846 child protection referrals in eight local authority areas in the early 1990s. The researchers found that 25% of all referrals were closed without the need for a direct visit, and that a further 51% were closed following investigative visits. Twenty four per cent of the cases resulted in child protection conferences, of which about half were registered and a quarter received no follow-up services at all. The child protection system was seen to be operating as a giant filter in which the worst cases in terms of risk to children were left for focused intervention. The concern of the researchers was that there were large numbers of families referred, many of which had more general child care and other problems warranting some form of service or intervention, but which received no attention.

The response of the Department of Health to these and other findings has been to encourage health and welfare professionals to adopt a lighter touch when carrying out child protection investigations. The aim is to engineer a shift back towards a more family supportive approach with less emphasis on child protection and more on working in partnership with parents. This has prompted much debate about getting the balance right between a family-focused and a child-protective approach (see for instance reports on the Rikki Neave case, e.g. Elliott & Mullin 1996).

6.3 COMMUNITY NURSING AND CHILD PROTECTION

Several commentators have pointed to the key role that health visitors and to a lesser extent other community nurses, notably school nurses, have in relation to child protection, particularly in a preventive capacity (Dingwall *et al.* 1983, Browne 1995). Health visitors have a responsibility for the health surveillance of all children up to the age of five and may sustain contact beyond that age if necessary. It is argued that they are in a unique position to pick up indicators of all forms of abuse, but particularly physical abuse, neglect and failure to thrive, because of their health training, and because of their universally accepted role of visiting and supporting all families. Their close network links with various aspects of the health service, is seen as another strength.

In some respects, however, these strengths have not been fully utilised in the past by the child protection system, partly because until the late 1980s health visitors as a body were ambivalent about their child protection role. It was felt that close association with the system might deleteriously influence the nature of relationships with their clients, and have a negative impact on the supportive and preventive work they could carry out. Another factor has been the primacy of the social work profession in child protection work, which has not made enough use of health visitor expertise in carrying out its duties. These issues were very evident in the handling of the Jasmine Beckford case, the inquiry into which recommended a much more central role for health visitors in child protection work with the under-fives (Brent 1985). While this has not yet happened, health visitors have now clarified their position more fully and, despite remaining committed to carrying out a supportive preventive function, are unequivocal about their responsibilities to child protection (Smart 1992). This has been aided by better internal supervision and the appointment of senior nurses with health visiting qualifications to liaise between community health services and the child protection system, as recommended by the Working Together guidelines (DoH 1991b, para. 4.20).

6.4 INVESTIGATING CHILDREN AT RISK

Making child abuse referrals

The conduct of making referrals and responding to them is dealt with in the 1991 Working Together guidelines and in Part IV of the 1989 Children Act, particularly section 47. The guidelines do not have the full force of law, but 'must be complied with, unless local circumstances indicate exceptional reasons which justify a variation' (Lyon 1995, p. 54). They require that concerns about child abuse be referred to social services departments, which have the main responsibility for conducting inquiries where they have reason to believe that a child in their area is suffering, or is likely to suffer, significant harm. (The NSPCC have similar powers, but have now greatly reduced their investigative role in many parts of the UK.) The grounds for intervention are very broad and generalised. Defining child abuse or significant harm for operational practice is an exceptionally difficult task (see Hardiker 1996). The official definitions in the Working Together guidelines include physical abuse, physical neglect, emotional abuse and sexual abuse. Munchausen's syndrome by proxy and failure to thrive are explicitly mentioned. However, these definitions merely label the categories of concern. They do not solve the issue of what degree of harm justifies referral and subsequent intervention. One strategy would be for community nurses to refer all concerns to social services department workers and

leave it to them to make the judgement. The down side of this is that it could lead to social workers feeling that health professionals are dumping their problems. There is also the possibility of loss of faith with a client/patient of long-standing, who finds herself and her family unexpectedly the subject of a child protection investigation. There are no easy answers to these problems. There is an obvious need for nurses and health visitors to consult with their supervisors. Informal consultation with social workers is also advisable. In some cases decisions to refer could be aired with parents themselves, with the caveat that such discussions are not likely to place the child concerned at further risk. In the case of concerns about sexual abuse, such discussions should be avoided.

Filtering out referrals

Gibbons *et al.*'s (1995) research demonstrates that social services departments in England deal with approximately 180,000 child abuse referrals annually. The first action normally taken by social workers in these departments is to check their own records including the child protection register, and to seek information from police, health and other welfare agencies. Information derived from these checks, together with the content of referrals, is seen as sufficient to satisfy concerns in about a quarter of all referrals without the need for home visits. Those referrals likely to be filtered out at this stage include a combination of the following factors: families where the suspicions of ill treatment are vague, where parents are considered by other professionals to be reasonable carers and about which there have been no previous referrals or concerns.

Following up referrals

According to Gibbons *et al.*'s (1995) research, direct contact is made by investigating agencies with the remaining 75% of cases. The form of intervention varies with the nature and extent of the concerns.

General concern cases
There are many cases referred to social services departments where there is no direct evidence of abuse, but general concerns that a child may be likely to suffer significant harm. For instance, the presence of a convicted child-offender in the home, cases where

mental illness on the part of one or both of the parents is thought to be placing a child at risk, and cases where there is resistance on the part of a parent or both parents to work with health and welfare professionals to tackle issues that are of concern to the latter. Usually, cases such as these will be visited by social services department social workers as a result of the referral. In cases where there are concerns about the health of younger children, social workers may be accompanied by health visitors depending on local agreements.

Where there is resistance by parents to intervention at this stage, statutory means of gaining access to a child for the purpose of assessment may be considered. The Child Assessment Order under section 43 of the 1989 Children Act, which must be applied for through the courts, can be used to meet this need. If the applicant is successful, parents are required to present named children for a period of specified assessment for up to seven days. It has to be stressed, however, that this order has been little used since it came on to the statute books (Dickens 1993); the procedure is seen to be cumbersome in comparison with that for obtaining an emergency protection order (see below), which may be used to achieve the same sort of goal.

The vast majority of cases being considered in this section are satisfactorily dealt with without the need for statutory orders. The current message from the Department of Health is that many of these cases should be more carefully considered for help and assistance under section 17 and schedule 2 of the 1989 Children Act. Such assistance includes the possibility of accommodation being provided for a child, referral to a family centre, help with financial and material concerns, and ongoing assistance from social workers. However, as has been seen, until recently, the focus of social services departments on prevention has been limited as has the allocation of resources to this area of work (Aldgate & Tunstill 1995). It remains to be seen whether encouragement from the Department of Health to shift the emphasis to family support will be sufficient in itself to bring about change in this area.

Serious abuse allegations

All serious cases are discussed between social services professionals and the police. These include:

■ most cases where there is evidence of physical abuse;

■ most cases of serious and chronic neglect, particularly those where there are major concerns about standards of parenting because of drug and alcohol misuse resulting in chaotic life styles which are harmful to children; and

■ virtually all cases where there is an allegation of intra-familial sexual abuse.

The police must be notified so that they can decide whether to commence criminal proceedings in relation to the alleged abuser. Where a child is perceived to be at immediate risk if he or she remains at home, an emergency protection order may be sought from the family court (or from a single magistrate) under section 44 of the Children Act. This empowers the applicant, (usually the social services department social worker), to remove the child concerned to a place of safety. The police also have powers of emergency protection under section 46 of the Act without the requirement of court backing. However, it should be noted that emergency protection orders are being used much less frequently since the implementation of the 1989 Children Act. More efforts are now being made to effect the removal of the alleged abuser from the household. This can be done voluntarily with financial assistance from the social services department under schedule 2 paragraph 5 of the 1989 Children Act, or it can be made a condition of a bail agreement if the alleged abuser is charged with an offence (Cobley 1995, pp. 55–7). In either circumstance, considerable emphasis is placed by social workers on the attitude of the non-abusing parent (Waterhouse & Carnie 1992). It should be noted that such an approach is less likely to happen in cases of physical abuse and neglect, where it might not be clear which of the carers is the alleged abuser.

Joint interviews

Where the police believe that an offence has been committed against a child, and that there is the possibility of pursuing a successful prosecution of an alleged offender, it is usually decided to hold a joint interview of the child who has alleged the abuse or who is alleged to be the victim of abuse. Joint interviews are carried out by social workers and the police, the latter of whom tend to specialise in family violence and abuse work. Research points to the police taking the lead role in these interviews (Fielding & Conroy 1992). Non-abusing parents and relatives may also be in attendance (see Corby 1998). Detailed guidance for the conduct of such interviews is set out in the Memorandum of Good Practice (Home Office 1992). The aim of the guidance is twofold – firstly, to reduce the amount of interviewing that children may be subjected to in an investigation, a specific concern of those who conducted the Cleveland inquiry report, and, secondly, to provide a means whereby children's main evidence can be presented in court without their having to restate their experiences openly and in public. All interviews are required to be videotaped using high quality technology, and questioning is expected to adhere to the rules of evidence that are customary in court proceedings. The guidance has been criticised by Wattam (1992) for being too artificial and formalised and as a result not meeting the emotional needs of children. Research by the Social Services Inspectorate (DoH 1994) has also shown that the chances of evidence derived from these interviews being used in criminal proceedings is very limited. In cases where the police do not feel that there is the likelihood of a prosecution (which is increasingly seen to be true in respect of younger children), investigations are carried out by social workers as described in the previous section.

Child protection conferences

Procedural rules

In nearly all cases where a joint interview is held, and in some of those where it is not but where continuing concerns persist, a child protection conference results. According to Gibbons et al.'s (1995) research this happens in about a quarter of all cases initially referred. The expectation is that conferences will be held no later than 15 days after the initial allegation. In reality, many conferences take much longer than this to arrange. The average number of people attending child protection conferences is around ten (Gibbons et al. 1995, p.69). Some attenders are regulars, including the chairperson, police representatives, the health visitor manager, and the city solicitor (in some areas). Other attenders are case-specific – social workers, school teachers, school nurses, health visitors, probation officers, GPs, foster parents and so on. Parents have the right to attend these conferences in most cases as well as older children. The Working Together guidelines place the onus on the conference participants to justify the exclusion of parents from conferences (DoH 1991b, para. 6.15). Initially,

concerns that the attendance of parents and children at child protection conferences would inhibit free professional discussion were raised. But most of the evaluative research into this topic suggests that professionals do not feel that this has happened (Thoburn et al. 1995, pp.1–12). Indeed, many are of the view that parental presence at conferences is likely to enhance work carried out with them at the post-conference stage. However, there is some doubt as to whether attendance at child protection conferences is seen by parents as enabling them to participate more fully in the process (Corby et al. 1996). The main gain for parents seems to be that they come out of the conference with a clear idea of what the concerns of the professionals are.

Functions

The functions of the child protection conference are set out in the Working Together guidelines (DoH 1991b, paras. 6.1–6.8). In brief they are to assess the risk to the subject child (or children) and to determine a plan to reduce/eliminate that risk. There are many factors to be taken into account:

- the nature and severity of the alleged abuse;
- the evidence available for criminal and care proceedings;
- the current situation in the household (e.g. does the alleged abuser still have access to the child concerned?);
- the attitude of the non-abusing parent to the child, and the degree of co-operativeness with health and welfare officials.

The conference is empowered to place a child's name on the child protection register and, if it does so, to appoint a named key worker, usually a social worker, to co-ordinate an agreed child protection plan which will normally involve other health and welfare agencies. Gibbons et al. (1995) found that this decision was reached in about half of all child protection conferences. In cases where the ongoing risk is considered so great that the child should be removed from his or her parents or, more usually at this stage, continue to be separated from them, the social services department or the NSPCC may initiate care proceedings (provided also that there is sufficient evidence for court) or it may provide accommodation for a child if the parents agree. Gibbons et al. (1995) found in their study that some form of care provision was made in 15% of the child protection conferences. The need for care proceedings in these circumstances may be obviated by relatives seeking section 8 orders under the 1989 Children Act. There are other possible outcomes of a child protection conference:

(1) A recommendation to the social services department to seek a supervision order through the courts. Such orders may have additional conditions attached to them, such as a requirement placed on the parents to bring a child to a clinic or family centre (see schedule 3 of the 1989 Children Act).
(2) A decision to take no (or very limited) further action with a family.

Follow-up work after the conference

It needs to be stressed again that for large numbers of children who are the subject of child protection conferences, the outcome is that they remain in the care of one or both of their natural parents. A quarter of the families that were subject to conferences in Gibbons et al.'s (1995) study received no ongoing support afterwards. There are concerns that, as with those families which are filtered out at the initial investigation stage (see above), opportunities to work in a preventive capacity may be being missed.

Those families whose children's names are placed on the child protection register are most likely of all to receive ongoing community-based resources and surveillance. As pointed out in the previous section, a key worker is appointed in these circumstances to carry out the requirements of a child protection plan. In many areas the mechanism for achieving this is via what are termed core group meetings, involving those professionals who might be directly involved with the families – health visitors, school teachers, school nurses, education welfare officers and probation officers in addition to the key workers – and the parents, children (depending on their age and understanding) and possibly other relatives. The working of these groups has not been closely researched (Calder 1991). In theory these group meetings offer better settings for parental and child participation than do child protection conferences, which are more formal, have more attenders and take place at a time when the potential for conflict and disagreement between professionals and parents is probably greatest (Mccallum & Prilleltensky 1996). They also provide

professionals from different disciplines with the opportunity to work constructively together.

Farmer and Owen (1995) in their study found that an important factor in successful follow-up work was the quality of the protection plan agreed upon at the child protection conference. More specific, clear goal-oriented plans were associated with better outcomes. There is little doubt that parents welcome clarity and straightforwardness from professionals with whom they are involved (Thoburn et al. 1995, pp. 215–7)). Thus plans and ongoing work should as far as possible be simple, clear, outcome-focused and time-limited. Having said this, the child protection system may well have identified some families who are likely to need ongoing support and involvement over a long period of time, particularly where neglect and emotional abuse are the causes for concern (Stevenson 1996). Longer-term involvement can be just as purposefully organised as can short-term work.

The following list is typical of the sort of ongoing work that can be required in a child protection plan agreed upon at a conference:

(1) The need for fuller assessment of the family.
(2) The need for help with parenting skills with the support of a family aide or via attendance at a family centre.
(3) The need for anger management or sex offender treatment.
(4) The need for nursery or respite services to reduce stress on parenting.
(5) The need for therapeutic input to help the child and non-abusing parent cope with the consequences of abuse.
(6) The need for regular health checks.

The work is clearly a mixture of support and monitoring in most cases, a combination that needs to be openly shared with, and explained to, families. It requires professionals from different disciplines to work co-operatively with each other. It also requires considerable resource allocation in order to be effectively carried out. Oversight of ongoing work is maintained by the requirement to review progress at least every six months. Children's names may only be deregistered at a full child protection conference, preferably attended by those present at the initial conference. The current trend is for shorter periods of registration than was the case until the mid-1980s. National child protection registration figures point to there now being as many deregistrations as registrations per year. Hopefully, bearing in mind the caveat raised by Stevenson above, shorter registration is correlated with more purposeful intervention. It should be stressed that if children who are on the register are abused again, either during the time that they are registered, or following deregistration, then the whole process of investigation starts again.

Evaluating child protection work

This concluding section will examine the effectiveness of the British system of child protection and consider the implications of the new developments for community nursing practice.

Effectiveness

Evaluating the effectiveness of child protection interventions is a very difficult process indeed. What counts as an adequate measure? Since 1974 the British child protection system has uncovered a whole range of abuses that previously were not publicly acknowledged. As has been seen, initial concerns about physical abuse were partially eclipsed by the growth of awareness of sexual abuse in the 1980s. Currently we are revealing abuse of children in residential homes on a scale which would not have been believed before (Dobson 1996). This process of discovery is an achievement in itself, but the size of the discovered problems far outweighs the resources that our society is prepared to put into responding to them. In these circumstances it is hard to know what effectiveness means because we are not dealing with a static situation. Another dynamic element not yet discussed is the growth of child poverty. The 1979–87 period saw a massive increase in unemployment in the UK with a consequent effect on children's material standards. While the rate of pauperisation of children has levelled off to some extent since that time, it was estimated in 1993 that between 30% and 40% of children in Britain were living at very low income levels in poor housing conditions in socially deprived environments (Kumar 1993). The potential for neglect of children is much greater in these circumstances than in times of greater affluence.

Thus the child protection system is now faced with a much wider and more numerous range of problems than was the case in the early 1970s. Attempts have been made to assess effectiveness in reducing the extent of physical abuse by looking at child mortality statistics, but the evidence is flimsy (Lindsey & Trocme 1994). In the recent research carried out by the Department of Health it is suggested that between a quarter and a third of children who come to the attention of child protection professionals are re-abused within two years. Serious re-abuse is, however, relatively rare (DoH 1995, Farmer & Owen 1995, pp. 311–18). There is no way of knowing whether they represent an improvement on what was achieved before the child protection system was brought into being. With regard to sexual abuse there is some evidence that children who have made allegations and been through the system, are glad overall that they did so (Roberts & Taylor 1993). However, the discovery of the extent of abuse in state care is a major concern – how many children have been rescued from abusive family situations only to be placed in abusive care situations? Certainly many more than was thought before.

Strengths and weaknesses

Rather than think of its effectiveness, therefore, it is probably more sensible to consider the strengths and weaknesses of the child protection system.

First, the strengths. As pointed out above, there is now much greater awareness than before of the fact that children are subject to abuse from adults and older more powerful children. We are also much more aware of the fact that such abuse can have long-term negative consequences, which include mental ill-health, low self-esteem and in some a propensity for violence or neglect (Finkelhor 1986). At the very least, the experience of being abused, physically, emotionally or sexually, makes it that much harder to develop trusting relationships with others throughout life. The consequences of child abuse can, therefore, be costly for society and painful for individuals.

Second, professionals do work better together in tackling child abuse than they did in the early 1970s (Corby 1995). There does seem to be more mutual understanding of each other's tasks, and more preparedness to focus on children's needs in carrying out professional duties. Earlier research into health visitors' and social workers' perceptions of what constitutes child abuse (Fox & Dingwall 1985) showed a high level of agreement. A more recent small-scale study by Wheeler (1992) demonstrated that these two professions had good understanding of each other's roles.

Third, children's wishes and needs are more likely to be taken into account than was the case ten years ago. Also there is more awareness of the rights of parents to be informed about, and involved in, the process of child protection investigations. How much that awareness is being translated into action is still an open question.

As regards weaknesses, many critics feel that the British child protection system is too inflexible and tends to be over-bureaucratic (Howe 1992). Individual professionals are considered to be given too little discretion in deciding on best courses of action and, as a result, tend to operate in a mechanistic and defensive way. A direct consequence of this, as recent research has suggested, is that families' needs for help can be overlooked because of a too narrow focus on child abuse.

Another major criticism is that the child protection system concentrates too much on the discovery and investigation of abuse, and not enough on treatment and the aftermath. Ideally, of course, there should be sufficient resources to do both adequately. The lack of resources available in child protection work is a key issue. There is greater societal intolerance of child abuse in Britain now than ever before, and very high demands placed on health and welfare professionals to do something about it. However, there is little preparedness to meet the costs of this enterprise, and, as a result, many needs are identified but little provision is made for following them up.

A final criticism is that not enough attention is paid to primary prevention of abuse in our society. There is very little done in terms of parent-preparation or sex education in Britain. There are no laws against hitting children as there are in Scandinavia. On a broader level, maternity leave and nursery provision are at lower levels than in most West European countries. There have been some encouraging developments in two of these areas though. Firstly, a government green paper 'Supporting Families' has been published which stresses the government's commitment to educating and helping new families, and specifically refers to health visitors as possible key agents in this process. Secondly, it has been announced that the government intends to change the law in relation to the punishment of children following a European Court of Human Rights ruling that a nine year old boy beaten by his stepfather with a garden cane had had his rights violated (*The Times*, 28 September 1998).

The future role of community nurses in child protection work

The shift in emphasis in child protection work, currently being backed by the Department of Health, in theory offers more opportunities for health visitors and other community nurses to contribute in a way which is in tune with their professional goals. Health visitors have traditionally been heavily involved at the preventive end both of health work in general and child protection work in particular. They have played a key role in identifying problems at an early stage and passing on their concerns to child protection agencies (Gilardi 1991). Often, they have been frustrated because of their inability to secure more social work support at this stage. According to Gibbons *et al.*'s research, 1995, the child protection system has been putting all its focus on identifying the worst cases and on concentrating its resources on them. The current trend back to broader family support approaches for those families whose children are not seen to be at serious risk, if properly implemented and resourced, could be greatly enhanced by health visitor input at both referral and ongoing work stages. Greater emphasis on working with deprived families, rather than filtering them out of the system, could make for more meaningful inputs and effective outputs. However, although health visitors, in conjunction with social workers, could play an important role in working with families with young children identified in this way, Browne (1995) is not encouraging in this respect – he points to a lack of emphasis placed by government on health visiting, and a shift away from home visiting to a more clinic-based approach. Much, it seems, will depend on local arrangements to secure continuing co-operation within tight budgets and working constraints. The government green paper, referred to above, suggests that currently there is room for more optimism than before.

6.5 CONCLUSION

Over the past two decades the community nursing profession has gained considerable experience and expertise in working with families where there are child protection concerns. It is to be hoped that this experience will not be lost at a time when their expertise seems to be in tune with the current policy developments. Though somewhat dated and a little idealistic, Joy Hendry's account of health visiting in the 1970s (Hendry 1977) gives some idea of the potential that lies within the community nursing role for helping families whose children are perceived to be at risk.

REFERENCES

Aldgate, J. & Tunstill, J. (1995) *Section 17 – the first 18 months of Implementation*. HMSO, London.

Brent, London Borough of (1985) *A Child In Trust: The Report of the Panel of Inquiry into the Circumstances Surrounding the Death of Jasmine Beckford*. Brent.

Browne, K. (1995) Preventing Child Maltreatment through Community Nursing. *Journal of Advanced Nursing*, **21** 57–63.

Butler-Sloss, Lord Justice E. (1988) *Report of the Inquiry into Child Abuse in Cleveland 1987*. cmnd.412. HMSO, London.

Calder, M. (1991) Child protection: core groups: beneficial or bureaucratic? *Child Abuse Review*, 5, 26–9.

Clyde, Lord (1992) *The Report of the Inquiry into the Removal of Children from Orkney in February 1991*. House of Commons Papers no.195, London.

Cobley, C. (1995) *Child Abuse and the Law*. Cavendish, London.

Corby, B. (1993) *Child Abuse: Towards a Knowledge Base*. Open University Press, Milton Keynes.

Corby, B. (1995) Interprofessional cooperation and inter-agency coordination. In: *The Child Protection Handbook*, (eds K. Wilson, A. James), Baillière-Tindall, London.

Corby, B. (1998) *Managing Child Sexual Abuse Cases*. Jessica Kingsley, London.

Corby, B., Millar, M. & Young, L. (1996) Parental participation in child protection work: rethinking the rhetoric. *British Journal of Social Work*, 26, 475–92.

Department of Health (1991a) *Child Abuse: A study of Inquiry Reports 1980–89*. HMSO, London.

Department of Health (1991b) *Working Together under the Children Act 1989 – A Guide to Arrangements for Inter-Agency Co-operation for the Protection of Children against Abuse*. HMSO, London.

Department of Health (Social Services Inspectorate) (1994) *The Child, the Court and the Video: A study of the Implementation of the Memorandum of Good Practice on Video Interviewing of Child Witnesses*. Available from the Health Publications Unit, Heywood.

Department of Health (1995) *Messages from Research*. HMSO, London.

Department of Health and Social Security (1974) *Report of the Committee of Inquiry into the Care and Supervision Provided in Relation to Maria Colwell*. HMSO, London.

Department of Health and Social Security (1982) *Child Abuse: A Study of Inquiry Reports 1973–1981*. HMSO, London.

Dickens, J. (1993) Assessment and the control of social work: an analysis of the reasons for the non-use of the Child Assessment Order. *Journal of Social Welfare and Family Law*, **15**, 88–100.

Dingwall, R., Eekelaar, J. & Murray, T. (1983) *The Protection of Children: State Intervention into Family Life*. Blackwell, Oxford.

Dobson, R. (1996) 3000 in new abuse scandal. *The Independent*, 11 Decrmber 1996, p.1.

Elliott, C. & Mullin, R. (1996) A short and brutal life. *Guardian* 31 October 1996, pp.1, 6.

Farmer, E. & Owen, M. (1995) *Child Protection Practice: Private Risks and Public Pain*. HMSO, London.

Fielding, N. & Conroy, S. (1992) Interviewing child victims: police and social work investigations of child sexual abuse. *Sociology*, **26**, 103–24.

Finkelhor, D. (1986) *A Sourcebook on Child Sexual Abuse*. Sage, Newbury Park, California.

Fox, S. & Dingwall, R. (1985) An exploratory study of the variations in social workers' and health visitors' definitions of child mistreatment. *British Journal of Social Work*, **15**, 467–77.

Gibbons, J., Conroy, S. & Bell, C. (1995) *Operating the Child Protection System*. HMSO, London.

Gilardi, J. (1991) Child protection in a south London district. *Health Visitor*, **64**, 225–7.

Hardiker, P. (1996) The legal and social construction of significant harm. In: *Child Welfare Services: Developments in Law, Policy, Practice and Research*, (eds M. Hill & J. Aldgate) Jessica Kingsley, London.

Hendry, J. (1977) Lady from the 'welfare'. *New Society*, 22–29 December, pp. 622–4.

HMSO (1989) *Children Act*. HMSO, London.

Home Office (with the Department of Health) (1992) Memorandum of good practice on video recorded interviews with child witnesses for criminal proceedings. HMSO, London.

Howe, D. (1992) Child abuse and bureaucratisation of social work. *Sociological Review*, **40**, 491–508.

Kumar, V. (1993) *Poverty and Inequality in the UK: The Effects on Children*. National Children's Bureau, London.

Lindsey, D. & Trocme, N. (1994) Have child protection efforts reduced child homicides?: an examination of the data from Britain and North America. *British Journal of Social Work*, 24, 715–32.

Lyon, C. (1995) Child Protection and Civil Law. In: *The*

Child Protection Handbook. (eds K. Wilson & A. James) Baillière-Tindall, London.

Lyon, C. & de Cruz, S. (1993) *Child Abuse*, 2nd ed. Family Law, Bristol, pp. 55–7.

Mccallum, S. & Prilleltensky, I. (1996) Empowerment in child protection work: values, practice and caveats. *Children & Society*, 10, pp.40–50.

Parton, N. (1985) *The Politics of Child Abuse*. Macmillan, London, pp. 48–64.

Roberts, J. & Taylor, C. (1993) Sexually abused children and young people speak out. In: *Child Abuse and Child Abusers: Protection and Prevention*. (ed. L. Waterhouse) Jessica Kingsley, London.

Smart, M. (1992) Professional ethics and participation - nurses, health visitors and midwives. In: *Participation in-*

Practice – Involving Families in Child Protection. (ed. J. Thoburn). University of East Anglia, Norwich.

Stevenson, O. (1996) Emotional abuse and neglect: a time for reappraisal. *Child and Family Social Work*, 1, 13–18.

The Times (Law Reports) 28 September 1998.

Thoburn, J., Lewis, A. & Shemmings, D. (1995) *Paternalism or Partnership? Family Involvement in the Child Protection Process*. HMSO, London.

Waterhouse, L.& Carnie, J. (1992) Assessing child protection risk. *British Journal of Social Work*, 22, 47–60.

Wattam, C. (1992) *Making a Case in Child Protection*. Longman, Harlow.

Wheeler, S. (1992) Perceptions of child abuse. *Health Visitor*, 65, 316–19.

Part 2

The Child and Nutrition

7

Breast Feeding: the Art and Science
Soraya Meah

7.1 INTRODUCTION

Breast feeding is the natural method of infant feeding, and, as such, offers numerous physical and social benefits to both mother and child (Renfrew et al. 1990; Minchin 1993, Inch et al. 1995; Henschel & Inch 1996; Stanway & Stanway 1996). However, despite evidence to support the benefits of breast feeding, nationally only 64% of women choose to breast feed at birth, and by the end of six weeks only 40% of women in England and Wales are still breast feeding (DoH, 1996) despite national guidelines encouraging women to continue for at least the first three months (DoH 1994). It has been suggested (on the basis of survey data) that six weeks marks a watershed in the course of breastfeeding and that if surmounted a mother is likely to continue to breast feed fully for the recommended period of time (Wright 1990). Clearly, this has implications for health professionals, in terms of their role as promoters of breast feeding and in facilitating mothers to develop the skills required to breast feed successfully.

This chapter presents an overview of the evidence which supports the short-, medium- and long-term benefits of breast feeding; the evidential basis of factors shown to affect successful breast feeding and organisational issues relating to breastfeeding and health care.

7.2 THE BENEFITS OF BREAST FEEDING

Infants

Breast milk is species specific, as such it contains a variety of components each one of which contributes to the immunological protection of the infant (Henschel & Inch 1996). Research has demonstrated that the breast fed infant receives significantly more protection from disease than infants who receive substitute milks (see Fig. 7.1). It is widely accepted that breast feeding is a priority in developing countries, where mortality is high among babies fed on formula milk (Victoria et al. 1987); in contrast, a somewhat laissez-faire attitude to breast feeding has emerged among industrialised nations, with low rates of infant mortality (Minchin 1993). Whilst it is accepted that infant deaths in the UK are unlikely to be attributed to diarrhoea or respiratory infection, it should be remembered that such conditions may cause unnecessary suffering and anxiety for many infants and their families.

Protection from infection
It has been reported that infants fed on formula milk in the UK are at greater risk of experiencing gastro-intestinal disease than breast fed infants (Howie 1990). The findings of this study, examining the relationship between infant feeding and infectious illness, indicated that babies who were exclusively breast fed for 13 weeks or more were five times less likely to develop gastrointestinal disease than formula fed infants. Breasts fed infants in the same study were also found to have a reduced incidence of respiratory

Research indicating that breast fed babies are at reduced risk of:	
Gastrointestinal illness e.g.	
Inflammatory bowel disease	Glassman *et al.* 1990
Gastroenteritis	Howie *et al.* 1990
Coeliac disease	Greco *et al.* 1988
Idiopathic hypertrophic pyloric stenosis	Rollins *et al.* 1989
	Habbick & Khanna 1989
Crohn's disease	Koletzko *et al.* 1989
Obstructive bowel disease	Wales *et al.* 1989
Food allergy and intolerance e.g.	
Insomnia	Kahn *et al.* 1985
Colic	Lothe & Lindberg 1989
Colitis	Israel *et al.* 1989
Respiratory disease e.g.	
Bronchiolitis	Welliver *et al.* 1986
Bronchitis pneumonia	Watkins *et al.* 1979
Ear infections	Pokander *et al.* 1985
Other illnesses e.g.	
Urinary tract infections	Pisacane *et al.* 1992
Diabetes	Mayer *et al.* 1988
Childhood lymphoma	Davies *et al.* 1988
Meningitis	Simmons *et al.* 1989
Autism	Tanoue & Oda 1989
Cot death	Mitchell *et al.* 1991

Figure 7.1   The benefits of breast feeding for infants. (Adapted with permission from Minchin 1998.)

infection compared with infants fed formula milk as a sole diet. Duncan *et al.* (1993) concluded that breast fed infants are at reduced risk from acute and recurrent otitis media in the first year of life. From a total of 1013 children Duncan found that 47% had at least one episode of otitis media in the first year of life, and 17% experienced recurrent otitis media. However, infants who were exclusively breast fed for at least four months were found to have 50% fewer episodes of otitis media; while infants who had received other foods as well as breast milk reported 40% fewer episodes. These findings may have long-term ramifications, in that otitis media is a cause of deafness.

Allergies

Breast feeding may also reduce the risk of children developing allergies. In particular, there is a growing body of evidence to link feeding infants cows' milk with adverse health outcomes in infancy (Atherton *et al.* 1978; Host *et al.* 1988; Burr *et al.* 1993). Cows' milk allergy and cows' milk intolerance are both problems common to infancy and childhood. Cows' milk allergy manifests itself in the form of childhood asthma, eczema and allergic rhinitis; while cows' milk intolerance often presents as a general failure to thrive. It has been hypothesised that a genetic predisposition and exposure to allergens, particularly cows' milk, is responsible for the development of these conditions (Host 1991). Chapter 13 considers atopic eczema and feeding advice in more detail.

Preterm babies

Breast milk has been shown to offer substantial benefits to vulnerable preterm babies in terms of morbidity and mortality (Lucas *et al.* 1984). Necrotising enterocolitis is a life threatening condition for infants in western societies, although it is rare in babies over 30 weeks gestation. Lucas *et al.* (1990), in a well designed, prospective, multi-centre, rando-mised controlled trial, found that the condition was 20 times more common among formula fed babies, reporting that 51 infants from a total of 926 in the study developed the condition, with a mortality rate of 26%. Pasteurised donor breast milk was found to be as protective as mothers' own milk. Lucas *et al.* (1990) have suggested that the falling use of breast milk in Britain's neo-natal intensive care units may account for an extra 500 cases of necrotising enterocolitis each year.

Neurological development

A body of evidence is also emerging that suggests that breast feeding can have positive effects on the neurological and cognitive development of infants (Lucas *et al.* 1990; Lucas *et al.* 1992; Lucas *et al.* 1994; Williams 1994; Lanting *et al.* 1994). The brains of formula fed babies have been found to differ in physical appearance from breast fed babies, which may be important in neuro-developmental outcomes (Williams 1994). Lucas and colleagues have con-ducted a series of randomised control trials to evaluate the cognitive development of breast fed and formula fed preterm infants (Lucas *et al.* 1990; Lucas *et al.* 1992; Lucas *et al.* 1994). Their findings consistently favour preterm infants who receive breast milk. Provision of mothers' own milk was associated with higher developmental scores at 18 months compared to infants who had received formula suitable for full-term babies. The same infants were followed up at seven to eight years of age and were found to have a higher intelligence quotient than infants who did not receive maternal milk. Children who had received their mothers' milk had an 8 point advantage in intelligence quotient after adjustments for differences between groups in mothers' education and social class (Lucas *et al.* 1990; Lucas *et al.* 1992; Lucas *et al.* 1994). This advantage was associated with being fed maternal milk by tube rather than the process of breast feeding. Lucas *et al.* (1992) also report a dose-response relation between the proportion of mothers' milk in the diet and subsequent intelligence quotient. It must be acknowledged that the work of Lucas and colleagues is concentrated on preterm infants, and it could be argued that such vulnerable infants are less able to cope with the shortcomings of formula milk. However, the research conducted by Lucas and his team is robust, and their findings are consistent with those of other researchers (Lanting 1994). In a

retrospective study, Lanting found a small advanta-geous effect of breast feeding in the neurological development of children at nine years of age.

Figure 7.1 is a summary of the benefits of breast feeding for infants.

Advantages of breast feeding for mothers

There are both physical and emotional advantages for women in breast feeding (Renfrew *et al.* 1990; Henschel & Inch 1996; Stanway & Stanway 1996). In general women often find that when they breast feed:

- involution of the uterus occurs rapidly;
- their lochial loss is completed more quickly;
- they lose weight more easily;
- they experience lactational amenorrhoea (which may be used as a natural form of contraception where the baby is breast fed exclusively on demand);
- they are more likely to experience a general feeling of calm and wellbeing because of the hormones they secrete whilst breast feeding.

In the long-term there is some evidence to suggest that women who breast feed are less likely to suffer from osteoporosis and breast cancer in later life (see Fig. 7.2). However, the relationship between breast feeding and these conditions is not fully understood.

Emotional benefits of breast feeding

In breast feeding the emotional and physical welfare of mother and infant are interconnected. Infants benefit not only from receiving breast milk but also from the skin-to-skin contact, which occurs during feeding. It has been suggested that this skin-to-skin contact comforts and soothes the infant, and in turn, has an effect on sleep patterns, and ability to self-comfort (Renfrew *et al.* 1990). The nurturing which takes place during breast feeding provides a founda-tion for a good relationship between mother and baby, which may contribute to healthy relationships within the family as a whole.

The health benefits to mother and child associated with breast feeding can only be enjoyed when breast feeding works well. Breast feeding is a natural process and some mothers learn to breast feed quickly, but for others it takes time and support. Some mothers need a great deal of professional and social support until they

Research indicating that breast feeding is associated with less risk of maternal	
Pre-menopausal breast cancer	McTiernan *et al.* 1986
Ovarian cancer	Cancer and Steroid Hormone Study 1987
Cervical cancer	Brock *et al.* 1989
Osteoporosis	Koetting & Wardlaw 1988

Figure 7.2 The benefits of breast feeding for mothers. (Adapted with permission from Minchin 1998.)

acquire the skills and confidence to breast feed successfully.

7.3 FACTORS AFFECTING SUCCESSFUL BREAST FEEDING

Promoting breast feeding will only promote health if it is accompanied by practical help, and, in western society, women rely predominantly on health professionals to provide this. It is beyond the scope of this chapter to provide a detailed description of the practical skills required to help women breast feed. Guides to best practice in helping women to breast feed are widely available; these include texts by Henschel & Inch (1996), the Royal College of Midwives (1991) and Renfrew *et al.* (1990).

It has been suggested that, to be effective in helping women to breast feed, health professionals need to be able to demonstrate the correct positioning of the baby at the breast, a comprehensive knowledge of the anatomy of the breast and a thorough understanding of the physiology of lactation (Renfrew & Lang 1995). This is essential to eliminate the problem of conflicting advice conveyed to women when breast feeding (Henschel & Inch 1996; RCM 1991).

In order for midwives, health visitors and general practitioners to work as a team in the promotion and management of breast feeding it is important that only those practices which have been demonstrated to be effective are passed on to mothers (Inch & Garforth 1989). Factors which have been shown to be important in establishing and maintaining breast feeding include:

- ante-natal care;
- correct positioning of the baby at the breast;
- timing and duration of feeds;

- supplements for mother and baby;
- support for breast feeding.
  (Inch & Garforth 1989; Inch & Renfrew 1989).

Ante-natal education

Attendance at ante-natal classes has been reported to range from 30 to 50%, with many failing to complete the full course (Black *et al.* 1984). Despite reports of low attendance, evidence from a systematic review of breast feeding education (Renfrew 1994a) indicates that ante-natal classes can have a positive effect in promoting breast feeding in general. However the evidence also indicates that giving women information about breast feeding has little effect on their choice of feeding method, although it may offer benefits to women who have already decided to breast feed. Renfrew (1994a) suggests there is a need for more research to assess the type of ante-natal classes women prefer and to establish which elements of the information given to women are most beneficial.

Ante-natal preparation of the breasts

The idea that women's breasts need to be prepared for breast feeding is not supported by current research (Inch & Garforth 1989; Renfrew *et al.* 1990; RCM 1991). Several studies have examined various forms of nipple conditioning, none have found any significant differences between the methods of conditioning, or between the use of masse cream, expression of colostrum, or the unprepared nipple (Alexander *et al.* 1992; Renfrew 1994b).

Correct positioning of the baby at the breast

Breast feeding has been described by Renfrew *et al.* (1990) as a combination of instinct, reflex and learning. Clinical practice suggests the act of positioning a baby correctly at the breast is one which has to be learnt. Correct positioning may be broken down into three elements: the mother's posture; holding the baby correctly; and alignment of the baby with the breast.

Good positioning means getting the mother into a comfortable position, sitting or lying, avoiding strain on her neck, back or arms. The mother needs to be made aware of the importance of holding her baby close to her, so that the baby can reach the breast without straining. The baby needs to be facing the mother, the baby's head, neck and back should be aligned and well supported. Initially, the mother will require practical help and skilled assistance when positioning the baby. It is important to remember that the mother cannot see where the baby's lower lip and jaw are in relation to her nipple, and must rely on observation of the baby's sucking pattern and the sensations she feels to confirm that the baby is positioned correctly.

Timing and duration of feeds

The feeding patterns of individual babies will be determined by their individual body rhythms. Current research highlights the importance of flexibility in care practices, indeed, evidence suggests that babies left to regulate themselves gain weight more quickly and breast feed for longer than babies who have external limitations imposed on them (Inch & Garforth 1989, Mathews 1989, Renfrew et al. 1990; Renfrew 1994c). Furthermore, there is no evidence to support limiting the duration of each breast feed or the use of breast feeding schedules (Renfrew 1994c). It is important that the milk produced in the breast is removed effectively by the baby feeding. If the milk is not removed the mother may experience breast problems which may hinder her ability to breast feed (Table 7.1).

Artificially imposed limitations on the duration of breast feeds can be detrimental to the baby. The rate and flow of milk during the course of the feed varies as does the fat content; at the start of the feed the baby takes a large volume of low calorie foremilk, this changes to high calorie hindmilk at the end of a feed. Therefore the length of the feed is likely to be determined by effectiveness and rate of milk transfer between mother and baby (Inch & Garforth 1989).

Consequently interference with the spontaneous feeding pattern of the baby may deprive him or her of essential vitamins, vitamin K for example is concentrated in colostrum and hindmilk.

Limiting the duration of feeds may also have a detrimental effect on the mother's milk supply. Insufficient milk supply has been reported as the most common reason given by mothers for discontinuing breast feeding (RCM 1991). Objective assessment of milk supply is difficult to obtain. However, observations in traditional societies suggest that less than 5% of women are likely to be physiologically incapable of producing an adequate amount of milk, which suggests over-diagnosis of the condition in western society (Inch & Garforth 1989). It is suggested that an effective means of preventing an insufficient supply of milk is unrestricted feeding by a well positioned baby.

Fluid supplements for mother and baby

A common misconception has arisen since the 1970s that mothers who breast feed require extra fluids in order to maintain their milk supply. There is no evidence to support a correlation between milk supply and fluid intake; the amount of fluids consumed by a mother who is breast feeding should be determined by her level of thirst (Renfrew et al. 1994d).

The practice of supplementing breast fed infants with water or formula milks is also unsupported by the available evidence (Renfrew 1994e; 1994f). In her systematic review of this practice, Renfrew concludes that a healthy baby has no need of large volumes of fluid other than those available physiologically from the breast. There is no evidence to suggest that additional fluids prevent or resolve physiological jaundice. However, the practice of giving fluids to breast fed babies is associated with an increase in the chances of the mother discontinuing breast feeding within the first few weeks of delivery (Inch & Garforth 1989; Renfrew 1994e,1994f).

Supporting breast feeding mothers

The relationship between support and breast feeding outcomes remains unclear (Beske 1982; Barronowski et al. 1983; Cronwett & Reinhardt 1987). It would appear that health care professionals exert minimal

Table 7.1 Breast problems commonly experienced by breast feeding mothers.

Problem	Description	Cause	Prevention	Action	Reference
Cracked nipples	Skin surrounding the nipple cracks and may bleed. Feeding the baby is painful.	Incorrect positioning of the baby at the breast. Curtailing feeds prematurely. Incorrect technique used when removing the baby from the breast.	Keep the breast clean and dry. Avoid nipple creams, shields etc.	Feed the baby on demand. The mother should feed sitting upright or lying down, she should be comfortable. The mother should be shown how to hold her baby. The baby should be well supported, so that it can reach the breast without effort. The baby should be positioned so that he/she can take a good mouthful of the breast without having to pull at the nipple. Allow the baby to determine the length of the feed. The mother must learn to rely on the sensations she herself feels in order to determine the baby is positioned correctly.	Inch et al. 1995 Renfrew et al. 1990 RCM 1991
Breast Engorgement	Extremely full and painful breasts.	Incorrect positioning of the baby at the breast. Limiting the frequency of feeds. Limiting the duration of feeds.	Feeding on demand. Allow the baby to empty each breast. Allow the baby to determine the length of each feed.	Correct positioning of baby at the breast. Feeding on demand. Allowing the baby to empty each breast during the feed. Allowing the baby to determine the length of each feed.	Inch et al. 1995 RCM 1991

Blocked milk duct	A hard red patch on the outside of the breast where the milk duct lies.	May be the result of breast engorgement or an ill fitting bra.	Wear loose clothing and a well fitting maternity bra. Feed baby frequently and encourage the baby to empty each breast.	Check correct positioning of the baby. Continue feeding on demand. Very gentle massage of the affected lobe may produce a thin strand of solidified fat.	Silverman 1993
Infective mastitis	A wedge shaped area of the breast becomes red, swollen, and painful to the touch. Mother may experience rise in pulse and temperature, aching flu-like symptoms.	Restriction of milk flow, causes build up of pressure in the alveoli of the breast, this may force substances from the milk into surrounding tissue, setting up an inflammatory reaction.	Correct positioning of the baby at the breast. Encouraging the baby to empty the breasts regularly.	Women who are diagnosed as having an infection should receive antibiotic therapy. Hand expression of milk from the infected breast should be conducted regularly.	Silverman 1993
Breast abscess	Infection in a breast lobe develops into a discrete painful swelling.	Untreated mastitis.	Continued breast feeding to relieve milk stasis and to prevent an abscess developing.	Antibiotic therapy and possible surgical incision and drainage of the abscess. Feeding should continue on the affected side to promote speedy resolution of the problem.	Silverman 1993 RCM 1991

influence on womens' choice of feeding method (Inch & Garforth 1989). However, there is some evidence to suggest that the duration of breast feeding can be increased by regular contact between the mother and the same care giver, in person or by telephone (Renfrew 1994g, Renfrew & Lang 1995). Although it must be remembered that the advice given can only have a positive effect on breast feeding outcomes if it is sound. Renfrew (1994g) suggests that support from health care professionals should take the form of early practical help with positioning of the baby at the breast, also that those health care professionals should be skilled at solving the problems associated with incorrect positioning.

It is unlikely that there is one form of support that will meet the needs of all breast feeding mothers. Support systems need to be planned on an individual basis, taking into account the social, cultural and ethnic background of mothers and their families (Cronwett & Reinhardt 1987; Higginbottom 1998). The most effective way of achieving this has yet to be identified and provides fertile ground for future research.

7.4 ORGANISATIONAL ISSUES

Increasing the number of women who breast feed would bring health gains to mothers and babies in the short and long term, in so doing the community as a whole would benefit. Aside from health gains in terms of quality of life and life years, there are also potential cost benefits to the National Health Service to be had by increasing the number of mothers who breast feed. The Department of Health has estimated that if all babies were breast fed the average health district could save £300,000 a year in the form of reduced hospital admissions from infants with gastroenteritis (DoH 1996).

Despite the potential health gains associated with breast feeding the number of mothers breast feeding their infants at the time of birth between 1980–1985 in England and Wales fell from 67% to 65%. This trend was repeated in the numbers of mothers breast feeding their infants at six weeks of age, with a fall from 42% in 1980 to 40% in 1985 (Martin & White

1988; 1982). The findings in the OPCS 1985 survey (Martin & White 1988) were that many mothers reported abandoning breast feeding prematurely because of problems which appeared preventable or easily solved. Mothers also indicated that health professionals were ineffective in providing satisfactory solutions to their difficulties. In response to this data, the government lent its support to the Joint Breast Feeding Initiative, a four-year project designed to raise the profile of breast feeding nationally, and to encourage local health authorities to set up breast feeding working groups. The objectives of these groups included the collection of data (e.g. numbers of mothers breast feeding) and the design and implementation of strategies to improve care for breast feeding mothers and their infants.

Following the Joint Breast Feeding Initiative further initiatives have been supported by the government to promote breast feeding and these include: the National Breast Feeding Working Group (1993); the UNICEF/WHO Baby Friendly Hospital Initiative UK (1994); Invest in Breast Together (1995); and National Network of Breast Feeding Coordinators (1995). These initiatives have sought to direct actions that may lead to successful breast feeding by addressing issues related to:

- policy and staffing within health care organisations;
- structure and functioning of services;
- education and training for health professionals;
- health education for service users.

The impact of national and local breast feeding initiatives on womens' experiences of breast feeding is uncertain as there appears to be an absence of any systematic evaluation of past or present initiatives. However Henschel and Inch (1996) report that three of the four UK hospitals assessed for Baby Friendly Hospital status in 1995 failed to meet the criteria. It is clear that, if the potential health gains of breast feeding are to be realised, a concerted effort is required from policy makers, health care providers and service users to enable women to breast feed successfully. How this can be achieved effectively is uncertain. It is sufficient to point out that the issue of breast feeding exceeds the boundaries of current health policy, and requires examination within a wider social, cultural and environmental context.

7.5 CONCLUSION

Existing evidence demonstrates that breast feeding offers health benefits to mothers and infants in the short, medium and long term. In turn, there are also potential cost benefits for health services in facilitating women to breast feed successfully. However, benefits can only be enjoyed when breast feeding works well, and current evidence casts doubt on the effectiveness of health professionals in meeting the needs of breast feeding mothers. Breast feeding needs to be placed prominently on the national research agenda. A systematic investigation is warranted, to explore the needs of mothers who breast feed; to identify strategies effective in meeting these needs, and to evaluate implementation in terms of health outcomes. The challenge for all health professionals is to convey breast feeding as a viable option to all mothers.

REFERENCES

Alexander, J.M., Grant, A., Campbell, M.J. (1992) Randomized controlled trial of breast shells and Hoffman's exercises for inverted and non protractile nipples. *British Medical Journal*, **304**, 1030–32.

Atherton, D.J., Sewell, M., Soothill, J.F., Wells, R.S. & Chilvers, C.E. (1978) A double blind controlled crossover trial of antigen-avoidance diet in atopic eczema. *Lancet*, **1**, 401–3.

Barronowski, T., Bee, D.E., Rassen, D.K. *et al.* (1983) Social support, social influence, ethnicity and the breastfeeding decision. *Social Science Medicine*, **17**, 1599–1611.

Black, P.M., Faulkner, A.M., Thomson, A.M. (1984) Antenatal classes: a selective review of the literature. *Nurse Education Today*, **3**, 130–3.

Beske, E.J., Garvis, M.S. (1982) Important factors in breastfeeding success. *Maternal Child Nursing*, **7**, 174–9.

Brock, K.E., Berry, G., Brinton, L.A., Kerr, C., Maclennan, R. & Mock, P.A. (1989) Sexual, reproductive and contraceptive risk factors for carcinoma-in-situ for the uterine cervix. *Sydney Medical Journal Australia*, **150** (3), 125–30.

Burr, M.L., Limb, E.S., Maguire, M.J., Amarah, L., Elridge, B.A., Lazell, J.C. *et al.* (1993) Infant feeding, wheezing and allergy: a prospective study *Archives of Diseases in Childhood*, **68**, 724–8.

Cancer and Steroid Hormone Study, CDC/NICHHD (1987) The reduction in risk of ovarian cancer associated with oral contraceptive use. *New England Journal of Medicine*, **316**, 650–5.

Cronenwett, L. & Reinhardt, R. (1987) Support and breastfeeding: a review. *BIRTH*, **14** (4), 199–203.

Davies, M.K., Savitz D.A. & Graubard, B.I. (1988) Infant feeding and childhood cancer. *Lancet*, **2**, 365–8.

Department of Health (1994) *Report on Health and Social Subjects 45: Weaning and The Weaning Diet. Report of the Working Group on the Weaning Diet of the Committee on Medical Aspects of Food Policy.* HMSO, London.

Department of Health (1996) *Good Practice Guidance to the NHS.* HMSO, London.

Duncan, B., Ey, J., Holberg, C.J., Right, A.L., Martinez, F.D. & Taussig, L.M. (1993) Exclusive breast feeding for at least four months protects against otitis media. *Paediatrics*, **915**, 867–72.

Glassman, M.S., Newman, L.J., Berezin, S. & Gryboski, J.D. (1990) Cows milk protein sensitivity during infancy in patients with inflammatory bowel disease. *American Journal of Gastroenterol.*, **85**, 838–4.

Greco, L., Auricchio, S., Mayer, M. & Grimaldi, M. (1988) Case control study on nutritional risk factors in celiac disease. *Journal of Pediatric Gasteroenterol Nutrition*, **7**, 395–9.

Habbick, B.F., Khanna, C. & To, T. (1989) Infantile pyloric stenosis: a study of feeding practices and other possible causes. *Canadian Medical Association Journal*, **140**, 401–4.

Henschel, D. & Inch, S. (1996) *Breast Feeding A Guide For Midwives.* Books For Midwives Press. Haigh Hochland Publications, Cheshire England.

Higginbottom, G. (1998) Breastfeeding and black women: a UK investigation. *Health Visitor*, **71**: 1,12–15.

Host, A. (1991) Importance of the first meal on the development of cow's milk allergy and intolerance. *Allergy PROC*, **12**, 227–332.

Host, A., Husby S. & Osterballe, O.A. (1988) A prospective study of cows' milk allergy in exclusively breast fed infants. Incidence, pathogenetic role of early inadvertent exposure to cows milk formula, and characterization of bovine milk protein in human milk. *Acta Paediatrica Scandanavia*, **77**, 663–70.

Howie, P.W., Forsyth, J.S., Ogston, S.A., Clark, A. & Flory, C. du V. (1990) Protective effects of breast feeding against infection. *British Medical Journal*, **300**, 11–16.

Inch, S. & Garforth, S. (1989) Establishing and maintaining breast feeding. In: *Effective Care in Pregnancy and Childbirth*, (eds I. Chalmers, M. Enkin & M.J.N.C. Keirse) Vol. 1, Chapter 80, 1349–74, Oxford University Press, Oxford.

Inch, S. & Renfrew, M.J. (1989) Common breast feeding problems. In: *Effective Care in Pregnancy and Childbirth*.

(eds I. Chalmers, M. Enkin & M.J.N.C. Keirse), Oxford University Press, Oxford, Vol. 1, Chapter 81, 1375–87.

Inch, S., Garforth, S. & Renfrew, M.J. (1995) Breast feeding. Chapter 46, In: *A Guide to Effective Care in Pregnancy & Childbirth*, (eds M. Enkin, M.J.N.C. Keirse, M.J. Renfrew & J. Neilson), 2nd edn. Oxford University Press, Oxford, England.

Israel, D., Levine, J., Pettei, M. & Davidson, M. (1989) Protein induced allergic colitis in infants. *Paediatric Research*, **25**, 116a.

Kahn, A., Mozin, M.J., Casimir, G. Montauk, L, Blum, D. (1985) Insomnia and cows' milk allergy in infants. *Paediatrics*, **76** (6), 880–4.

Koetting, C.A. & Wardlaw, G.M. (1988) Wrist, spine and hip bone density in women with variable histories of lactation. *American Journal of Nutrition* **48**, 1478–81.

Koletzko, S., Sherman, P., Corey, M., Griffiths, A., Smith, C. (1989) Role of infant feeding practices in the development of Crohn's Disease in childhood. *British Medical Journal*, **298**, 1617–8.

Lanting, C.I., Fidler, V., Husman, M., Towen, B.C. & Boersma, E.R. (1994) Neurologial differences between 9 year old children fed breast milk and formula milk as babies. *Lancet*, **344** (8933), 1319–22.

Lothe, L. & Lindberg, T. (1989) Cows milk whey protein elicits symptoms of infantile colicky behaviour in colicky formula fed infants a double blind cross over study. *Paediatrics*, **84**, 262–6.

Lucas, A., Morely, R., Gore, S.M., Cole, T.J. & Bamford J.F.B. (1984) Multi centre trial on feeding low birthweight infants: effects of diet on early growth. *Archives of Diseases in Childhood*, **58**, 722–30.

Lucas, A., Morely, R., Cole, T.J., Gore, S.M., Lucas, P.J., Crowlie, P. *et al.* (1990) Early diet in preterm babies and developmental status at 18 months. *Lancet*, **335**, 1477–81.

Lucas, A., Morley, R., Cole, T.J., Lister, G. & Leeson-Payne, C. (1992) Breast milk and subsequent intelligence quotient in children born pre term. *Lancet*, **339**, 261–4.

Lucas, A., Morely, R., Cole, T.J., Gore S.M., (1994) A randomized multi center study of human milk versus formula and later development in pre term infants. *Archives of Diseases in Childhood*, **70**, 141–6.

Lucas, A. & Cole, T.J.(1990) Breast milk and neonatal necrotizing enterocolitis. *Lancet* **336**, 1519–23.

McTiernan, A. & Thomas, D.B. (1986) Evidence for a protective effect of lactation on risk of breast cancer in young women. *American Journal of Epidemiology* **124**, 353–8.

Martin, J. & Monk, J. (1982) *Infant Feeding*. Office of Population Census and Surveys, HMSO, London.

Martin, J. & White, A. (1988) *Infant Feeding*. Office of Population Census and Surveys, HMSO, London.

Mathews, M.K. (1989) The relationship between maternal labour analgesia and delay in the initiation of breast feeding in healthy neonates in the early neonatal period. *Midwifery*, **5**, 3–10.

Mayer, E.J., Hamman, R.F., Gay, E.C. Lezotte, D.C., Savitz, D.A. & Klingensmith, G.J. (1988) Reduced risk of IDDM among breast fed children. The Colorado IDDM Registry. *Diabetes*, **37** (12), 1625–32.

Minchin, M. (1993) *Breast Feeding: Advantages For Developed Countries*. Independent Booklet. ALMA Publications. Armadale, Victoria, Australia.

Minchin, M. (1998) Artificial Feeding: Risky For Any Baby? Independent booklet, ALMA Publications, Victoria, Australia.

Mitchell, E.A., Scragg, R., Stewart, A.W., Becroft, D.M., Taylor, B.J., Ford *et al.* (1991) Results from the first year of the New Zealand Cot Death Study. *New Zealand Medical Journal*, **104** (906), 71–6.

Pisacane A., de Luca, U., Impagliazzo, N., Russo, M.D. & Caracciolo, G. (1992) Breastfeeding and acute appendictis. *British Medical Journal*, **310** (6983), 836–7.

Pokander, J., Luotonen, J., Timonen, M. *et al.* (1985) Risk factors affecting the ocurrence of acute otitis media among 2–3 year old urban children. *Acta Otolaryngol* **100**, 260–65.

Renfrew, M.J. (1994a) Antenatal breastfeeding education. In: Pregnancy and Childbirth Module (eds M.W. Enkin, M.J.N.C. Keirse, M.J. Renfrew & J.P. Neilson), Cochrane Database of Systematic Reviews: Review No. 04171, 13 April 1993. Published through Cochrane Updates on Disk, Oxford Update Software, Disk issue 1.

Renfrew, M.J. (1994b) Antenatal expression of colostrum. In: Pregnancy and Childbirth Module. (eds M.W. Enkin, M.J.N.C. Keirse, M.J. Renfrew & J.P. Neilson), Cochrane Database of Systematic Reviews: Review No. 04028, 13 April 1993. Published through Cochrane Updates on Disk, Oxford Update Software, Disk issue 1.

Renfrew, M.J. (1994c) Restricted schedule of breastfeeding. In: Pregnancy and Childbirth Module (eds M.W. Enkin, M.J.N.C. Keirse, M.J. Renfrew & J.P. Neilson), Cochrane Database of Systematic Reviews: Review No. 04178, 13 April 1993. Published through Cochrane Updates on Disk, Oxford Update Software, Disk issue 1.

Renfrew, M.J. (1994d) Extra fluids for breastfeeding mothers. In: Pregnancy and Childbirth Module (eds M.W. Enkin, M.J.N.C. Keirse, M.J. Renfrew & J.P. Neilson), Cochrane Database of Systematic Reviews: Review No. 04189, 13 May 05l 1994. Published through Cochrane Updates on Disk, Oxford Update Software, Disk issue 1.

Renfrew, M.J. (1994e) Provision of water supplements to breastfed newborns. In: Pregnancy and Childbirth Module (eds M.W. Enkin, M.J.N.C. Keirse, M.J. Renfrew & J.P. Neilson), Cochrane Database of Systematic Reviews: Review No. 04174, 13 April 1992. Published through Cochrane Updates on Disk, Oxford Update Software, Disk issue 1.

Renfrew, M.J. (1994f) Provision of formula supplements to breastfed newborns. In: Pregnancy and Childbirth Module (eds M.W. Enkin, M.J.N.C. Keirse, M.J. Renfrew & J.P. Neilson), Cochrane Database of Systematic Reviews: Review No. 04175, 13 April 1992. Published through Cochrane Updates on Disk, Oxford Update Software, Disk issue 1.

Renfrew, M.J. (1994g) Postnatal support for breastfeeding mothers In: Pregnancy and Childbirth Module (eds M.W. Enkin, M.J.N.C. Keirse, M.J. Renfrew & J.P. Neilson), Cochrane Database of Systematic Reviews: Review No. 04173, 13 May 1994. Published through Cochrane Updates on Disk, Oxford Update Software, Disk issue 1.

Renfrew, M.J. & Lang, S. (1995) Feeding techniques and breastfeeding success. In: *A Guide to Effective Care in Pregnancy & Childbirth*. (eds M. Enkin, M.J.N.C. Keirse, M.J. Renfrew & J. Neilson) 2nd Edn. Oxford University Press, Oxford. England.

Renfrew, M.J., Fisher, C. & Arms, S. (1990) *Breastfeeding: Getting Breastfeeding Right for You*, Celestial Arts. California.

Rollins, M.D., Shields, M.D., Quinn, R.J.M. & Wooldridge, M.A. (1989) Pyloric stenosis: congenital or acquired. *Archives of Diseases in Childhood*, 64 (1), 138–9.

Royal College of Midwives (RCM) (1991) *Successful Breastfeeding* Churchill Livingstone, London.

Silverman, L. (1993) *The Art and Science of Midwifery*, Prentice Hall, U.K.

Simmons, B.P., Gelfand, M.S., Haas, M. Metts, L. & Ferguson, J. (1989) Sakazaki infections in neonates associated with intrinsic contamination of a powdered milk formula. *Infection Control Hospital Epidemiology*, 10 (9), 398–401.

Stanway, P. & Stanway, A. (1996) *Breast is Best*, Pan Books, London, England.

Tanoue, Y. & Oda, S. (1989) Weaning time of children with infantile autism. *Journal Autism Development Discord*, 19, 425–34.

Victoria, C.G. Smith, P.G., Vaughn, J.P., Noble, L.C., Lamardi, C., Texeura, A.H. *et al.* (1987) Evidence of protection by breast feeding against infant deaths from infectious diseases in Brazil. *Lancet*, 2, 319–22.

United Kingdom National Case Control Study (1993) Breast feeding and risk of breast cancer in young women. *British Journal of Medicine*, 307, 17–20.

Wales, J.K., Milford, D. & Okorie, N.M. (1989) Milk bolus obstruction secondary to the early introduction of a premature baby milk formula: an old syndrome re-emerging in a new population. *European Journal of Paediatrics*, 148, 676–8.

Watkins, C.J., Leede, S.R., Corkhill, R.T. (1979) The relationship between breast and bottle feeding and respiratory illness in the first year of life. *Journal of Epidemiology Community Health*, 33, 80–2.

Welliver, R.C., Wong, D.T., Sun, M. McCarthy, M. (1986) Parainfluenza virus bronchitis. *American Journal of Diseases in Childhood*, 140, 43–40.

Williams, A.F. (1994) Is breast feeding beneficial in the UK? Statement of the Standing Committee on Nutrition of the British Paediatric Association. *Archives of Diseases in Childhood*, 17, 376–9.

Wright, P. (1990) Early feeding behaviour. In: *Excellence in nursing the research route: Midwifery*. (eds A. Faulkner & T. Murphy-Black) Scutari Press, London.

8

Infant Feeding and Early Weaning: Principles and Practice

Soraya Meah and Steven Ryan

8.1 INTRODUCTION

Nutrition in the early years of life is a major determinant of growth and development. Initially newborn infants are solely reliant on a milk diet, breast milk being the optimum choice of milk. However, breast milk is not necessarily a mother's preferred choice. It has been estimated that only 27% of babies born in the UK in 1995 were breast fed for four months or more (ONS 1995), as recommended by the World Health Organization (WHO 1990). For some years now a variety of milk formulae have been available to mothers and it is widely accepted that such infant formulae are a safe alternative to mother's own milk for infants born in western countries.

Currently mothers are exposed to a plethora of complex information about breast milk and infant formulae and within this context health visitors are the most likely health professionals to advise and support mothers, both in their initial choice of feeding method and as the infant develops and is introduced to a weaning diet. Thus an evidential basis for the nutritional advice provided by health visitors is crucial if they are to be effective in supporting mothers to be confident in their own judgement in relation to providing a nutritionally sound diet for their infant. It is against this background that the following chapter has been written.

8.2 INFANT FEEDING: MILK FORMULA

Milks available

Modified cows' milk formulae

When a mother chooses not to breast feed, she is able to provide milk for her baby as a 'modified cows' milk formula'. These products are supplied by a number of manufacturers who attempt to mimic the major nutrient composition of mature human milk (see Table 8.1). The products have to adhere to the compositional guidelines produced by the European Union. As technology has evolved, so has the nutritional composition of milks. 'Synthetic milk adapted' (SMA) was the first of the modern modified formulae designed to mimic the carbohydrate, fat and protein composition of human milk.

Nowadays, further nutrients lower down the nutritional scale are being added to formula. Most are added on theoretical grounds rather than on grounds of scientific evidence of benefits in an infant population. It is thought that long-chain essential fatty acids are beneficial in the diet but there is currently no direct evidence that this is so (Farquharson et al. 1992; Agostini et al. 1995). The addition of nucleotides to formula milk is another example, where similarly only small clinical studies support a large amount of evidence from animal work.

Since human milk protein is predominantly whey, the modified milks most closely resembling it are *whey predominant*. An alternative is a casein predominant formula, where the curd content is greater

Table 8.1 Composition of human milk and cows' milk formula: compositional guidelines for infant formula and follow-on formula (per 100 ml). From Weaning and the Weaning Diet, RHSS 45 (DoH 1994).

	Unit of measurement	Mean values for mature human milk	Infant formula	Follow-on formula
Energy	KJ	293	250–315	250–335
	Kcal	70	60–75	60–80
Protein	g	1.3	1.2–1.95	1.5–2.9
Carbohydrate	g	7	4.6–9.1	4.6–9.1
Fat	g	4.2	2.1–4.2	2.1–4.2
Vitamins				
A	μg	60	39–117	39–117
D	μg	0.01	0.65–0.63	0.65–1.95
E	μg	0.35	≥0.33	≥0.3
K	μg	0.21	2.6	ns*
Thiamin	μg	16	265	ns
Riboflavin	μg	30	39	ns
Niacin	μg	620	163	ns
equivalent	μg	620	163	ns
B6	μg	6	22.8	ns
B12	μg	0.01	0.07	ns
Total folate	μg	5.0	2.6	ns
Panthothenic acid	μg	260	195	ns
Biotin	μg	0.8	1.0	ns
C	mg	3.8	5.2	5.2
Minerals				
Sodium	mg	15	13–39	ns
Potassium	mg	60	39–94	ns
Chloride	mg	43	32.5–81	ns
Calcium	mg	35	19.5	ns
Phosphorous	mg	15	16.3–58.5	ns
Magnesium	mg	3	3.3–9.8	ns
Iron	μg	76	325–975	650–1300
Copper	μg	39	13–52	ns
Zinc	μg	295	325–975	325
Iodine	μg	7	3.3	3.3

ns: not specified

than that of whey – more like cows' milk. Other than the different protein composition these latter milks must comply with the regulations mentioned above. It has been suggested that there may be differences in amino acid balance but as there is no evidence of a clinically meaningful difference, whey predominant and casein predominant milk are considered nutritionally the same.

Follow-on milk

Follow-on milks are based on standard cows' milk formulae as above, but they contain additional minerals, vitamin C, protein and iron. They are not suitable for a newborn baby but are designed for use in the second half of the first year (DoH 1994; 1995).

Soya milk

Commercially available soya milks differ from modified cows' milk formulae in having soya protein as the protein source. They contain no lactose, using glucose polymers as the carbohydrate source, and to make up for compositional deficiencies they contain more protein and are supplemented with methionine. To overcome a relative reduction in mineral bioavailability they contain additional calcium and phosphorus. Soya milks are available over-the-counter, on prescription and with milk tokens. They appear to be nutritionally adequate, although questions still remain about content and availability of minerals (Lonnerdal 1994).

Protein hydrosylates

Commercially available since 1942, protein hydrosylates contain cows' milk protein hydrosylate. The protein is chemically or enzymatically broken down into smaller particles, single amino acids and short chains of amino acids known as oligopeptides. Protein hydrosylates were initially thought to be non-immunogenic (that is, they could not initiate an allergic response), but now it is thought that there may be some immunogenicity and so even more pre-digested (elemental) formulas are available. Protein hydrosylates differ from standard cows' milk formulae in having a higher protein, higher carbohydrate and lower fat content. The fat may contain medium chain triglycerides. Such specialised formulae should only be used after confirmation of a medical diagnosis, and are only available on prescription. Babies who are prescribed such milks require ongoing medical and dietetic supervision. There is an increasing range of such formulae.

Unmodified cows' milk

Unmodified cows' milk is not a safe or effective milk in the newborn period. This is because of its high content of curd protein, making it indigestible in the newborn. It also has a high salt content and a particularly high calcium and phosphorus content. In some early modified formulae, failure to overcome all of these problems during modification led to a number of complications, such as hyperphosphataemic tetany and hypernatraemic dehydration. These deficiencies in unmodified cows' milk for the newborn period change to an advantage later on when a high mineral, high protein drink is very advantageous. Iron content is however low and bioavailability poor.

The use of formula milks

Modified cows' milk formulae

Most formula-fed infants are started on a whey predominant formula as this is how the milks are pro-

moted by the manufacturers; a first milk, with casein predominant formula being promoted as second milks. Given the tight compositional guidelines and the lack of evidence for the benefits of more recent additional nutrients, no single milk can be more highly recommended than any other. For instance, although benefits in animals and temporary effects in humans have been observed, there is no evidence that enhancement with long-chain polyunsaturated fatty acids has a meaningful long-term beneficial effect in the human infant. (Neuringer *et al.* 1986; Farquharson *et al.* 1992; Agostini *et al.* 1995).

Casein milks are suggested for older 'hungry' babies. The idea is that the casein, on contact with acid and enzymes within the stomach, becomes semi-solid curds, which give a 'fuller' feeling to the stomach and take longer to digest and thus diminish the babies' hunger.

Follow-on milk

Follow-on formulae are designed to complement the weaning diet in later infancy. It has been suggested that they can overcome specific nutritional problems with lack of iron.

A randomised replacement with a follow-on formula has shown that a high incidence of iron deficiency seen in babies fed on cows' milk formula from six months can be mostly prevented (Daly *et al.* 1996). The evidence for the use of such a formula compared to a standard infant formula is still based on theoretical considerations. In one trial of a follow-on formula supplemented with iron versus a formula without additional iron, there was no evidence of enhancement of iron status, although this was a study of a population at low risk of iron deficiency (Stevens & Nelson 1995).

Soya milk

Soya milks are primarily designed to be used in children with gastroenteritis complicated by either lactose intolerance or cows' milk protein allergy (Lonnerdal 1994). Some health professionals believe that soya milk fed infants are less likely to develop allergies to cows' milk, and others that this can be useful for treating colic where it is believed that this is a manifestation of cows' milk protein allergy. They can also be used for infants with galactosaemia.

Protein hydrosylates

These milks can be used for all of the above conditions mentioned for soya milk, and in addition for certain absorptive and digestive disorders such as short bowel enteropathy, and pancreatic insufficiency (cystic fibrosis).

Unmodified cows' milk

There is a consensus that the introduction of unmodified cows' milk should be delayed until 12 months of age. This is because of the association between unmodified cows' milk and anaemia (DoH 1994). This may have two causative factors; poor iron constant/absorption together with occult intestinal bleeding, an immunological (and hence allergic) phenomenon. (Although widely quoted, the theory of intestinal blood loss has not been confirmed in all studies (Fuchs *et al.* 1993).) However, early introduction of such milk is associated with lower social and educational status, so that other confounding factors in the diet may be responsible.

Common problems

The hungry dissatisfied baby

A majority of mothers change their child's infant formula at least once, and most commonly from a whey to a casein predominant formula. Mothers usually do this because their baby is unsettled, or appears hungry or dissatisfied with the whey milk.

There seems, however, to be no evidence from randomised studies for the effectiveness of a casein-based formula in ameliorating 'excess hunger' (Thorkelsson *et al.* 1994). This is also borne out in our clinical practice. The repeated changing of milks by mothers is so common that it can be described as a normal event. Changing between nutritionally similar formulae is of no nutritional disadvantage to the baby, although taste and palatability problems have been suggested.

Implications for practice

The available evidence suggests that repeated changing of the milk formula by mothers who consider their baby to be hungry is unlikely to compromise the nutrition of the infant. It is also unlikely to address the underlying reasons for the baby being unsettled.

Infant colic

The repeated episodes of crying and distress in the otherwise healthy infant have been called infant colic.

It is generally believed that the behaviour represents abdominal pain and following this assumption, changing the baby's milk has been a popular intervention.

The pathophysiology of colic is still not understood as can be seen from theories as diverse as abnormal colonic fermentation and treatment such as cranial osteopathy. The evidence that effective drug treatment, including dicyclomine, is available is lacking (Oggero *et al.* 1994). However, mothers may be reassured that the distress associated with colic is resolved spontaneously in most instances, and only rarely do isolated symptoms ascribed to colic represent an important pathology.

Hill *et al.* (1995) have suggested that milk protein intolerance/allergy is responsible for colic, and that use of a soy or protein digested formula will be beneficial. There is much anecdotal and little empirical evidence to support this (Thomas *et al.* 1987; Hill 1995). Indeed, one study reported that parental counselling was more effective than changing milks (Taubmann 1988). In conclusion there is insufficient evidence that either soya milks or pre-digested formulae are necessary or appropriate for this poorly understood condition.

Implications for practice

There is not enough evidence to suggest that milk should be changed for uncomplicated infant colic (Thomas *et al.* 1987). Such changes are unlikely to be successful and if there are other symptoms such as diarrhoea or vomiting, it may not be simple colic and further investigation is warranted.

Allergies

Both soya milks and protein digested formulae have been recommended for treatment and prevention of allergies since cows' milk protein is considered an important allergen in these conditions.

Since a small number of children become allergic to soy protein as well as cows' milk protein, some have advocated that children with putative cows' milk protein allergy should receive a semi-elemental formula from the outset.

High risk of allergy is usually defined by a family history, especially in first-degree relatives of severe atopy, and with a history of cows' milk protein being an important allergen.

There are two important randomised controlled trials which show that use of a protein hydrosylate formula will reduce manifestations of allergy in infancy. In their study, Mallet & Henocq (1992) also showed a reduction in allergic problems such as eczema, but not asthma later in childhood. Reduction in prevalence was by between one third and one half. A study of 453 infants using soya milk failed to show any benefit in preventing the emergence of allergic phenomena, compared to standard cows' milk formula (Burr *et al.* 1993).

Implications for practice

Currently there are no reliable tests for cows' milk allergy. The diagnosis is made on the basis of clinical manifestations of allergy (vomiting, diarrhoea or eczema) which is worsened by challenge with cows' milk protein and alleviated by its withdrawal from the diet. Ideally this should be done on a blind basis (i.e. in a hospital, where clinical signs can be observed) since the symptoms are frequently subjectively reported.

If cows' milk protein allergy is diagnosed a cows' milk protein free diet should be advised for at least six months, after which a challenge is arranged. In most children the clinical allergy is temporary and by school age has usually resolved. If the child is on solid food then a full dietetic review is required so that advice is appropriate to ensure the diet is free of cows' milk protein. It is also important to ensure it is nutritionally adequate, especially in respect to calcium intake.

Gastroenteritis

Complications of gastroenteritis include lactose and cows' milk intolerance and delayed recovery. The use of soy, pre-digested formulae, reduced strength milks and delay in milk feeding have all been suggested as ways of avoiding some or all of these problems (Chew *et al.* 1993).

Even in very young infants early re-feeding within six hours (compared to 24 hours) after cessation of vomiting is not disadvantageous. This helps to avoid additional under-nutrition (Gazala *et al.* 1988). There also appears to be no benefit from using half-strength as opposed to full-strength formula. Both strengths are equally likely to result in persisting diarrhoea, which is four times more likely if lactose is found in the stool (Chew *et al.* 1993).

The study by Allen (Allen *et al.* 1994) showed that although diarrhoea persisted longer in infants randomised to cows' milk formula than in infants re-fed with soya milk (by an average of two days), by 14 days there was no difference in bowel habit or weight gain.

Implications for practice

In formulafed infants with gastroenteritis, persistent vomiting is likely to lead to dehydration and should be treated with oral rehydration solution until the vomiting stops. Such solutions should not be used for more than 24 hours, since the gut mucosa becomes malnourished and has difficulty recovering. They should be used until vomiting stops, when most infants should be recommenced on full-strength formula, which should be continued even in the ongoing presence of diarrhoea.

Soya milk or a pre-digested formula is considered if enteropathy persists with continuing weight loss, persistent lactose intolerance or, if secondary cows' milk protein tolerance is diagnosed. The latter may present with weight loss and persistent lactose intolerance as well as a return to vomiting. If lactose intolerance is suspected, stool samples should be sent for tests for either reducing substances or sugar chromatography. Lactose intolerance is a temporary phenomenon and lactose should be reintroduced into the diet after six weeks. A relapse of diarrhoea suggests that the underlying diagnosis is cows' milk protein intolerance, when a non-cows' milk formula will be required for several months.

Table 8.1 compares composition of human milk with that of infant formula and follow-on formula.

Preparing formula feeds

The preparation of infant formula has become more sophisticated over the past two decades. This has led some people to assume that formula feeding is a simple, safe method of feeding to rival breast feeding (Hill 1968); this assumption is not supported by empirical evidence. It has been documented that formula fed infants are disadvantaged in many ways (Henschel & Inch 1996). In particular they are exposed to a greater risk of infection even in industrialised societies (DoH 1994).

The formula fed infant may be compromised by:

- the possibility of errors during manufacture of the formula (Minchin 1985);
- incorrect preparation of feeds, which alter the concentration of the feed (Lucas 1991, Lucas *et al.* 1992); and

■ contamination with bacteria during preparation of the feed at home, due to poor domestic hygiene.

In view of these risks it is imperative that parents receive clear and precise instructions in the preparation of feeds. All infant formulae come with full instructions on how to reconstitute the milk formula correctly, however it is the responsibility of the health professional to assess parents' understanding and compliance with the manufacturers' instructions. All too often this is over looked and well-intentioned parents make serious errors when feeding their baby. Anecdotal examples include parents adding extra amounts of formula to a bottle because they have a 'big baby', or swapping the correct measuring scoop for another because they feel the colour is more appropriately matched to the child's gender. Coupled with the need for good practice in making up formula feeds is the appropriate use of sterilising agents for kitchen utensils. Once again the role of the health professional must be stressed in ensuring that parents are fully informed of the necessity to sterilise equip-

ment, and are competent in the techniques used. The need for only cooled boiled water to be used to make up the formula milk feeds is even more important given recent government advice to people with weak immune systems and those immunosuppressed not to drink any water without boiling it first then allowing it to cool. This advice followed on from the discovery in drinking water of unacceptable levels of a microbe, *Cryptosporium*, that can cause life-threatening gastroenteritis in people with weak immune systems, and diarrhoea, vomiting and stomach pains in less vulnerable people (*Guardian*, 4 November 1998).

The pre-term baby

The nutritional requirements of pre-term and growth-retarded infants differ greatly from those of a term baby. It is beyond the scope of this chapter to provide an in-depth discussion of the nutritional management of such infants. However an outline of available pre-term milk formulas and their current use in practice is given in Table 8.2.

Table 8.2 The pre-term infant.

Pre-term milk	Pre-term post-discharge milk	Implications for practice	Weaning pre-term infants
Only used in hospital.	Major nutrient composition lies between that of a hospital pre-term formula and a standard milk.	Pre-term and growth-retarded infants may exhibit spectacular catch-up growth between the equivalent of full term and 3–4 months.	There is no consistent advice or research findings to determine when to wean a pre-term baby.
High nutrient composition compared to standard milks e.g. 80 kCal/ 100 ml.	Contains increased calcium and phosphorus and protein and energy.	They should be allowed to take feeds on demand, as volumes above those routinely recommended (Lucas *et al.* 1992).	A pragmatic approach is taken in most situations with weaning commencing somewhere between 4 months of age and 4 months after 'full term'.
Designed to provide adequate nutrition and to prevent specific nutritional difficulties in the pre-term, e.g. metabolic bone disease, sodium deficiency.	Not currently prescribable or available on milk tokens in the UK.	Changing milks, especially to casein-based formulas does not appear to be effective. Pre-term infants should receive a post-discharge formula for at least 3 months after discharge (Lucas *et al.* 1992; Bishop *et al.* 1993).	

8.3 WEANING

Weaning is the process during which the infant and young child change from milk (breast milk or formula) to a fully mixed diet. It is often viewed by mothers as a landmark in the development of a baby's life and the relationship between mother and baby. Government guidelines recommend that the majority of infants should not be introduced to solid foods until four months of age, and that a mixed diet should be offered by six months of age (DoH 1994). However, there is some evidence that these guidelines do not mirror common practice. A national survey of diet and nutrition in children aged one and a half to four and a half years of age, conducted in 1990, indicated that 16% of mothers reported giving food other than milk to their infants by eight weeks of age, and over 50% of mothers had introduced solids to their infants by three months of age. The extent to which these findings represent an accurate depiction of national practices of infant weaning is questionable; as the reports of some mothers may refer to small 'tasters' of pureed food, while maintaining a predominantly milk diet, alternatively some infants may have received rapidly increasing amounts of solid food in their diet.

The authors of the report 'Weaning and the Weaning Diet' (DoH 1994), highlight the difficulties in producing national guidelines of equal relevance to breast fed and formula fed infants based on the available evidence. The basis for their recommendations is that infants of between four and six months of age are physically and developmentally mature enough to cope with a weaning diet, irrespective of whether they have received breast or formula milk.

The weaning process

By four months of age infants have developed sufficient co-ordination to eat semi-solid foods, and most will be able to maintain a sitting posture while supported in a chair, to facilitate feeding. At five months they will readily accept pureed foods from a spoon. The action of chewing food is developed by six months. Infants at this age will actively seek out objects to put into their mouths, this natural tendency may be used to encourage infants to develop skills in chewing, and this can be done by offering them foods

to hold. It is worthy of note that by seven months of age children have developed the ability to close their mouths and turn their heads as an act of refusal, and this may be used as a ploy to delay weaning, if an infant is reluctant to accept the new tastes and textures of solid food.

Teething often coincides with weaning, at about six months. Teeth are an important factor in children's ability to develop the skill of chewing and exploring the texture of different foods, but at this point they are not essential to good nutrition, or to the introduction of solid foods. However it is important to warn parents against introducing foods and drinks that can predispose to dental caries.

Introducing a weaning diet: practical steps

Weaning foods differ in both taste and texture from breast or formula milk, they also require different techniques of feeding. Successful weaning is dependent on overcoming the child's natural aversion to experiencing the alien smells and tastes of new foods. The most effective means of achieving this will depend on the individual child, and on parental preference. An example of a weaning programme is given in Figure 8.1.

Problems of weaning

Weaning too early

Early weaning is sometimes thought to be associated with a number of problems including obesity, gastroenteritis and allergy. A large, prospective, observational study has not supported this contention, although its authors did note that allergic diseases may be more common in susceptible individuals (Forsyth *et al.* 1993). Gastroenteritis susceptibility is probably more related to cessation of breast feeding than introduction of solids, even in a population with a high incidence of diarrhoeal disease (Molbak *et al.* 1994). The link between excessive weight gain in infancy and prolonged obesity is lacking (Zive *et al.* 1992).

Weaning too late

Although breast milk alone is an adequate source of nutrition in early infancy, growth failure begins to be seen around six months of age if it is continued (Ahn & MacLean 1980) and protein requirements are not

---

- Introduce one new taste at a time.
- A baby cereal or baby rice is a good food to start with, progressing to pureed vegetables, fruit and meat.
- To begin with, a small amount of food should be offered to the infant, e.g. one small teaspoon of cereal made up to a runny consistency.
- The food should be given at a specific time each day, e.g. 10 a.m. When the infant enjoys the cereal and eats it readily, a new taste may be introduced. This should be offered at a second time of the day, e.g. 2 p.m. feed.
- It may take 1–2 weeks to establish each taste.
- The weaning diet is gradually established at all day time feeds and is increased in amounts.
- Feeding times may be changed to fall in line with family meal times by the eighth or ninth month.

Figure 8.1　Weaning programme. (Lewer & Robertson 1983; Stoppard 1990.)

met (Whitehead 1995). Debate continues on this point, since, in some infants, exclusive breast feeding until nine months can sustain adequate weight gain (Borresen 1995).

Nutritionally inadequate weaning foods

Although many health professionals advocate the use of home prepared foods as the basis of an infant's diet, there is a risk that the ensuing food may have a deficient nutrient composition. In one large study (Stordy *et al.* 1995), many home prepared food samples had an energy density below that of human milk, with low values also for fat, iron, calcium and zinc, and excess sodium and non-starch poly-saccharides (fibre). Particular practices leading to some of these problems were initial weaning with pureed fruit alone, avoiding red meat (a good source of zinc and iron), but having a large amount of vegetables.

The avoidance of red meat has also been associated with public concern about the impact of bovine spongiform encephalopathy (BSE) on the human population (see Chapter 9). This has led some parents to resort to providing a vegetarian diet for their infant without being aware of the need to provide alternative sources of iron in the diet (Belton 1995; Seymour 1996). Fears associated with the emergence of BSE are likely to persist for sometime. This is a unique incident and in view of the lack of clear evidence on which to base advice, health visitors would be advised to keep abreast of emerging research findings while taking steps to ensure that parents are fully aware of the nutritional needs of their infants and how these can be met.

Further problems arise from the popular mis-

conception that an ideal diet should be high in fibre and low in fat, while this type of diet may offer health benefits to adults it is not designed to meet the nutritional requirements of infants and young children (Morgan *et al.* 1995). Clearly health visitors are best placed to address this type of problem, in that they may employ a family-centred approach to nutrition and diet.

Specific allergies

The delay in first feeding of gluten to babies is felt to be important in the observed reduction in the incidence of coeliac disease (Stevens *et al.* 1987). Mothers may have difficulty in ensuring that their child's diet is truly gluten free until the recommended age of six months, and frequently select gluten-free products while inadvertently giving gluten in other foodstuffs (van den Boom *et al.* 1995).

Ethnicity, culture and diet

It is beyond the scope of this text to provide an account of the various cultural differences between the ethnic groups which make up a multicultural society such as our own; or to discuss the issues related to health care and culture. However, health professionals need to be aware that cultural differences between service users and providers is likely to have consequences for health outcomes (Amandah 1994). This is particularly important in relation to weaning practices where there is growing evidence to point to possible tensions between advice given by health professionals and traditional cultural practices (Corbett 1989; Seymour 1996; Thomas & De Santis 1995).

8.4 CONCLUSIONS

Government guidelines recommend that weaning should generally begin between four and six months of age in term babies. However, evidence that early weaning is damaging is not strong and if a mother has commenced early weaning, advice should be given to ensure that correct foods are used – for example to delay gluten. For most parents the health visitor is the lead professional in providing advice on the weaning process, as such, it is imperative that he or she interacts with parents to formulate a weaning programme that is based on the available evidence, but is still sensitive to parental choice. The key to this is to assess parents' existing knowledge of nutrition and the weaning process, in order to prevent any of the dietary misconceptions mentioned above, and to ensure that a home prepared diet is adequate.

REFERENCES

Agostini, C., Trojan, S., Bellu, R., Riva, E. & Giovannini, M. (1995) Neurodevelopmental quotient of healthy term infants at 4 months and feeding practice: the role of long-chain polyunsaturated fatty acids. *Pediatric Research*, **38**, 262–6.

Ahn, C.H. & MacLean, W.C. (1980) Growth of the exclusively breast-fed infant. *American Journal of Clinical Nutrition*, **33**, 183–92.

Allen, U.D., McLeod, K. & Wang, E.E. (1994) Cow's milk versus soy-based formula in mild and moderate diarrhoea: a randomized, controlled trial. *Acta Paediatrica*, **83**, 183–7.

Amandah, L. (1994) Nursing in today's multicultural society: a transcultural perspective. *Journal of Advanced Nursing*, **20**, 307–13.

Belton, N. (1995) Paediatric nutrition: iron deficiency in infants and young children. *Professional Care of Mother and Child*, **5** (3), 69–71.

Bishop, N.J., King, F.J. & Lucas, A. (1993) Increased bone mineral content of preterm infants with a nutrient enriched formula after discharge from hospital. *Archives of Diseases in Childhood*, **68**, 573–8.

Borresen, H.C. (1995) Rethinking current recommendations to introduce solid food between four and six months to exclusively breastfeeding infants. *Journal of Human Lactation*, **11**, 201–4.

Burr, M.L., Limb, E.S., Maguire, M.I. *et al.* (1993) Infant feeding, wheezing and allergy: a prospective study. *Archives of Diseases in Childhood*, **68**, 724–8.

Chew, F., Penna, F.J., Peret Filho, L.A. (1993) Is dilution of cows' milk formula necessary for dietary management of acute diarrhoea in infants aged less than 6 months. *Lancet*, **341**, 194–7.

Corbett, K.S. (1989) An ethnographic field study of infant feeding practices in St Croix, United States Virgin Islands. PhD Thesis. The University of Texas.

Daly, A., MacDonald, A., Aukett, A., Williams, J., Davidson, J. & Booth, I.W. (1996) Prevention of anaemia in inner city toddlers by an iron supplemented cows' milk formula. *Archives of Diseases in Childhood*, **75**, 9–16.

Department of Health (1994) *Report on Health and Social Subjects 45: Weaning and The Weaning Diet*. Report of the Working Group on the Weaning Diet of the Committee on Medical Aspects of Food Policy. HMSO, London.

Department of Health (1995) *A Guide to Dietary Reference values for Food Energy and Nutrients for the United Kingdom*. HMSO, London.

Farquharson, J., Cockburn, F., Patrick, A.W., Jamieson, E.C. & Logan, R.W. (1992) Infant cerebral cortex phospholipid fatty acid composition and diet. *Lancet*, **340**, 810–13.

Forsyth, J.S., Ogston, S.A., Clark, A., Florey, C. du V. & Howie, P.W. (1993) Relation between early introduction of solid foods to infants and their weight and illnesses during the first two years of life. *British Medical Journal*, **306**, 1572–6.

Fuchs, G., DeWier, M., Hutchinson, S., Sundeen, M., Schwartz, S. & Suskind, R. (1993) Gastrointestinal blood loss in older infants: impact of cows' milk versus formula. *Journal of Pediatric Gastroenterology and Nutrition*, **16**, 4–9.

Guardian (1998) Water warning to people with weak immune systems. 4 November.

Henschel, S. & Inch, D. (1996) *Breastfeeding: A Guide For Midwives*. Books For Midwives Press, Hale, England.

Hill, A.F. (1968) A salute to La Leche League International. *Journal Pediatrica*, **73**, 161–2.

Lonnerdal, B. (1994) Nutritional aspects of soy formula. *Acta. Paediatrics*, **S402**, 105–8.

Lucas, A. (1991) Letter. *British Medical Journal*, **302**, 351–1.

Lucas, A. *et al.* (1992) Randomised trial of a ready to feed compared with powdered formula. *Archives of Diseases in Childhood*, **67**, 935–9.

Mallet, E. & Henocq, A. (1992) Long-term prevention of allergic disease by using protein hydrosylate formula in at-risk infants. *Journal of Pediatrics*, **121**, S95–S100.

Minchin, M. (1985) *Breastfeeding Matters*. Alma Publications and George Allen and Unwin, Australia, pp. 11, 150.

Molbak, K., Gottschau, A., Aaby, P., Hojlyng, N., Ingholt, L. & da Silva, A.P.J. (1994) Prolonged breast feeding, diarrhoeal disease, and survival of children in Guinea-Bissau. *British Medical Journal*, 308, 1403–6.

Morgan, J.B., Kimber, A.C., Redfern, A.M. & Stordy, J.B. (1995) Healthy eating for infants – mothers' attitudes. *Acta. Paediatrics*, 84, 512–15.

Neuringer, M., Connor, W.E., Lin, D.S., Barstad, L. & Luck, S. (1986) Biochemical and functional effects of prenatal and postnatal omega-3 fatty acid deficiency on retina and brain in rhesus monkeys. *Proc. Natl. Acad. Sci. USA*, 83, 4021–5.

Office For National Statistics (1995) *Breastfeeding in the United Kingdom in 1995*. ONS, London.

Seymour, J. (1996) Weaning: dietary advice for parents. *Nursing Times*, 92 (25), 56–58.

Stevens, F.M., Egan-Mitchell, B., Cryan, E., McCarthy, C.F. & McNicholl, B. (1987) Decreasing incidence of coeliac disease. *Archives of Diseases in Childhood*, 62, 456–68.

Stordy, B.J., Redfern, A.M. & Morgan, J.B. (1995) Healthy eating for infants – mothers' actions. *Acta. Pediatrica*, 84, 733–41.

Thomas, J.T. & De Santis, L. (1995) Feeding and weaning practices of Cuban and Haitian immigrant mothers. *Journal of Transcultural Nursing*, 6 (2), 32–4.

Thorkelsson, T., Mimouni, F., Namgung, R., Fernandez-Ulloa, M., Krug-Wispe, S. & Tsang, R.C. (1994) Similar gastric emptying rates for casein- and whey-predominant formulas in preterm infants. *Pediatric Research*, 36, 329–33.

van den Boom, S.A.M., Kimber, A.C. & Morgan, J.B. (1995) Weaning practices in children up to 19 months of age in Madrid. *Acta. Paediatrics*, 84, 853–8.

Whitehead, R.G. (1995) For how long is exclusive breast-feeding adequate to satisfy dietary energy needs of the average baby? *Pediatric Research*, 37, 239–43.

Zive, M.M., Salmenpera, L., Siimes, M.A., Perheentupa, J. & Miettinen, T.A. (1992) Infant feeding practices and adiposity in 4-year-old Anglo- and Mexican-Americans. *American Journal of Clinical Nutrition*, 55, 1104–8.

World Health Organization (1990) Innocenti Declaration. WHO/UNICEF meeting 1990. Breastfeeding in the 1990s: A Global Initiative. WHO.

FURTHER READING

Gazala, E., Weitzman, S., Weizman, Z., Gross, S.J., Bearman, J.E. & Gorodischer, R. (1988) Early vs. late refeeding in acute infantile diarrhea. *Israeli Journal of Medicine and Science*, 24, 175–9.

Hill, D.J., Hudson, I.L., Sheffield, L.J., Shelton, M.J., Menahem, S. & Hosking, C.S. (1995) A low allergen diet is a significant intervention in infantile colic: results of a community-based study. *Journal of Allergy and Clinical Immunology*, 96, 886–92.

Lucas, A., Bishop, N.J., King, F.J., Cole, T.J. (1992) Randomised trial of nutrition for preterm infants after discharge. *Archives of Diseases in Childhood*, 67, 324–7.

Lucas, A., King, F. & Bishop, N.B. (1992) Postdischarge formula consumption in infants born preterm. *Archives of Diseases in Childhood*, 67, 691–2.

Oggero, R., Garbo, G., Savin, F. & Mostert, M. (1994) Dietary modifications versus dicyclomine hydrochloride in the treatment of severe infantile colic. *Acta. Paediatrics*, 83, 222–5.

Robertson, L. (ed) (1983) *The Essentials of Nursing*. Macmillan, London.

Stevens, D., Nelson, A. (1995) The effect of iron in formula milk after 6 months of age. *Archives of Diseases in Childhood*, 73, 216–20.

Stoppard, M. (1990) *New Baby Care*, 2nd edn. Dorling Kindersley, London.

Taubmann, B. (1988) Parental counselling compared with elimination of cow's milk or soy milk protein for the treatment of infant colic syndrome: a randomized trial. *Pediatrics*, 81, 756–61.

Thomas, D.W., McGilligan, K., Eisenberg, L.D., Lieberman, H.M. & Rissman, E.M. Infantile colic and type of milk feeding. *Am. J. Dis. Child*, 141, 451–3.

9

Nutrition in Childhood: Advice and Dilemmas

Carmel Mary Flanagan and Lynne Kennedy

9.1 INTRODUCTION

The association between diet and health has been widely accepted and is the subject of much research both past and present. Substantial health gains can be demonstrated by increasing the nutritional quality of the diet, whilst on the other hand, the impact of a poor diet during childhood is particularly pronounced. Sociological determinants have an impact on the development of eating behaviour and subsequent food choices. These important influences are recognised but are beyond the scope of this chapter. For further reading see Mennell (1992) or Fieldhouse (1995). Much of the evidence presented in the chapter comes from empirical evidence following quantitative analytical research on the type of foods comprising children's diet.

The health profile of developed countries has changed dramatically since the turn of the century. In 1906 the infant mortality rate in the UK was 118 deaths per 1000 live births, compared to less than 20 deaths per 1000 in 1990. This decline is in part due to advances in health care, preventative measures such as immunisation, and better nutrition. Malnutrition, due to hunger and nutrient deficiencies, has been replaced by problems associated with over-consumption and imbalances in nutrient intake. A healthy diet and optimal nutrition intake is important to children's growth and development. Furthermore a poor diet may influence the development of certain health related problems, including dental caries, low

bone mass, nutritional anaemia, overweight and obesity.

9.2 PATTERNS OF CONSUMPTION

The need to develop healthy eating habits

The links between dietary factors and chronic diseases such as cardiovascular disease, obesity, certain cancers and adult diabetes, are widely documented (e.g. WHO 1990). The typical British diet is high in total fat, saturated fat and sodium, and low in complex carbohydrates and fibre. Dietary fat intake is estimated to contribute to 30% of premature deaths due to coronary heart disease and cancers (Bingham 1991). Although coronary heart disease mortality and morbidity is falling, trends for obesity have risen sharply. The prevalence of obesity in England is on the increase. In 1980 6% of men and 8% of women were obese, by 1993 these figures had risen to 13% of men and 16% of women. Increasing scientific evidence highlights the need for dietary changes in the population, starting in childhood. Dietary Reference Values (DRVs) and guidelines to individuals have subsequently been revised (DoH, 1991), and nutrition targets aimed at reducing mortality and morbidity associated with diet have been set to improve the health of the nation (DoH 1992). Between 1992 and 1996 the Nutrition Task Force (DoH) existed to implement these targets. Their strategy outlined for each sector in the food chain a role in promoting nutrition (DoH 1994a).

Childhood is a period of rapid growth and development during which diet and nutrition have an important role in promoting optimal health. Food preferences developed during infancy and childhood are shown to have an impact on health in adult life (e.g. Barker 1990; Whincup 1996). Furthermore, food preferences established during infancy and childhood are thought to continue into adulthood, becoming more resistant to change. Encouraging young children to eat a wide variety of foods can lead them to develop a taste for a varied and healthy diet, which might improve overall nutritional adequacy. Early development of good eating habits is therefore important.

Nutritional requirements

Infants and young children have the highest energy and nutrient requirements. Capacity for food is, however, limited during the early years. Diets therefore should contain foods that are nutrient dense to satisfy the important growth and development requirements. Thus, low energy, bulky foods recommended as part of general healthy eating guidelines for adults are unsuitable for babies or young children. Adult guidelines should only be introduced beyond two, and only then with caution, gradually increasing consumption of starch and non-starch polysaccharides with a corresponding fall in the proportion of dietary energy from fats. Whilst the Department of Health (1991) consider adult guidelines applicable to children above the age of five, a recent survey showed many mothers to be misguided in thinking healthy eating guidelines for the adult population are directly applicable to children (Morgan 1995). Overzealous application of healthy eating advice may lead to energy deficiency and hence failure to thrive in young children (Stordy 1995).

Nutritional requirements across age groups are detailed in the Coma Report on Dietary Reference Values (DoH 1991). The dietary energy requirements of children aged 0–14 are shown in Table 9.1 and Table 9.2 shows dietary nutrient intakes for vitamins and minerals for children aged 0–10.

Table 9.1 Reference nutrient intakes for energy – estimated average requirements (EAR) for energy of children 0–14 years (Department of Health 1991).

Age	EAR MJ/d (Kcal/d)	
	Boys	**Girls**
0–3 months	2.28 (545)	2.16 (515)
4–6 months	2.89 (690)	2.69 (645)
7–9 months	3.44 (825)	3.20 (765)
10–12 months	3.85 (920)	3.61 (865)
1–3 years	5.15 (1230)	4.86 (1165)
4–6 years	7.16 (1715)	6.46 (1545)
7–10 years	8.24 (1970)	7.28 (1740)
11–14 years	9.27 (2220)	7.92 (1845)

Dietary Reference Values RHSS 41 Crown copyright material is reproduced with permission of the Controller of Her Majesty's Stationery Office.

9.3 HEALTHY EATING

Current intakes

If advice to change the eating habits of children is to be developed, we must first have some idea of current food and nutrient intakes across different age groups. At the time of writing, however, information about the intakes of children at a national level is incomplete. Nelson (1993) provides a useful summary of the major studies into children's dietary patterns conducted during the 1980s and 1990s. Only four of the ten studies available had samples above 1000. Recent attempts to produce a more comprehensive assessment of the nutritional and dietary status of adults, and now children in the UK has resulted in a series of national surveys completed or under way. Information on current intakes of children aged between $1\frac{1}{2}$ to $4\frac{1}{2}$ is complete (Gregory et al. 1995), whilst results of the survey into children aged 4–18 years in 1997 are due in 1999.

The picture for children is no better than that for adult trends. Children of pre-school age are eating poor diets resulting in high intakes of salt, sugar and dietary fat. This group are failing to consume sufficient amounts of fruit, vegetables or iron providing foods (Gregory et al. 1995). Although the mean

Table 9.2 Reference nutrient intakes (RNI) for vitamins and minerals (Department of Health 1991).

	Age (in months)				Age (in years)		
	0–3	4–6	7–9	10–12	1–3	4–6	7–10
Vitamins							
Thiamin mg/d	0.2	0.2	0.2	0.3	0.5	0.7	0.7
Riboflavin mg/d	0.4	0.4	0.4	0.4	0.6	0.8	1.0
Niacin (nicotinic acid equivalent) mg/d	3	3	4	5	8	11	12
Vitamin B6 mg/d[1]	0.2	0.2	0.3	0.4	0.7	0.9	1.0
Vitamin B12 µg/d	0.3	0.3	0.4	0.4	0.5	0.8	1.0
Folate µg/d	50	50	50	50	70	100	150
Vitamin C mg/d	25	25	25	25	30	30	30
Vitamin A µg/d	350	350	350	350	400	500	500
Vitamin D µg/d	8.5	8.5	7.0	7.0	7.0	–	–
Minerals							
Calcium mg/d	525	525	525	525	350	450	550
Phosphorus mg/d[2]	400	400	400	400	270	350	450
Magnesium mg/d	55	60	75	80	85	120	200
Sodium mg/d[3]	210	280	320	350	500	700	2000
Potassium mg/d[4]	800	850	700	700	800	1100	2000
Chloride mg/d[5]	320	400	500	500	800	1100	1800
Iron mg/d	1.7	4.3	7.8	7.8	6.9	6.1	8.7
Zinc mg/d	4.0	4.0	5.0	5.0	5.0	6.5	8.7
Copper mg/d	0.2	0.3	0.3	0.3	0.4	0.6	0.7
Selenium µg/d	10	13	10	10	15	20	30
Iodine µg/d	50	60	60	60	70	100	110

[1] Based on protein providing 14.7% of EAR for energy.
[2] Phosphorus RNI is set equal to calcium on molar terms.
[3] 1 mmol sodium = 23 mg.
[4] 1 mmol potassium = 39 mg.
[5] Corresponds to sodium; 1 mmol = 35.5 mg.

Dietary Reference Values RHSS 41 Crown copyright material is reproduced with permission of the Controller of Her Majesty's Stationery Office.

energy intake of those surveyed was below the estimated average requirement, growth rates appear normal. Mean fat intake was shown to be in the region acceptable for adults and older children (34–36%), (DoH 1991). This suggests however that sugar, rather than fat, in the form of sugary drinks and snacks is a major source of energy for this group. For infants approximately half their energy comes from dietary fat, and it is only after the age of two that this gradually shifts towards adult guidelines of 35%. Indeed the government report into weaning for infants states that a fat-restricted diet is not appropriate for children under two (DoH 1994b). Snacking is typical for young children. Whilst snacks can be a useful means of ensuring nutritional adequacy, particularly for children with poor appetites or those who are small eaters, foods that are high in salt, sugar and

fat but low in other nutrients should be restricted. For these reasons Buttriss (1995) recommends that parents should offer:

- small chopped fruit and raw pieces of vegetables;
- bread, breadsticks and crispbreads;
- sandwiches made with low fat fillings;
- a drink of milk and a plain biscuit;
- yoghurt or fromage frais;
- plain popcorn instead of crisps;
- limit fruit juice and squash to mealtimes;
- keep sweets and chocolates for special treats.

In developed countries micronutrient deficiency is now rare, due mainly to improvements in the food supply. For select groups of the population, however, intakes of vitamins and minerals essential for physiological functions are below recommended levels. Gregory *et al.* (1995) found that the $1\frac{1}{2}$ to $4\frac{1}{2}$ age group contained one in twelve children who were anaemic; 84% of the children under four years old had intakes of iron below the recommended nutritional intake (RNI); this reduced to 57% above the age of four. Iron deficiency is a particular risk for children, especially those on low incomes, those following vegetarian diets and for teenage girls who embark on unsupervised slimming diets. Foods rich in iron, such as red meat and fortified cereals, bread and dark green vegetables can help reduce the risk.

In terms of actual food intake, cereals and cereal products make the largest contribution to energy intake. Milk and milk products, also significant sources of energy, are the main sources of protein ahead of meat and meat products (Table 9.3).

Likewise schoolchildren's diets are reportedly high in fat and sugar, with relatively fewer sources of complex carbohydrates, and a lack of fresh fruits and vegetables. According to Nelson's review (1993) the percentage energy from fat and from total sugars for UK schoolchildren exceeds the recommended levels. Not surprisingly then, the main nutritional problem for this age group is overweight or obesity, due in part to this imbalance and a lack of physical activity. Similarly the DHSS survey in 1989 also found that energy intakes from fat (not from total sugars) for children aged 11–12 and 14–15 ranged between 37% and 39% against recommended levels of 35%. The high proportion of foods rich in fat and sugar, and soft drinks containing sugar remains a significant problem in schoolchildren's diets with consequences in subsequent years. Nelson's study (1993) showed that children between the ages of $10\frac{1}{2}$ and 12 were exceeding recommended levels of energy from fat and almost doubling recommended levels of energy from total sugars.

Although less significant than in previous generations of schoolchildren, the problem of insufficient calcium and iron intake, particularly amongst teenage girls, still remains. Children and adolescents who drink milk regularly are reportedly more likely to have higher bone mass and thus less risk of osteoporosis in later life. A recent study (Cadogan *et al.* 1997) reported that increased milk consumption significantly enhances bone mineral acquisition in adolescent girls.

School meals

For many British school children, school meals provide their main meal of the day. In recent years there has been increasing criticism of the ad hoc quality and management of school meals. The government has however put forward proposed legislation to establish minimum nutritional standards for school meals, and place a duty on local education authorities and on schools managing their own school meals arrangements to meet these standards. It is hoped this will address consequences resulting from the abandonment of nutrition guidelines in 1980. Schools need to adopt a whole day approach, addressing breakfast provision, and healthy mid-morning snacks as well as mid-day meals. In addition to this, some studies have suggested that children who regularly skip breakfast, or who have a low nutritional status, may obtain benefits from regular breakfast consumption in terms of cognitive benefits (Simeon *et al.* 1989). It is thus essential that a holistic approach to education is adopted which includes nutrition education as well as the provision of healthy foods to meet recommended dietary requirements. In response to such concerns some areas have formulated School Nutrition Action Groups (SNAGS). The overall aims of such groups is to bring the appropriate people together in order to respond to education and health issues, in particular nutritional needs, ensuring what is provided is consistent with what is taught in the classroom.

9.4 VARIATION IN FOOD INTAKE

As seen in adult surveys, regional and socio-economic variations in food intake exists amongst pre-school children. Compared with non-manual households, children from manual and lower socio-economic households tend to have higher intakes of starch, lower intakes of total sugars, vitamins E, C, B12, beta-carotene and most minerals. With increasing interest in the role of dietary antioxidants in protecting against diseases such as coronary heart disease, such variations warrant action.

According to one survey 5% of children (aged 11–16) go to school without eating breakfast (Gardner Merchant 1994), the greatest proportion seeming to be those children from low income households. In Liverpool, on Merseyside, a survey of children's health and life style found that 10.8% of year 6 (10–11 year olds) children go without breakfast, and over

Table 9.3 Percentage contribution of foods to the energy and nutrient intakes of children aged $1\frac{1}{2}$–$4\frac{1}{2}$ years (Adapted from Gregory *et al.* 1995 and Buttris & Gray 1995).

	Energy	Protein	Iron	Calcium	Zinc	Vitamin C	Vitamin A	Riboflavin	Vitamin B12	Folate
Cereal & cereal products	30	23	48	19	23	2	8	24	11	36
Milk & milk products	20	33	6	64	33	8	34	51	47	17
Vegetables, potatoes & savoury snacks	12	8	14	3	9	19	17	3	1	21
Meat & meat products	10	22	14	3	25	2	20	8	20	5
Egg & egg dishes	1	3	3	1	2	0	3	2	5	2
Sugars, preserves & confectionery	8	2	3	3	2	0	1	4	1	1
Beverages	8	1	2	2	1	50	4	2	6	8
Fat spreads	3	0	0	0	0	0	9	0	0	0
Fruit & nuts	3	1	3	1	2	1	0	2	0	4
Fish & fish dishes	2	4	2	1	0	0	1	1	7	1

With permission from the National Dairy Council, London.

60% eat chocolates and sweets three or more times a week (Balding 1995). Again, nutritionally, children from households in lower socio-economic groups suffered most. According to the Child Poverty Action Group and a report by the National Children's Home (NCH 1991) one in four children live in poverty. Not surprisingly children of these families often went without meals and are, therefore, nutritionally at risk. In order to develop a further understanding of the factors involved in the links between food, health and low income readers can follow up the sources at the end of this chapter.

Differences in food and nutrient intake can be explained by social, cultural and economic factors. Research has shown that families are already aware of the types of food they should eat, but social and cultural influences are a strong force in determining the types of food eaten in the home (Health Education Authority 1989). Several studies have highlighted the significant influences of the male partner in determining what foods are served at the table. In addition, where the family's income is low, resistance and inability to carry out changes to improve the family diet is high (Kennedy & Hunt 1994). There is evidence that children themselves may have their own priorities with 'health' almost at the bottom of the list (Gardner Merchant 1991; Health Education Authority 1995).

Impact of inequitable wealth

Income levels can affect the types of food consumed in a variety of ways. Given that a high percentage of those in the lowest income group do not have access to a private car, they also have restricted access to many of the large out-of-town food retailers where healthy food (fresh fruit and vegetables for example) can be purchased more cheaply. Low income also limits the ability to buy food rich in protective nutrients (James *et al.* 1997). Improving the diet can offer substantial health gains. The poor diets of children from lower socio-economic groups, can have short-term consequences (for example, high rates of dental caries) as well as long-term consequences (for example limited bone accretion, or the future development of atherogenesis) (James *et al.* 1997).

In a recent review of nutrition strategies at a regional level (Kennedy & Dawson 1996), health professionals were clearly concerned about the quality of children's diets and the increasing proportions of overweight and inactive children. A wide range of factors influencing food consumption patterns were recognised (Figure 9.1). Districts were advised to consider how these may be incorporated into future strategies to promote better nutrition using a health promotion approach.

Impact of advertising

The food and drink industry spends millions of pounds, using various methods to target children. One hundred and forty new products launched in the UK in 1990 were aimed at children; of these products, over 70 were sugar and chocolate confectionary, soft drinks and snack foods (Leatherhead Food Research Association 1991). Few of those products advertised will encourage a healthy diet, and furthermore, may act to undermine healthy eating messages. National policies of advertising need to be developed which promote rather than undermine healthy eating, particularly with a focus on young children.

The study of factors influencing choice of food is a complex area., and understanding why people choose certain foods can help in giving appropriate advice. Health professionals are referred to Fieldhouse (1995) to extend their insights in this area.

As Bingham (1991) warns, nutrition education *alone* will not bring about the changes required to improve the health of the nation: access, availability and affordability are equally important. Thus a more holistic approach based on the principles of the health promotion approach of the World Health Organization (WHO 1988) is useful if variations in nutritional status are to be eradicated (Vaandrager 1995; Vaandrager *et al.* 1993).

9.5 SPECIAL DIETS

Vegetarianism

Vegetarian diets have been adhered to by certain cultures for many hundreds of years and nutritional requirements have been adequately met. The government's committee on medical aspects of food (COMA) have stated that a vegetarian diet is appropriate for children of all ages and can meet all the necessary requirements for normal growth and

---

Main health and nutrition related problems perceived locally

(1) Obesity in adults and young children.
(2) Heart disease and stroke.
(3) Diabetes and high blood pressure.

Related factors

(1) The high cost of a healthier diet in inner city areas.
(2) Inadequate access to a choice of reasonably priced healthy food, resulting from a general growth in out-of-town retailing and a decline in local shopping facilities.
(3) A general decrease in public interest towards healthy eating.
(4) Lack of skills required to prepare healthy food and a failure of the school curriculum to teach basic food skills.
(5) Dietary problems among ethnic minority groups and sub groups such as infants, children and the increasing elderly.
(6) Lack of nutritional training among Primary Health Care teams.
(7) Tooth decay in young children.
(8) Lack of nutrition policies or nutrition standards for schools.
(9) Limited opportunities for choosing healthy foods in settings such as schools and workplace.

Wider factors influencing elements of food supply and demand

(1) Changes in food and agricultural policies, methods of food production, food retailing and marketing and advertising industries.
(2) Changes in local shopping facilities resulting in higher costs, reduced access and availability and quality in less affluent areas.
(3) Changing food cultures and preferences for less healthy foods; popularity of fast food and convenience foods.

Figure 9.1   Reported factors influencing trends in food consumption in the North West (Reproduced with permission from *The Health of the North West of England* (1996). The Report for the Regional Director of Public Health, 1995).

development (DoH 1994b). Nevertheless, vegetarian diets require careful planning and consideration to ensure a variety of nutrients, particularly protein, are obtained from various sources including both dairy and plant food. Particular attention towards dietary quality is needed. Alternative sources of nutrients need to be incorporated into the diet to ensure adequate intake of iron, B12 and vitamin D, which are primarily found in animal produce. Given the relatively high energy density of some vegetarian foods, particularly dairy, cheese or nut products, fat and energy intake should also be monitored.

Vegan diets

Vegan diets are far more restrictive than vegetarian diets, with all meat or fish and dairy or animal products excluded. Children following a vegan diet need careful monitoring to ensure nutritional requirements are being adequately met. Vegans tend to have lower vitamin B12 and vitamin D intakes (The Vegetarian Society 1995); vegan diets, therefore, may need to be supplemented with foods that are fortified with these vitamins. The Vegetarian Society has noted that infants are particularly at risk of vitamin D, calcium and iodine deficiencies when following a vegan diet. Both calcium and vitamin D are required in relatively high amounts for optimum bone development during childhood years when peak bone mass is being developed. Concern has arisen that vegan and vegetarian diets are potentially affecting peak bone mass and therefore increasing the risk of weak bones and the formation of osteoporosis in later life. Information and education of parents in addition to surveillance is therefore vital.

9.6 EATING DISORDERS

For most people eating can be associated with enjoyment, but for some it can provoke painful experiences. Health and nutrition professionals have an important role to play in the development of healthy eating behaviours and habits at the earliest possible age. The promotion of appropriate eating habits in childhood, nutrition intervention programmes and health education all have an equally important role in addressing such problems.

In order to present a more global picture of the main nutrition disorders currently seen in children, this section addresses both obesity and the problems of anorexia nervosa and bulimia nervosa.

Some evidence suggests that both obese and anorexic subjects have a reduced ability to recognise hunger (Brone & Fisher 1988). Further work suggests that early feeding experiences are important, and that parents not having been responsive to hunger communications may contribute to this deficit in hunger recognition (Brone & Fisher 1988).

Childhood obesity

According to the 1990 Office of Population Census and Survey Study, 45% of men and 36% of women in the UK are overweight. The vast majority of evidence suggests that overweight children are likely to become overweight adults. One of the 1992 Health of the Nation targets (DoH 1992) was to reverse this trend to the levels of obesity seen in 1980, however, achievement seems increasingly unlikely. A positive association between being overweight in childhood and long-term mortality has been shown (Javier *et al.* 1992). Avoidance of obesity and of eating disorders such as anorexia nervosa is thought to reduce morbidity and mortality in later life.

The effects of obesity on ill health have been widely accepted, and the purpose of this section is to emphasise the importance of prevention and long term control strategies. Eating disorders need to be tackled early as their effects extend beyond the short term towards major health risks in the long term. The best solution remains one of prevention. In children it is difficult to develop an index to diagnose being overweight, because of the growth spurts unique to childhood and adolescence. The actual point at which

one changes from being overweight to obese is also subject to various definitions, and the evidence suggests it is more common to react to problems of eating disorders than to adopt a preventative approach. The necessity for early management appears to be a key issue. Sherry *et al.* (1992) reiterated the need for early intervention and suggested initiatives such as growth screening, as well as information on weight management and physical fitness programmes, to be incorporated into school settings, the need being not only to identify, but further to avert childhood obesity.

Obesity may establish itself as early as the first twelve months of infancy (Poskitt 1986). Furthermore, infants also develop eating habits and eating environments which they will carry into adulthood. Early infancy seems the most obvious time to consider obesity prevention.

Prevention of obesity

Evidence from studies into the formation of eating disorders and problems associated with energy balance presents a complex picture of the potential risk factors involved. Current life style patterns need to be carefully incorporated into the planning of any advice on nutrition.

Recent research showed that 47% of GPs in the UK had dietary advice clinics in existence (Kopelman & Venables 1991). The introduction of health pro motion clinics into many general practices has provided an opportunity for primary care teams to provide a substantial role in nutrition education and, consequently, the opportunities to change eating behaviour patterns.

There is some disagreement as to whether it is the population or the individual who should be targeted with nutrition advice. The number of young children who risk becoming overweight is considerable, thus measures to improve diet and activity as a nation have long been suggested (Poskitt 1986). The development of profiles to identify high-risk groups, using predictors, has also been argued (DoH 1992). A number of predictors already identified include factors such as parental weight (Garn and Clark 1976), 'adiposity rebound' at less that six years of age (Rolland-Cachera *et al.* 1987), and eating behaviour. Actual clinical causes of overweight and obesity such as Cushing's Syndrome, genetic or endocrine causes are relatively rare, but obviously such causes need to be excluded.

The alarming increase in obesity in the UK has been largely attributable to people becoming less active. Activity levels have declined at a faster rate than the fall in the same period of food or energy intakes. The proportion of energy derived from dietary fat has also increased. The response is therefore to address these two factors in terms of reducing fat in the diet and increasing physical activity. The Royal College of Physicians (1983) argue that given there has been little done in the way of trials towards examining prevention of obesity, it may be damaging to offer poorly researched advice which may later need modification. Nevertheless, a consensus exists that energy balance is a major part of the solution. Recognising the scale of the problem, the Department of Health (1996) has called for priority research into the *prevention* and treatment of obesity.

Such mass change requires the co-ordinated efforts of the different sectors involved in the food chain, from producer or manufacturer down to retailer and the promotion industry and not just individuals. Factors known to influence food choice, such as the availability and accessibility of affordable health foods, must also accompany any nutrition advice programmes for change to be possible. Improved food policy and legislation will go some way towards tackling the current conflict of interest which exists between commercial profit and nutrition and health.

Treatment of obesity

Obesity is often misconceived as an incurable chronic disease. However much evidence suggests this is not the case. Once obesity is recognised, and the severity of the problem is established by a dietician or general practitioner, appropriate action can take several forms. Different skills are required for the treatment of severe obesity, and therefore are unlikely to be the sole responsibility of a community nurse.

Poskitt (1986) states that the majority of obese infants, as well as a considerable number of older children, undergo 'spontaneous resolution' of their obesity as they grow up. A decade later obesity experts now warn against allowing children to grow into their weight and stress the importance of physical activity and diet in the prevention of overweight at an early age. Understanding the mechanisms of this process may offer further hope to effective management of obesity in the future.

There has been much research carried out into the predisposition of some children to be overweight.

While factors have been examined, with variable levels of certainty, there remains the fact that *nutrition intake and energy expenditure still remain important variables and ones which can be altered.* Consequently, excessive food intake needs to be considered as well as other causes of obesity when providing nutrition advice.

Limited research has been undertaken regarding the most appropriate type of diet for overweight children. The Royal College of Physicians (1983) however states that a diet 'low in sugar and fat but high in a variety of cereals, vegetables and fruit can, in conjunction with the development of sound behavioural patterns, achieve a progressive loss of body fat as growth continues'.

At the end of the first year, children's energy requirements increase (Table 9.1) and, therefore, so should their intakes (Platon & Collipp 1980). It is the preferred method to give children too little, and allow them to ask for more, than to put too much on the plate. Many young children who are 'plump' during the second year soon become more active and will eventually attain a normal weight (this applies only to the child who is not fat at 12 months) (Craddock 1973).

Some overweight children may have underlying emotional problems, which influence or lead to their current problems. Eating as a form of comfort or control over their parents is one example. Factors in both the environment and heredity have been examined for their role in contributing to the development of overweight children. Current research suggests that hereditary factors have a more significant role than environmental factors in children under 10 years whilst the reverse applies for environmental factors (Brooke *et al.* 1985). A stark example of environmental influence is the increasing evidence of a link between excessive television viewing and development of obesity largely due to both the consumption of energy rich food and reduced physical activity (Dietz & Gortmaker 1985). Consideration of such factors as part of any treatment programme is therefore necessary.

Rigid diets, in which exact foods to be eaten are given on diet sheets, are often unrealistic, especially for the younger child. They also do little to re-educate the eating habits of the individual. Behaviour modification is aimed at changing the acquired eating patterns, which have been learned over time, and sustained by the environment. The overall principle applied is that the learned eating behaviours be re-learned in a more appropriate and healthy way. The use of diaries to record eating has been shown to be important for a number of reasons. Firstly, accurate diaries initially act as a good way to convince the overweight individual or appropriate parent that too many calories are being consumed. Secondly, the diaries act to record the environment and circumstances in which the food was consumed, and can, therefore, provide important information in behaviour modification. The involvement of other family members in making changes to eating patterns themselves is also critical to success.

A calorie-controlled diet is essential as the basis for treatment combined with increased physical activity. Other methods are available for dealing with being overweight and more commonly obesity, although more rigorous methods, similar to those applied to adults, are generally thought to be unsuitable for children, for example jaw wiring. Generally doctors have avoided using appetite-suppressing drugs mainly because of their side effects and potential for addiction. Invasive surgical techniques are generally also thought to be inappropriate for children.

Management methods using family-based approaches have shown significant success (Mellin & Frost 1992). Follow-up surveys at five and ten year intervals have shown that the weight loss is maintained over time. However, it is recognised that this management style is largely unavailable, due to a shortage of suitably qualified nurses. Further success may be achieved if the role of nurses in this area were to be further investigated and developed. Figure 9.2 lists variables related to successful treatment of overweight children.

Summary on obesity concerns

Some consider that obesity is a condition for which there is no effective treatment, the situation is com-pounded by the high risk of relapse. There remains some disagreement as to the most effective and accurate methods to detect weight problems in children. The fact remains that, with modern management methods, overweight people *can* be treated and the target weights *can* be achieved and sustained.

Weight control programmes offered in schools are often directed at the individual, and are rarely successful, or, at best, offer short-term solutions. Given that many children do not have direct control over the type of food purchased for family consumption and are subject to great pressure from peers, nutrition education programmes directed only at children will have a limited impact because they ignore much of the social practices and practical aspects surrounding eating behaviours.

Choices about food are bound up in the family culture and environment. Studies conducted outside the UK have shown that efforts to control dietary intake in children by controlling school meals can have significant effects on the control of obesity (Saito & Taatsumi 1994). Davis and Christoffel (1994) suggest that many of the methods used to manage early obesity can be adopted for prevention and intervention on early obesity during pre-school years.

In the light of the difficulties of treating obesity, prevention clearly offers the best approach to dealing with this increasing problem, and any recommendations aimed at the population in general must address the requirements of children also.

Childhood anorexia nervosa

Anorexia nervosa, a problem of compulsive slimming, is a behavioural deviance which is demonstrated by the rejection of food. Anorexia nervosa as seen in children is different to that of adolescents or adults. Gerbaka and Karam (1992) have noted how anorexia nervosa can occur during infancy. Despite the fact

---

- Active participation of parents and siblings.
- Inclusion of physical activity.
- Examination of family motivational structures (regarding behaviour control and modification (Epstein 1993).
- Continued support for maintenance of achieved weight.
- Annual or biannual visits to dietary advice clinics (Kopelman *et al.* 1991).

It remains difficult to develop a model to predict successful outcome of treatment programmes.

Figure 9.2 Variables related to successful treatment of overweight children.

that clear evidence has shown anorexia nervosa to occur both in infancy and childhood, prevalence studies are lacking. Studies have shown however, that there is limited awareness in recognising the condition of anorexia nervosa in young children (Bryant-Waugh *et al.* 1992). This is particularly important given that any delay in treatment is likely to have adverse consequences.

The development of anorexia nervosa has been attributed to many factors. All factors need to be thoroughly addressed in order for a treatment programme to be effective. Studies of children as young as nine and ten have highlighted problems related to the fear of being overweight and subsequent eating restrictions (Gustafson-Larson & Terry 1992). Differences in early feeding patterns may influence the underlying factors involved in the manifestation of anorexia nervosa (Steiner *et al.* 1991). Clearly more research needs to be carried out to examine the impact of early feeding methods on later development of anorexia nervosa, and any potential scope for prevention.

The *actual reasons* for the development of eating disorders are not clearly understood. Many factors have been attributed, such as media portrayal of slim women as being successful, and a general acceptance of slimness in the western culture. This is in stark contrast to the prejudices applied to those who are obese. Other factors put forward as relevant to the development of anorexia nervosa are underlying psychological problems, possibly of inharmonious family units, insecurity, other emotional problems, or evidence of sexual abuse. A further broad category is the drive to resist bodily changes and to deny 'growing up' by maintaining a child-like figure.

Deprivation of food can have long-term consequences resulting from energy and nutrient deficiency, especially affecting the cardiovascular and gastrointestinal systems (Fairburn 1988), and nutritional anaemia is frequently observed.

Prevention of anorexia nervosa

Many health professionals have important roles in the identification and treatment of both anorexia and bulimia nervosa. The dental practitioner is in a good position to identify possible warning signs, for example erosion of enamel due to vomiting (Robb & Smith 1996). Community nurses are in a good position to be able to assess and, if necessary, refer children showing signs of rapid weight loss. The

development of the role of the nurse, particularly the school nurse, to be alert to warning signs needs to be examined (Figure 9.3).

> ■ Refusal to maintain normal body weight.
> ■ Slow pulse rates.
> ■ Over 25% loss of pre-illness body weight.
> ■ Distorted eating patterns.
> ■ Specific nutritional deficiencies.
> ■ No other condition to account for symptoms.

Figure 9.3 Warning signals that may be picked up at the practice level.

Social forces play a very important part not only in producing the eating disorder but also in maintaining it. Many non-medical agents exert a great deal of influence over eating behaviour and social pressure; these include industry, government, schools, and the media. A history of teasing has been shown to be significantly related to body image (Thompson *et al.* 1995). This may be an area which schools, with the encouragement or support of nursing professionals, could look towards addressing. Further research may be important to understand the causal sequences and implications involved in the development of eating disturbances. There has been a disappointing lack of research addressing the problem of how practically to approach behaviour change, particularly for children.

Management and treatment of anorexia nervosa

The initial barrier to the treatment of an eating disorder is the unwillingness of the patient to accept that a problem exists. Diagnosis, particularly in males, initially depends on eliminating possible organic causes, as well as on an assessment of mental and psychiatric status. A thorough understanding of the level of severity is essential for the effective planning and management of treatment. Nursing staff in primary health care need to be aware of initial warning signs. Overall primary care nurses and health visitors are more likely to be managing sub-clinical cases in the community. The treatment process with the more severe clinical disease is more specialised.

The establishment of good relations between the health professional and the patient during the initial stages is necessary for progress. Opportunities also need to be created to allow the patient to learn more about his or her condition. Treatment can normally be carried out with the anorexic person attending treatment as an outpatient. The overall aim is to address the underlying problems and eventually to enable the client to take control and maintain responsibility for his or her weight gain and ultimately control it. Prescribed drugs have not been particularly effective in controlling this eating disorder, although anti-depressants may initially be prescribed (to address emotional problems thought to be linked) as part of the overall treatment package.

Behaviour modification has an important role to play in both the treatment of anorexia nervosa and of obesity; this is particularly important for the management of eating disorders in children. Due to the relatively minor control children have over family meals, and the essential role of family dynamics in the manifestation of many cases of anorexia nervosa, a holistic approach is preferred. Rost and Molinari (1992) recommend that in cases of anorexia nervosa which are seen in young patients family therapy is particularly important. This can later be followed by psychotherapy. The influence of family interaction patterns is repeatedly stressed in the literature. Though it has been generally accepted that family interaction is important in treatment, the type of interaction which is most effective is less certain. The most widely reported family technique for the treatment of anorexia nervosa was designed by Minuchin and Rosman (1978). This focuses on the disengaging of the family and establishing for each member their individuality, worth and competence.

Summary of anorexia nervosa

Childhood experiences, particularly with regard to the family arrangements and discord, have been shown to be important factors in the development of eating disorders (Schmidt et al. 1993).

Also identified as being important are the social pressures towards a desire to be thin. Environmental pressures such as those perpetuated by the media which suggest women will be more accepted and successful in western culture if they are thin are potential areas which could be modified as part of a prevention strategy.

Psychological, sociological and physical factors have all been identified as significant in the development of eating disorders. While some of these factors may be examined in terms of prevention strategies, others will be best approached by early diagnosis and

effective management programmes. Effective treatment delivered early provides the best prognosis. Success is dependent on the involvement of parents and/or significant others, for example guardians, siblings and close family members.

Bulimia nervosa

Bulimia is characterised by binge eating, followed by behaviours aimed to counteract weight gain, such as vomiting, excessive use of laxatives and extensive physical exercise. Bulimia has several features in common with anorexia. Bulimics also have an obsessional concern with their body weight and shape, although they may not be underweight, and it is therefore more difficult to detect. Furthermore, bulimics, like anorexics are secretive and effective at disguising any abnormal eating patterns.

Although bulimia is characterised as a separate eating disorder from anorexia, many anorexics go on to become bulimic. Treatment programmes are broadly similar to those of anorexia, namely the identification of the problem and the subsequent need for the individuals to accept that a problem exists. Management is aimed at addressing the underlying causes, as well as the maintenance of body weight and the development of healthy eating patterns with the co-operation and support of the family.

Without effective reporting procedures in place it has been difficult to establish current prevalence amongst children. The incidence rate for anorexia nervosa in the general population has been estimated to be 8 per 100,000 per year (Hoek 1993). The incidence of bulimia nervosa in the general population is thought to be greater; 11.4 new cases per 100,000 (Hoek 1993). Given the complex nature of eating disorders, the role of nurses, unless specialised, will lie more in identification or monitoring rather than treatment.

9.7 FOOD SCARES

Technological advances and changing methods of manufacturing and food production, such as genetic engineering, as well as some examples of sensationalised reporting have resulted in recent years in a number of scares relating to consumption of certain foods and associated illness. The most notable of these has been beef production and associated Bovine Spongiform Encephalopathy (BSE) and Creutzfeldt-Jakob Disease (CJD) which have received enormous media coverage.

CJD is a rare neurological disease which usually presents in late middle age with progressive dementia and is usually fatal within six months. It is characterised by spongiform changes in the brain only seen at post-mortem. The agent of this and related transmissible spongiform encephalopathy (TSE) diseases in animals, such as BSE and scrapie, is believed to be a protein highly resistant to physical and chemical inactivation. During the 1980s, the number of cows in Britain infected with BSE spiralled reaching a peak in the late 1980s and feed contaminated with animal protein was thought to be the agent of transmission of BSE.

In view of concerns that BSE in cows might be transmissible to humans, steps have been taken to remove infected animals and any suspected specific risk material (SRM) from the food chain. This process began in 1989 with a ban on the use of specified bovine offal (brain, spinal cord, thymus, tonsils, spleen and intestines), the tissues thought most likely to contain the infective agent, in products for human consumption. Since 1996, all British cattle older than 30 months have been destroyed and in 1997 the government introduced a ban on the sale of beef on the bone for human consumption.

In the 1990s there was an increase in the small number of deaths in Britain from CJD in people of a much younger average age than previously associated with CJD, believed to be due to a new variant of the classical CJD, (NVCJD).

In circumstances such as this, especially where the issues are ongoing with further developments likely to occur, it is extremely important to emphasise the need for parents to adhere only to information provided by official sources such as the Department of Health for guidance. Hearsay and media coverage should be avoided as a source of official and sound information. In some circumstances it may be difficult to establish the current risk to human health of a particular source of food. This calls for vigilance and the need to keep up to date with official sources of information.

Specific guidance can not be given for a particular food scare, as the action which will be needed will depend on the circumstances surrounding the event.

However the following general advice can be given in the event of a food scare:

- Try to avoid panic.
- Where possible avoid listening to hearsay. Follow advice provided by official sources. If there is difficulty accessing or following such guidelines contact your GP or health visitor for help.
- During food scares be extra alert, for example additional preparation may be important such as extra cooking of eggs to avoid *Salmonella* poisoning. Also be vigilant of the symptoms of ill health which may be associated with the particular food scare and do not delay in seeking medical attention.
- Advice should be sought from health professionals on the best approach for dealing with certain high risk groups, for example infants.
- It is also important to be able to distinguish between the risks associated with consuming potentially hazardous pathogens in food compared with the risks of contracting illness; certain levels of pathogens such as *Salmonella* may occur in foods and not be a risk to healthy individuals.
- Be aware that withdrawing a particular food from your child's or family's diet may result in a deficiency in certain essential nutrients. In such circumstances make sure the withdrawn food is replaced with another food to provide a balanced nutritional diet. Again, if in doubt seek advice from your GP, health visitor, or dietitian.

The impact of food scares must be highlighted. Sensationalisation, poor reporting and inadequate information availability can result in parents changing infants' diets with possible detrimental effects to their health.

9.8 CONCLUDING REMARKS

Recommendations for practice

Information gathered about the current eating patterns of children reveals the nature and extent of the action required. Dieticians are trained to deal with the clinical and health promoting aspects of diet. The Nutrition Task Force published a useful review of the range of initiatives by dieticians aimed at improving the health of the nation (DoH 1994a). The important role of health professionals in primary care in improving nutritional status of the population is however increasingly recognised. Given the significant influence of childhood dietary patterns on health in later life, nurses based in the community are increasingly expected to provide nutrition advice.

Nutritional requirements of children

- The development of eating patterns in childhood needs further research.
- Eating patterns extend into adulthood; this needs to be acknowledged and addressed.
- Accurate data relating to the prevalence of eating disorders and nutritional problems in childhood is needed.
- Children's nutritional requirements differ from those of adults and should be reflected in any nutrition or advice on healthy eating.
- A *proactive* approach to developing healthy eating patterns at an early age is needed.

Food choices

- Education has an important role in promoting better nutrition, particularly where special diets are followed (e.g. vegan).
- If healthy food choices are to be made, e.g. in school meals and tuckshops, the availability and affordability of fresh healthy food is primary.
- All organisations involved in the supply or provision of food should increase their support for the promotion of healthy eating.
- Provision of up-to-date, clear and consistent information to enhance awareness and acceptability of healthy eating and the credibility of health professionals as sources of healthy eating advice is vital.

Health professionals

Primary health care teams and health professionals in the community have a vital role to

- promote healthy eating messages;
- encourage appropriate eating patterns;
- identify nutrition related problems and eating disorders at an early stage;

- provide and maintain certain treatment programmes;
- refer to specialists as necessary.

Long term issues

- The link between dietary factors and chronic diseases such as cardiovascular disease, obesity, certain cancers, and late onset diabetes are widely documented. Risk factors develop and are therefore amenable to prevention from an early age.
- Weight management and prevention of obesity should be more proactive starting during early childhood.
- Eating disorders need to be recognised and managed early to achieve the best possible outcome.
- Continued research and development into improved surveillance systems, effective management and treatment programmes at the community level is needed.

REFERENCES

Balding, J. (1995) *Young People in 1994.* Schools Health Education Unit, University of Exeter.

Barker, D.J.P. (1990) The fetal and infant origins of adult disease. *British Medical Journal*, **301**, 111.

Bingham, S. (1991) Dietary Aspects of a Health Strategy for England. In: *The Health of the Nation, the BMJ View*, British Medical Journal Publications, London, pp. 19–26.

Brone, R.J. & Fisher, C.B. (1988) Determinants of adolescent obesity: a comparison with anorexia nervosa. *Adolescence*, V **XXIII** (89), Spring 1988, Libra Publishers Inc.

Brooke, O.G. & Abernethy, E. (1985) Obesity in children. *Human Nutrition: Applied Nutrition*, **39A**, 304–14.

Bryant-Waugh, R.J., Lask, B.D., Shafran, R.U.I. & Fosson, A.R. (1992) Do doctors recognise eating disorders in children? *Archives of Diseases in Childhood*, **67** (1), 103–5.

Buttriss, J.L. (1995) (ed.) *Nutrition in General Practice. Part 2: Promoting Health and Preventing Disease.* Royal College of General Physicians, London.

Buttriss, J.L. & Grey, J. (1995) *Nutrition of Infants and Pre-School Children.* Fact File 2. National Dairy Council, London.

Cadogan, J., Eastell, R., Jones, N. & Barker, M.E. (1997) Milk intake and bone mineral acquisition in adolescent girls: controlled intervention trial. *British Medical Journal*, **315**, 1225–60.

Craddock, D. (1973) *Obesity and its Management*. 2nd edn. Churchill Livingstone, Edinburgh, p. 180.

Davis, K. & Christoffel, K.K. (1994) Obesity in pre-school and school age children. Treatment early and often may be best. *Archives of Pediatric and Adolescent Medicine*, **148** (12), 1257–61.

Department of Health (1991) Committee on Medical Aspects of Food Policy. *Dietary Reference Values for Food Energy and Nutrients for the United Kingdom*. Report on Health and Social Subjects 41. HMSO, London.

Department of Health (1992) *Health of the Nation – A Strategy for Health in England*. HMSO, London.

Department of Health (1994a) *Eat Well! An action plan from the Nutrition Task Force to achieve the Health of the Nation targets on diet and nutrition*. Department of Health, London.

Department of Health (1994b) Committee on Medical Aspects of Food. *Weaning and the weaning diet*. HMSO, London.

Department of Health (1996) *The Health of the Nation, Obesity. Reversing the Increasing Problem of Obesity in England*. A report from the Nutrition and Physical Activity Task Force. HMSO, London.

Department of Health and Social Security (DHSS) (1989) Committee on Medical Aspects of Food Policy. *The Diets of British Schoolchildren*. Report on Health and Social Subjects 36. HMSO, London.

Dietz, W.H. & Gortmaker, S.L. (1985) Do we fatten our children at the television set? Obesity and television viewing in children and adolescents. *Paediatrics*, **75** (5), 807–12.

Epstein, L.H. (1993) Methodological issues and ten-year outcomes for obese children. *NY Acad. Sci.*, **699**, 237–49.

Fairburn, C. (1988) Eating disorders. Anorexia and bulimia. *Nutrition and Food Science*. September/October, pp. 11–13.

Fieldhouse, P. (1995) *Food and Nutrition Customs and Cultures*. 2nd edn. Chapman & Hall, London.

Gardner Merchant (1994) The Gardner Merchant School Meals Survey 'What are our children eating?' Gardner Merchant Educational Services, Kenley House, Kenley, UK. In: *National Dairy Council Nutrition Quarterly Review*, Summer, p. 27.

Garn, S.M. & Clark, D.C. (1976) Trends in fatness and the origins of obesity. *Paediatrics*, **57**, 433–56.

Gerbaka, B. & Karam, P. (1992) Infantile anorexia nervosa. *Journal Medical Libanais*, **40** (4), 211–15.

Gregory, J., Foster, K., Tyler, H. & Wiseman, M. (1990) *The Dietary and Nutritional Surveys of British Adults*. HMSO, London.

Gregory, J.R., Collins, D.L., Davies, P.S.W., Hughes, J.M. & Clarke, P.C. (1995) *National Diet and Nutrition Survey: Children aged $1\frac{1}{2}$–$4\frac{1}{2}$. Volume 1: Report of the Diet and Nutrition Survey*. HMSO, London.

Gustafson-Larson, A.M. & Terry, R.D. (1992) Weight-related behaviours and concerns of fourth-grade children. *J Am Diet Assoc.* **92** (7), 818–22.

Harvey, J. & Passmore, S. (1994) School Nutrition Action Groups (SNAGs) Birmingham Health Education Unit, 74 Balden Road, Birmingham B32 3CH.

Health Education Authority (1989) *Diet, Nutrition and Healthy Eating in Low Income Groups*. HEA, London.

Health Education Authority (1995) *Diet and health in school age children*. Nutrition Briefing Paper, HEA, London.

Hoek, H.W. (1993) Review of epidemiological studies of eating disorders. *International Review of Psychiatry*, **5**, 61–74.

James, W.P.T., Nelson, M., Ralph, A. & Leather, S. (1997) The Contribution of nutrition to inequalities in health. *British Medical Journal*, **314**, 1545–9.

Javier, N.F., Szklo, M. & Comstock, G.W. (1992) Childhood weight and growth rate as predictors of adult mortality. *American Journal of Epidemiology*, **136** (2), 201–3.

Kennedy, L. & Hunt, C. (1994) *Evaluation of a community based nutrition programme for low income groups – is there a role?* Report to the Health Education Authority. Mabledon House, London. Copies held @ Dept. of Public Health, University of Liverpool.

Kennedy, L. & Dawson, J. (1996) Health and Nutrition. In: *The Health of the North West of England*. The report of the Regional Director of Public Health 1995. North West Regional Health Authority, pp. 93–100.

Kopelman, P. & Venables, T. (1991) *Successful Management of Overweight*. Adis International Limited, Chester, England.

Leatherhead Food Research Association, July (1991) *Children's eating habits. An in-depth study of the attitudes and behaviour of children aged 6–11*. Leatherhead Food Research Association, Leatherhead.

Mellin, L.M. & Frost, L. (1992) Child and adolescent obesity: the nurse practitioner's use of the SHAPE-DOWN method. *Journal of Pediatric Health Care*, **6** (4), 187–93.

Mennell, S.J., Stephens, J., Murcott, A. & Otteslog, A.H. Van (1992) *The Sociology of Food; Eating, Diet and Culture*. Sage, London.

Minuchin, S. & Rosman, B.L. (1978) *Psychosomatic Families: Anorexia Nervosa in Context*. Harvard University Press, Cambridge, Mass.

Morgan, J.B. (1995) Healthy Eating for infants – mothers' attitudes. *Acta Paediatrica*, **85**, 512–15.

Murcott, A. (1982) The Cultural Significance of Food and Eating. Paper presented at a Symposium on Food habits and Culture in the UK. *Proceedings of Nutrition Society*. **41**, 203.

National Children's Homes (1991) *NCH Poverty and Nutrition Survey 1991*. NCH, London.

Nelson, M. (1993) Cause for concern. In: *National Forum for Coronary Heart Disease Prevention. Food for children. Influencing choice and investing in Health.* Tavistock Square, London.

Platon, J., Collipp, M.D. (1980) Obesity in childhood. In: *Obesity* (ed. A.J. Stunkard). Saunders, Philadelphia.

Poskitt, E.M.E. (1986) Obesity in the young child: whither and whence? *Acta Paediatrica Scandinavia*, Suppl. 332, 24–32.

Robb, N.D. & Smith, B.G. (1996) Anorexia and bulimia nervosa (the eating disorders): conditions of interest to the dental practitioner. *Journal of Dentistry*, 24 (1–2), 7–16.

Rolland-Cachera, M.F., Deheeger, M., Avons, P., Giulloud-Bataille, M., Patois, E. & Sempe, M. (1987) Tracking adiposity patterns from one month of age to adulthood. *Annals of Human Biology*, 14, 219–22.

Rost, B. & Molinari, M. (1992) Need for control and anxiety of loosing it – reflections on the treatment of anorexia nervosa. *Z-Kinder-Jugenpsychiatr.*, 20 (3), 155–9.

Royal College of Physicians (1983) Obesity. Reprinted from the *Journal of Royal College of Physicians of London*, 17 (1), 3–58.

Saito, K. & Taatsumi, M. (1994) Effect of dietary therapy in school health programs for obese children. *Nippon Koshu Eisea Zasshi*, 41 (8), 693–705.

Schmidt, U., Tiller, J. & Treasure, J. (1993) Setting the scene for eating disorders: childhood care, classification and course of illness. *Psychological Medicine*, 23, 663–72.

Sherry, B., Springer, D.A., Connell, F.A. & Garrett, S.M. (1992) Short, thin or obese? Comparing growth indexes of children from high and low poverty areas. *Journal of American Dietetics Association*, 92 (9), 1092–5.

Simeon, D.T. & Grantham-MacGregor, S. (1989) Effects of missing breakfast on the cognitive functions of schoolchildren of differing nutritional status. *American Journal of Clinical Nutrition*, 49, 646–53.

Steiner, H., Smith, C., Rosenkranz, R.T. & Litt, I. (1991) The early care and feeding of anorexics. *Child Psychiatry and Human Development*, Spring, 21 (3), 163–7.

Stordy, B.J. (1995) Healthy eating for infants – mothers' actions. *Acta Paediatrica*, 84, 733–41.

The Vegetarian Society (1995) *Vegetarian Vitality. A report on the health benefits of the vegetarian diet and the nutritional requirements of vegetarians.* The Vegetarian Society, Altrincham, Cheshire.

Thompson, J.K., Coovert, M.D., Richards, K.J., Johnson, S. & Cattarin, J. (1995) Development of body image, eating disturbance and general psychological functioning in female adolescents: covariance structure modelling and longitudinal investigations. *International Journal of Eating Disorders*, 18 (3), 221–36.

Vaandrager, H.W. (1995) Constructing a healthy balance. Action and research ingredients to facilitate the process of health promotion, PhD Thesis, Wageningen Agricultural University, The Netherlands.

Vaandrager, H.W., Koelen, M.A., Ashton, J.A. & Colomer Revuelta, C. (1993) A four step health promotion approach for changing dietary patterns in Europe. *European Journal of Public Health*, 3 (3), 193–8.

Walford, G. & McCune, N., (1991) Long-term outcome in early-onset anorexia nervosa. *British Journal of Psychiatry*, Sep. 159, 383–9.

Whincup, P. (1996) Cardiovascular risk factors in British children from towns with widely differing adult cardiovascular mortality. *British Medical Journal*, 313, 79–84.

World Health Organization (1986) *Ottawa Charter of Health Promotion.* WHO, Copenhagen.

World Health Organization (1988) *Healthy nutrition.* WHO Regional Publications, European Series No 24, Regional Office for Europe, Copenhagen.

World Health Organization (1990) *Diet, nutrition and the prevention of chronic disease.* Technical report series, WHO, Geneva.

FURTHER READING

Department of Health (1991) *Dietary Reference Values (DRVs) for energy and nutrients for the United Kingdom.* Report of the Panel on Dietary Reference Values to the Committee of Medical Aspects of Food Policy. HMSO, London.

Department of Health (1994) *Eat Well: An action plan from the Nutrition Task Force to achieve Health of the Nation targets on diet and nutrition.* Department of Health, London.

Department of Health (1996) *Low income, food nutrition and health: strategies for improvement.* A report by the Low Income Project Team for the Nutrition Task Force. HMSO, London.

Fieldhouse, P. (1995) *Food and Nutrition: Culture and Customer* (2nd edn). Chapman and Hall, London.

Health Education Authority (1992) *Scientific basis of nutrition education. A synopsis of dietary reference values.* Briefing Paper. HEA, London.

Health Education Authority (1993) *Nutrition interventions in primary health care. A literature review.* Briefing Paper. HEA, London.

National Forum for Coronary Heart Disease Prevention (1993) *Food for children. Influencing choice and investing in health.* A report of a conference on 'Diet and Schoolchildren' organised by the NFCHDP, Tavistock Square, London.

Williams, C., Dowler, E.A. (1994) Identifying successful
local projects and initiatives on diet and low income: a
review of the issues. A working paper for the Nutrition
Task Force Low Income Project Team. Department of
Health, London.

APPENDIX 9.1: LIST OF USEFUL CONTACTS

Local health authorities will be able to provide a list of contacts in the area such as the Community Dietetics or Health Promotion Departments. Credible and up-to-date information, resources, recent reports, advice and in some cases training is available. For more information on national issues:

British Dietetic Association
7th Floor, Elizabeth House
22 Suffolk Street
Queensway
Birmingham B1 1LS

Health Education Authority (England)
Trevelyan House
30 Great Peter Street
London SW1P 2HW

HEA Unit for Health Promotion in Primary Care
Nutrition Section
Block 10
The Churchill Hospital
Oxford OX3 7LJ

National Dairy Council Nutrition Service
5–7 John Princes Street
London W1M 0AP

10

Dental Health: A Practical Guide to Preventive Dentistry

A.S. Blinkhorn

10.1 INTRODUCTION

Dental ill health is a problem which begins in childhood and keeps us company for the rest of our lives. This slightly depressing message should, however, not concern most of us unduly. Significant advances have been made in our understanding of the aetiology and control of the two main oral problems, dental decay (caries) and gum (periodontal) problems. The dental profession can say with a great measure of confidence that, provided certain simple health education messages (Levine 1996) are put into practice, caries and periodontal disease can be kept under control.

The fact that there are straightforward practical oral health education messages highlights the importance of involving all health and education professionals in the fight against dental ill health. The dental team are not asking busy professional people to devote large amounts of time to dental health education but to take a general interest in oral health when interacting with children and adults. Simple advice given at the right time can often save people pain and sepsis in the future.

This book is concerned with the health of young children and this chapter will deal principally with this important target group. Nevertheless, dental disease is such an ubiquitous problem that some general points about adult oral health will be discussed to give a broader overall picture.

10.2 THE TEETH AND SURROUNDING TISSUES

During growth and development, two dentitions erupt, the primary (deciduous, baby) followed by the permanent (adult) (Sullivan 1994). This is to allow for changes in the size of the jaws as they grow and develop and hence the size and number of teeth they can accommodate (Stewart *et al.* 1982)

The primary teeth

These erupt between six months and three years of age, subject to considerable variation. There are 20 teeth in all. In each quarter (or quadrant) of the mouth there are two incisors, one canine and two molars. The lower central incisors are usually the first to erupt (Ten Cate 1980).

The permanent dentition

This erupts between six years of age and adulthood and the full complement of teeth is 32. However, the third permanent molars (wisdom teeth), which usually erupt between 17 and 21 years of age, sometimes fail to appear due to their lack of development or because of insufficient room in crowded jaws. In each quadrant of the mouth there are two incisors, one canine, two premolars and three molars in the complete dentition. The first to erupt are the first permanent molars which appear behind the primary molars at six years of age. These teeth are often mistaken by parents for primary teeth. The permanent incisors erupt shortly afterwards and replace the primary incisors. The next main group of teeth, the premolars, canines and second permanent molars, commence eruption at around 10 years of age and are usually in place by 13 years. The premolars replace the primary molars, as these are shed, and the permanent canines replace their primary predecessors. The second and third permanent molars erupt behind the first permanent molars as the jaws grow to accommodate them (Hägg & Taranger 1986).

Structure of teeth

All teeth consist of a crown and a root or roots. The crown is the part that is visible in the mouth, while the root is lodged in a socket in the bone of the jaw and serves to anchor the tooth more or less rigidly in place. The crowns are fully formed and mineralised before they erupt into the mouth, however, the roots are not fully formed until some three years after eruption is complete. The roots of the primary teeth are resorbed and disappear as part of the natural shedding process (Stewart *et al.* 1982).

Teeth vary in their shape according to function, but the reliance of twentieth century populations on processed and cooked foods has lessened the importance of teeth being an essential part of the digestive process. However, the teeth have important social functions in relation to appearance, facial expression and speech.

On a cursory examination teeth can be seen to consist of a white crown and a darker looking root. A tooth is, however, composed of a number of different structures (Figure 10.1):

- Enamel forms the outer part of the tooth crown. It is made up of millions of long, microscopic, crystalline prisms each consisting of a large number of crystals and is 96% inorganic in composition. The most common inorganic constituents are calcium and phosphate in the form of hydroxy- and fluor-apatite crystals. Enamel is the hardest, most mineralised tissue in the body (Thylstrup & Fejerskov 1994).

- Dentine is the inner hard tissue and forms the bulk of the tooth. It is 75% inorganic in composition. The microstructure is tubular, the tubes containing processes from the cells lining the central chamber of the tooth which contains the dental pulp.

- The pulp occupies the centre of the tooth and consists of a mass of blood vessels and nerves. It is

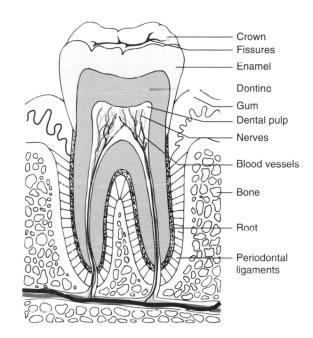

Crown
Fissures
Enamel
Dentine
Gum
Dental pulp
Nerves
Blood vessels
Bone
Root
Periodontal ligaments

Figure 10.1   Structure of a tooth.

the sensory organ of the tooth, detecting changes in temperature at the tooth surface and registering sensations from painful stimuli.

- Cementum is a thin layer of bone-like tissue that envelopes the dentine of the root of the tooth. It serves as an attachment for the periodontal ligaments which retain the tooth root in its socket.

- The periodontium consists of alveolar bone surrounding and supporting the root(s), the periodontal membrane, which is the fibrous tissue attaching the tooth in its socket, and gingiva (gum) which is the pink coloured mucous membrane and underlying fibrous tissue covering the alveolar bone in the mouth. The union of the epithelium covering the gum with the neck of the tooth forms a cuff, and the gingival crevice between the crest of the gum margin and the tooth surface is normally no more than 2 mm in depth. The epithelium lining the crevice joins the tooth surface to form the epithelial attachment. Immediately below the epithelial attachment there are ligament-like fibres. These represent the beginning of the periodontal membrane.

The structure of the teeth and supporting tissues is described in great detail by Berkovitz *et al.* (1977) in a well illustrated colour atlas.

10.3 THE ORAL ENVIRONMENT

If you relax, lick your teeth and then run your tongue over your lips an important component of the oral environment will become immediately obvious, saliva. This lubricates the mouth bathing the teeth and soft tissues. It is largely secreted from three pairs of glands which have ducts opening into the mouth. It serves a number of functions including the lubrication of the food bolus as it passes down the oesophagus to the stomach. It has bacteriocidal properties, hastens blood coagulation and assists the cleansing of the teeth along with the natural muscular action of the lips, cheeks and tongue. One of the most important functions of saliva lies in its ability to neutralise acid and maintain a slightly alkaline environment in the mouth for much of the time. This property arises from the presence of bicarbonate ions in saliva. The presence of calcium and phosphate also serves to reduce to some extent the demineralisation of the teeth during acid attack and to remineralise them when the acid is neutralised. This remineralisation process is facilitated by the presence of fluoride ions (Edgar & O'Mullane 1990).

Running the tongue over your teeth is a simple assessment of how well you are cleaning your teeth. A slight 'furry' feeling means that dental plaque is sticking to the teeth. It is a colourless film of material composed of masses of bacteria in a sticky polysaccharide matrix which adheres to the surfaces of teeth, particularly in locations which are inaccessible to natural or mechanical cleansing. New plaque forms within a few hours on teeth which are thoroughly cleaned and tends to accumulate and thicken with the passage of time unless regularly removed. Plaque is of great importance in the aetiology of dental disease. Some of the bacteria metabolise sugar and form acid whilst others produce harmful products which can cause inflammation of the gums (gingivitis) and destruction of the periodontal tissues (periodontal disease). Plaque which is allowed to remain in the gingival crevice between the gum margin and neck of the tooth, and that occurring on the tooth surfaces

above the gum margin can calcify and harden to form tartar (sub-gingival and supra-gingival calculus). This tends to retain further harmful accumulations of bacteria in contact with the periodontium (Pearce 1991).

10.4 COMMON ORAL DISEASES

We have discussed the common oral structures, the next step is to consider the common oral diseases. There are many diseases which can affect the mouth but two major problems are dental caries and periodontal disease.

Dental caries can occur within a few months of the teeth erupting. It is thus primarily a disease of childhood and early adult life. It first affects the tooth enamel at localised sites; notably in the fissures of the biting surface of the teeth. If allowed to progress, a cavity forms and the dentine underlying the demineralised enamel becomes softened and infected with bacteria so that eventually the pulp is threatened. The inflammatory response of the pulp, confined and contained within the pulp chamber gives rise to the symptoms of toothache. The eventual outcome is death of the pulp and the formation of an abscess in the bone surrounding the root tip (Whelton & O'Mullane 1997).

Periodontal disease includes gingivitis and periodontitis. It is primarily a problem for adolescents and adults but may have its origins in childhood. Gingivitis is inflammation confined to the epithelium and connective tissue around the tooth, while periodontitis is the inflammation of supporting structures of the teeth, that is to say bone, cementum and fibrous tissue. Periodontal disease can begin at any time after tooth eruption. The common form progresses slowly and, unlike caries, does not usually threaten the integrity of the dentition until middle life or later. It occurs at affected tooth sites as irregular bursts of destructive inflammatory activity interspersed with quiescent periods. The disease is usually preceded by inflammation of the gum (gingivitis) characterised by redness, swelling and a tendency to bleed easily. However, periodontal disease itself (periodontitis) is characterised by pocketing which occurs between the bone surrounding the tooth root and cementum, which has been degraded by the inflammatory process. This leads to progressive destruction of the tooth's bony support. The process continues down the root until eventually the tooth may lose a large part of its support. Eventual outcomes are suppuration, loosening of the tooth, and tenderness, soreness or pain. At this stage teeth are usually removed (Löe & Brown 1993).

The important point to emphasise is that both dental caries and periodontal disease can be controlled.

10.5 EPIDEMIOLOGY OF DENTAL DISEASE

In the nineteenth century dental caries was associated with considerable pain and sepsis. It was not uncommon for a dental abscess to be registered as a cause of death. Happily this state of affairs no longer exists and in modern times dental disease and the practice of dentistry are not usually associated with mortality in western countries (Hardwick 1969). Nevertheless some deaths attributable in part to dental ill health are recorded each year. For example, there are occasional fatalities in association with general anaesthesia for dental treatment (Murray 1993). Other fatalities resulting from bacteraemia following dental operative procedures in people with heart valvular defects, may also occur. There are also in the community children and adults with medical conditions for whom the consequences of dental disease and dental treatment are potentially so severe that special arrangements for their care are required in order to avoid hazardous situations. Individuals with haemorrhagic disorders, severe cardiac and respiratory conditions and patients receiving therapy with a number of specific drugs must, among others, be regarded as high risk groups, often in need of comprehensive preventive dental care throughout life (Blinkhorn & Mackie 1992).

For most other people, however, it is the pain and inconvenience of dental disease and the associated sepsis, dysfunction and disfigurement which causes it to be a troublesome health problem. In western countries, where the acute killer diseases of the past have for the most part been conquered, it is the

degenerative and chronic diseases, of which caries and periodontal disease are examples, which are receiving attention. As expectations rise and the value of a healthy, natural dentition is appreciated, people are becoming more interested in the possibility of avoiding dental disease and retaining their teeth for life. From the economic point of view, by 1995 over £1.5 billion was being spent on dental treatment in the UK. This represents one of the largest expenditures on any single group of diseases in the country. Again, days lost from work each year on account of dental disease represent an appreciable loss to the nation in terms of resources. However, the fact that both caries and periodontal disease are preventable means that their control in the community, although difficult, is not an insuperable challenge for those health professionals working in both primary and secondary care (Blinkhorn et al. 1994).

In westernised industrialised countries like the UK, sugar consumption may approach 50 kg per head of the population each year which is more than double the world average (Sreebny 1982). As a consequence, despite a general decline in levels of dental decay in many of these countries since at least the early 1970s, the occurrence of caries today still remains unacceptably high. Periodontal disease is also of almost universal occurrence although it may be more severe in some developing countries where dental awareness is low and the teeth are rarely cleaned. Caries and periodontal disease are among the commonest ailments to afflict people in the UK and between them, the two diseases and their sequelae are the major cause of tooth loss. Caries accounts directly for around 30% of dental extractions in all age groups, while periodontal disease probably accounts for some 20% (Kay & Blinkhorn 1987).

The prevalence of dental caries

The effects of dental caries are cumulative so that the prevalence of the disease, manifested by untreated cavities or restored or extracted teeth, increases with age. In five year old children in England and Wales, average numbers of decayed, missing and filled teeth (dmft, primary teeth) actually fell from 4.0 to 1.8 between 1973 and 1983. However, the prevalence of the disease in young children has remained more or less static at this reduced level since that time although recent evidence suggests that it may be increasing, notably in children from less privileged communities. Paradoxically the proportion of UK five year old children with no experience of dental decay has continued to increase (Downer 1994a).

Again, in 12 year old children, average numbers of decayed, missing and filled permanent teeth (DMFT, permanent teeth) fell from around 3.0 in 1983 to 1.4 in 1993 and have probably continued to decline. A similar accelerated decline has also occurred in young adults where, according to UK national surveys of dental health, average caries experience among 16–24 year old adults fell by over 30% between 1978 and 1988. Although dental health has improved steadily since the early 1970s, particularly in the younger sections of the population, many people still have high levels of caries (O'Brien 1994).

Prevalence of periodontal disease

As this disease is not directly related to the aims of this book only one fact which will be of personal interest to potential readers will be included. In 1988, 75% of young adults included in the Adult Dental Health survey (Todd & Lader 1991) had periodontal pockets around one or more teeth with 13% having deep pockets. So if you are in that age group make sure you remember to brush your teeth effectively and ensure your teeth are scaled/polished at regular intervals.

Risk factors for dental disease

Dental caries rates as measured by the decayed, missing and filled teeth (DMFT) index is related to age but not strongly associated with gender, race, socio-economic status or the degree of urbanisation. However, when the components of the DMFT are considered separately, differences do emerge. For example, females, whites, urban dwellers and higher social classes have higher filled scores and lower decayed and missing scores (Stamm *et al.* 1991).

The reasons for the differences have been put down to the indirect influence of behavioural patterns and life style. We know that toothbrushing habits, sugar intake and use of dental services have strong associations with socio-economic status (Downer 1994b).

10.6 AETIOLOGY OF DENTAL CARIES

The previous sections of this chapter have stressed that dental disease can be controlled, hence all health and education professionals can be confident that any advice they give on dental health will help patients – provided of course it is put into practice. However, in order to offer advice it is important to have a clear understanding of the causes of dental disease.

Dental caries (decay) is a particular problem for children. It destroys the hard tissues of the tooth and it is always associated with bacteria present in the mouth which colonise the surface of a tooth forming a sticky retentive film called dental plaque (Loesche 1986). Before the disease can progress the bacteria require the presence of readily fermentable carbohydrate. Ordinary dietary sugar is the most common form of refined carbohydrate (Rugg-Gunn 1988).

When considering sugars it is helpful to distinguish sugars naturally present in the cells of food (*intrinsic*) from those which are free in food or added to it (*extrinsic*). This difference in physical location influences the availability of the sugar for metabolism by the bacteria in the dental plaque. Intrinsic sugars are not metabolised by the bacteria whereas extrinsic sugars are. For example, glucose contained in fruit (intrinsic) does not cause dental caries but glucose added to foods or drinks (extrinsic) is cariogenic (causes dental caries). Sucrose appears to be the most cariogenic sugar, but glucose, fructose and maltose are only marginally less so. Natural syrups such as honey, maple syrup and concentrated fruit juices will cause dental caries, but starches are generally considered to be non-cariogenic (COMA 1991).

The non sugar sweeteners do not cause dental caries. A convenient classification for non-sugar sweeteners is to divide them into either bulk or intense sweeteners (Rugg-Gunn & Edgar 1985). Bulk sweeteners are substances with a similar sweetness to sucrose. They can be metabolised to supply energy but can also be used to provide bulk and physical structure to foods. All these sweeteners are insulin independent. They have the disadvantage of being poorly absorbed from the alimentary tract and can cause osmotic diarrhoea. Bulk sweeteners include isomalt, lactitol, malitol, mannitol, sorbitol, xylitol and hydrogenated glucose syrup (lycasin). Intense sweeteners are substances with a sweetness many times that of sucrose. They need only minute amounts to give an effect and provide no bulk or calories. Intense sweeteners include saccharin, aspartame, acesulfame K and thaumatin.

The caries process

When cariogenic sugars enter the mouth acid is produced by the bacteria in the plaque metabolising the sugar and this results in the demineralisation of the tooth surface. After a period of 20–30 minutes the acid will have been buffered by the saliva and remineralisation of the tooth surface will occur. This process can be demonstrated graphically by plotting the fall in pH within the dental plaque following the consumption of sugar. This is known as the Stephan Curve (Stephan 1940) (Figure 10.2).

When the pH goes below the critical pH (5.5) demineralisation occurs, and when the pH rises above 5.5 remineralisation occurs. This cycle of damage and repair has been called the 'ionic see-saw'. Decay only results if the demineralisation exceeds remineralisation, in which case the surface of the tooth eventually breaks down and a cavity appears.

The Stephan Curve can be used to illustrate how the ionic see-saw can be weighted in favour of demineralisation and hence increasing the chances of decay. When sugary foods and drinks are taken at meal times there will be approximately four acid demineralisation periods and there will be plenty of time for remineralisation to occur (Figure 10.3). However, if sugary foods and drinks are consumed regularly between meals the number of acid attacks increase and the scope for remineralisation is severely limited (Figure 10.4).

The early decay process is a contest fought at the tooth surface and is based on the movement of calcium and phosphate ions in and out of the dental enamel.

10.7 CONTROLLING DENTAL CARIES

Theoretically, any factor that influences the balance of the 'ionic see-saw' will affect the amount of decay that occurs. However, for all practical purposes only three need to be taken into account. These are: fluoride, sugar, and fissure sealants.

Fluoride

The presence of fluoride both during the development of the teeth and after their eruption has a marked effect on the progress of dental decay. The effect of fluoride is due partly to its incorporation into the developing tooth before eruption and to its direct topical contact with the tooth after eruption. The topical action of fluoride is now believed to be the most important effect, as its presence in the mouth encourages remineralisation of teeth which have been subjected to acid attack. Thus fluoride is a therapeutic agent as well as a preventive one (WHO 1994). There are a number of ways to bring the benefits of fluoride to communities and individuals, and these will be described.

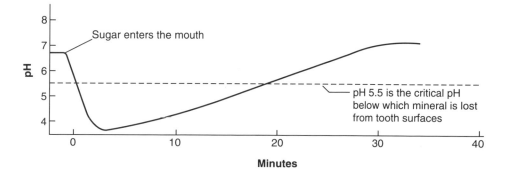

Figure 10.2 Stephan Curve, plotting pH within dental plaque against time.

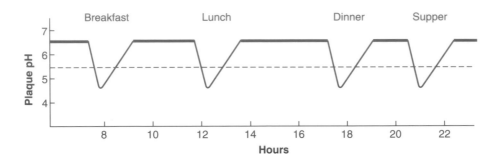

Figure 10.3   Sugar at meal times.

Water fluoridation

This is the most effective and efficient public health strategy, and is achieved by augmenting the level of fluoride in the public water supply. The fluoride ion exists naturally in all water supplies, but where the level is at or above one part of fluoride to every million parts of water (1 ppm or 1 mg/litre) life-long residents have much less decay than people living in areas where fluoride levels are low. Scientists were alerted to the beneficial effects of fluoride when it became clear that in communities where fluoride was naturally present at or above 1 ppm decay rates were low. This led to the idea that other communities could benefit if the concentration of fluoride was increased artificially to around 1 ppm. Some 250 million people world-wide now have the benefit of water fluoridation and reductions in decay of over 50% are the norm (Blinkhorn *et al.* 1981).

Unfortunately water fluoridation has attracted adverse publicity and considerable spurious allegations about its safety have been presented in the media. The safety of fluoride in public water supplies is one of the most intensely studied public health measures. To date all the evidence collected has found fluoridation to be safe and effective (Knox, 1985).

Toothpaste

The twice daily use of a fluoride toothpaste is a major factor in the control of dental caries. Although toothbrushing in itself has not been shown to prevent dental caries, it is a very important way of applying fluoride directly on to the tooth surface. Parents should be encouraged to begin brushing their children's teeth as soon as they erupt. Fluoride is highly effective as a topical agent, hence the great value of fluoride toothpastes (Konig 1993).

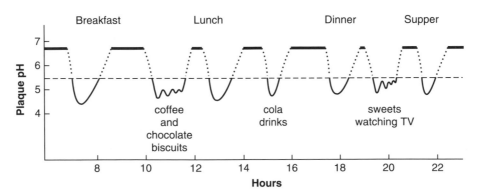

Figure 10.4   Sugar between meals.

Fluoride supplements

For some children, especially those who have experienced caries of their first dentition, fluoride supplements in the form of tablets/drops are of value (Stephen & Campbell 1978). Fluoride tablets or drops, taken daily, ensure that the appropriate amount of fluoride enters the developing tooth and is available topically as the teeth erupt. Fluoride supplements are given in the form of drops for younger children, moving on to tablets as the child gets older. The recommended dosages for fluoride supplements are dependent on the level of fluoride in the local water supply. Table 10.1 gives recommended dosages of fluoride for different age groups in an area where the fluoride level in the local water supply is less than 0.3 ppm. The local water company will be able to advise you on the fluoride ion concentration in your drinking water.

Table 10.1 Recommended fluoride doses (in mg of fluoride per day)*.

Age	mg of fluoride per day
6 months to 3 years	0.25
2–6 years	0.50
6 years and plus	1.00

* Fluoride level in local water supply less than 0.3 ppm.

At one time fluoride supplements were given last thing at night, just before bedtime. However, children usually brush their teeth last thing at night with a fluoride toothpaste, therefore they will not benefit greatly if the supplement is given at this time. Children should be given their fluoride supplement at a time other than when their teeth are cleaned, this maximises the preventive effect. It is often convenient to give the supplement at lunch time or when children come home from school.

It should be stressed that fluoride supplements are a long-term measure and should be given daily until adolescence. In areas with a low prevalence of caries the general use of fluoride supplements it is not justified.

The prescription for fluoride supplements is usually written out for sodium fluoride BP; 2.2 mg of sodium fluoride will provide 1 mg of fluoride ion, 1.1 mg of sodium fluoride will provide 0.5 mg of fluoride ion and 0.55 mg of sodium fluoride will provide 0.25 mg of fluoride ion (Holloway & Joyston-Bechal 1994).

Fluoride mouth rinses

These are indicated for adolescents who have recently started to develop dental caries (Blinkhorn *et al.* 1983). This is usually as a result of a change in snacking or drinking habits due to growing independence from parental influences. A fixed orthodontic appliance which is not being looked after properly will also encourage the development of dental caries. In this instance a fluoride mouth rinse is helpful and should be used at a time different from when a fluoride toothpaste is used. A daily rinse is more effective at controlling dental caries than a weekly rinse.

Dietary control of dental caries

It has been demonstrated that if sugars enter the mouth more than four times a day demineralisation may exceed remineralisation and caries will result. Thus the appropriate dietary advice is to encourage individuals to limit the frequency of sugar consumption. Only snacks and drinks that do not contain sugar should be recommended between meals, these include wholemeal bread, fresh fruit, cheese, cold meats, vegetables and low fat crisps. Sugar-free drinks include tap water, milk, diet drinks, bottled water, tea and coffee without sugar.

Infant drinks

In the UK over 25,000 children under five years of age have teeth extracted under general anaesthesia every year. The main reason for these extractions is pain caused by decayed teeth (Hinds & Gregory 1995). The main aetiological agent of dental caries in these young children is sweetened drinks. Concentrated syrups, fruit juices, cordials containing sugar and milk with sugar added can all cause dental caries if they constantly bathe the teeth.

Mothers of infants should be warned of the dangers of putting sugar-containing fruit drinks and juices into feeding bottles or reservoir feeders. Children should not have a bottle containing juice throughout the night nor use a bottle or a feeder cup continually throughout the day. Such practices result in almost continuous bathing of the teeth with a sugary solution causing severe tooth destruction called rampant caries.

Soya milk

This has been produced for infants who are allergic to cows' milk protein or have lactose intolerance. In order to try to copy cows' milk, baby formulae must have a minimum carbohydrate content, this is normally in the form of the sugar lactose, which is in breast milk and is safe for teeth. However in soya milk glucose syrup has to be used which is a non-milk extrinsic sugar and can cause dental caries.

Soya milk can be considered as a sugar containing 'drink'. Parents who have to use soya milk must be instructed on good feeding practices, by not allowing ad lib feeding from a bottle. This will help to reduce the risk of rampant caries. The soya milk should be used as a feed, not a drink. Bottles containing soya milk should not be used as a comforter especially at night time. The infant should graduate on to a cup as soon as one can be mastered.

Fissure sealants

These are plastic coatings that can be placed on the biting surfaces of back teeth. They exclude both sugar and bacteria from the deep fissures which are prone to decay. This form of protection is becoming increasingly important as fluoride is highly effective at controlling decay on all tooth surfaces except the fissured biting surface of the back molar teeth. Sealants should be applied to the permanent teeth soon after they erupt (Simonsen 1993).

10.8 COMMON DENTAL QUESTIONS ASKED BY PARENTS OF YOUNG CHILDREN

Does a child have weak teeth if the mother's diet is deficient in calcium during pregnancy?

No, teeth take calcium preferentially so are not affected by a diet that is low in calcium. Some children are more prone to dental caries than others, even when diet and exposure to fluoride are similar. This is probably related to the rate of flow and composition of saliva which affects its ability to neutralise plaque acids (Rugg-Gunn *et al.* 1984).

Will apples and carrots keep my children's teeth healthy and clean?

Yes, if substituted for sugar-containing snacks. Fruit and vegetables do not cause tooth decay. Apples and carrots do not keep teeth clean. Only regular and thorough toothbrushing will remove plaque effectively and so maintain gum health (Levine 1996).

Do teeth sometimes come through bad?

No, but they may appear to do so if the child is having a bottle or cup containing a sugared drink or concentrated fruit juice. Teeth which are continuously bathed in sugar in this way decay rapidly. This is known as 'bottle caries' or rampant caries (Winter 1980).

Will regular toothbrushing prevent tooth decay?

No, fluoride in toothpaste markedly increases the tooth's resistance but plaque removal does not in itself prevent caries. This is because plaque is deposited continuously, so that even a few minutes after teeth have been brushed, sufficient plaque will present on the teeth (particularly in the grooves on the biting surfaces and between the teeth) to cause an acid attack on the enamel when sugar is consumed. Reduction in frequency of sugar consumption will help to reduce tooth decay. Toothbrushing helps to control gum disease. Nevertheless, it is important to remember the importance of encouraging brushing with a fluoride toothpaste twice a day (Davies & Ellwood 1995).

Will bad baby teeth damage the adult teeth?

No, this is a parent's second chance, by reducing the sugar intake a child can have a perfect set of permanent teeth. The only caveat is that baby teeth which are abscessed can interfere with the development of the permanent successor so referral to a dentist is indicated (Blinkhorn & Mackie 1992).

Are all toothbrushes the same?

Toothbrushes vary greatly in cost and design. Currently the dental profession recommends that a brush should have a small head and multi tufted fibres packed densely together (Levine 1996). There is no convincing evidence that electric toothbrushes are more effective than hand operated brushes. They may however be very useful for people who have difficulty holding an ordinary brush.

On average, children should be encouraged to change brushes every four months as the bristles lose their resilience and do not remove plaque effectively. Manufacturers are constantly trying to stimulate demand by producing novel toothbrush designs. There is little evidence that one type of brush is better than another. The key factors are the small head and using the brush effectively.

Is wearing a brace really necessary?

The answer to this question is yes and no! (Shaw *et al.* 1991). Orthodontic care will be of value if the front teeth stick out a long way and could be traumatised or there is strain on the jaw joint as a result of the teeth coming into premature contact. In addition some children and their parents may become very concerned about irregularities of the front teeth.

On the other hand, some orthodontic care for minor irregularities is of questionable value and orthodontic specialists usually offer care on the basis of an index of treatment need in an effort to utilise scarce resources wisely. At one time children were referred for orthodontic care at an early age. However, with the advances in orthodontic technology most treatment is undertaken with braces which are actually fixed in place with a special bonding agent and treatment is undertaken from 12–14 years of age. Children with high decay rates and poor levels of toothcleaning are not usually offered orthodontic treatment as the brace may exacerbate the poor oral health.

Is one toothpaste more effective than another?

In the UK the widespread availability and use of fluoride toothpastes has been responsible for the dramatic reductions in dental caries. Fluoride is now present as an active ingredient in almost all toothpastes as either sodium fluoride, sodium monofluorophosphate, a combination of both or stannous fluoride. The maximum level of fluoride permitted by the EU Cosmetics Directive in cosmetic products is 1500 ppm fluoride. The efficacy of fluoride is concentration dependent and most products contain 1000 to 1500 ppm fluoride. Recently toothpastes containing lower levels of fluoride (400–500 ppm fluoride) have been developed for children under six years of age. Such toothpastes will not be as clinically effective as those containing 1000–1500 ppm fluoride. The low fluoride pastes have been produced because some young children have been eating toothpaste or brushing several times a day with large amounts of paste on the brush. In such instances there is a danger that the developing front teeth could become mottled because the large intake of fluoride interferes with the normal formation of tooth enamel. The manufacturers of fluoride toothpastes recommend that children under six years of age should only have a small pea sized amount of toothpaste placed on the brush and should clean their teeth just twice a day (Melberg 1991).

Are sugary medicines really bad for children's teeth?

Chronically sick children who take prescribed sugar-containing medicines on a long-term basis have been shown to develop more dental caries than similar children who took tablets or who took medicines in a sugar-free form. It is usually assumed that healthy children take medicines infrequently, therefore even if these contain sugar they will not cause dental caries. However, a high proportion of children do take medicines frequently. Children, on average, take medicines for one day in ten or one week in eight. Prescribed medicines account for 55% of drugs used, the other 45% being over-the-counter preparations, particularly paracetamol and cough medicines.

The time of day when children take their medicine is an important point to consider as it clarifies how they can cause dental caries. Medicines are often given just before bedtime. A sugar-containing analgesic is given to relieve pain or reduce fever. A night-time tickly cough is soothed by a sugary cough syrup to help the child go off to sleep. Giving a sugar-containing medicine as a child goes to bed is highly damaging to the teeth. During sleep the salivary flow into the mouth is reduced and this limits the buffering and cleansing action of the saliva. The sugary syrup clings to the teeth and the mouth remains acid for a considerable length of time.

The simplest way to prevent sugar-containing

medicines causing dental caries is to recommend a sugar-free variety instead (Mackie 1995).

What should parents do if their child's front tooth is knocked out?

Epidemiological reports show that by the age of 12 years over half of all children have suffered some trauma to their front teeth. All children who have damaged their teeth should be seen by a dentist. However, there is one instance where immediate treatment by any health professional is indicated; this is when a permanent tooth is knocked out. If a permanent tooth which has been knocked out is replaced straight back into its socket there is a 90% chance that this will be successful and the tooth saved (Blinkhorn & Mackie 1992).

A tooth which has been knocked out should be held by the crown and gently pushed back into its socket, making sure that it is the right way round. This is usually painless if done immediately after the accident. The child should then be instructed to bite on a handkerchief and go straight to a dentist so that a splint can be prepared and antibiotics prescribed.

If it is not possible to replace the tooth the child should go immediately to a dentist with the tooth placed in a suitable storage medium, such as milk or physiological saline. If the tooth has been kept in the right storage medium it can be successfully replanted several hours after the accident. On the other hand the chances of a dry tooth being successfully replanted are very poor (Blinkhorn & Mackie 1996).

Do not try to put a baby tooth which has been knocked out back into the socket as you may damage the developing adult tooth.

Is there any way to stop children teething?

Unfortunately the majority of young children do suffer discomfort as the baby teeth erupt and this often results in more trauma for the parents than the child. Several sleepless nights in succession taxes the endurance of most mothers and fathers. The first symptom of teething is the production of excess saliva and 'dribbling' occurs. Following on from this the child may be restless, have red cheeks and will not go off to sleep because of the discomfort. Teething is often accompanied by the urge to bite on fingers or on hard objects such as the edge of a cot or toys.

Other symptoms such as fever, upset stomachs and diarrhoea have been attributed to teething. A more likely explanation for these symptoms is that the child is coincidentally suffering from some other minor upset in addition to teething (Seward 1972).

We really know very little about teething so the treatment is palliative; giving the child something to bite on often alleviates the discomfort. Parents should be warned against letting the child chew on small unsecured objects which could be swallowed or inhaled. Several different designs and types of teething rings are available, but the ones which contain a viscous fluid and can be cooled in the fridge seem to be the most successful. Massaging the gums with a finger and a little topical anaesthetic paste in the form of one of the teething gels can bring some relief. A sugar-free paracetamol syrup will help relieve the child's discomfort and may help all the members of the family to get some sleep.

At what age should my child visit the dentist?

Some dentists are pleased to see a young child even before the teeth erupt whilst others prefer to wait until all the baby teeth have erupted, usually about two and a half to three years of age. However, most dentists like to register children before two years of age as an early visit will enable them to offer dietary advice, particularly on the dangers of giving the child a night time bottle containing juice or sugared milk (Levine 1996).

10.9 KEY DENTAL HEALTH EDUCATION MESSAGES

Health visitors, practice nurses, school nurses and midwives have an important role to play in making sure children do not suffer from dental caries because they are far more likely to interact with many families than dentists, who only offer care on demand.

This chapter has provided evidence that dental ill health is controllable through relatively simple measures. The main problem is making sure the appropriate messages are offered to parents.

The Health Education Authority in their publication *The Scientific Basis of Dental Health Education* (Levine 1996) have delineated the key messages that should be offered to the general public. These are:

(1) **Diet: reduce the consumption and especially the frequency of intake of sugar-containing food and drink.**
    The number of times that sugars enter the mouth is the most important factor in determining the rate of decay. They should be consumed as part of a meal rather than between meals. Snacks and drinks should be free of sugars. The frequent consumption of acidic drinks should be avoided.

(2) **Toothbrushing: clean the teeth thoroughly twice every day with a fluoride toothpaste.**
    Effective plaque removal is essential for the prevention of periodontal disease. The toothbrush is the only means of plaque removal that should be recommended on a public health basis; other oral hygiene aids, apart from disclosing agents, are a matter for personal professional advice. Thorough brushing of all surfaces twice every day is of more value than more frequent cursory brushing, and a gentle scrub technique should be advised. The toothbrush size and design should allow the user to reach all tooth surfaces and gum margins easily and comfortably. Toothbrushing by itself will not prevent dental decay, but a major benefit will be gained by the use of a fluoride toothpaste.

(3) **Fluoridation: request your local water company to supply water with the optimum fluoride level.**
    Fluoridation of the water supply is a safe and highly effective public health measure.

(4) **Dental attendance: have an oral examination every year.**
    Everyone, irrespective of age and dental condition, should have an oral examination once a year. Children and those at risk from oral disease may need to be seen more frequently, at intervals determined with professional advice.

If these were accepted by the public then the majority of dental problems would be of a minor nature and much pain and misery could be avoided.

10.10 THE PROVISION OF DENTAL SERVICES IN THE UNITED KINGDOM

The dental services in the UK are predominantly based in the primary care sector with only a very small proportion of care being offered in hospitals. The primary care sector is divided into general dental practitioners (GDPs) and the community dental service. The former are independent contractors whilst the latter is a salaried service.

Dentists have to be registered with the General Dental Council before they are allowed to practice. There are approximately 28,000 dentists on the register of whom 26,000 currently work in the UK. Around 20,000 of these dentists work in general dental practice and provide some, if not all, their patients with National Health Service dental care. There are no restrictions on where a dentist may practise (BDA 1997) which is reflected in the dentist to population ratio (Table 10.2).

The Community Dental Service (CDS) is much smaller with approximately 1400 dentists providing dental care. The role of the CDS is to ensure that

Table 10.2 Dentist/population ratio*.

Region	Population
Northern	3340
Yorkshire	3310
Trent	3595
East Anglia	3337
North West Thames	2426
North East Thames	3060
South East Thames	2802
South West Thames	2397
Wessex	3112
Oxford	3102
South Western	2793
West Midlands	3592
Mersey	3090
North Western	3071
Wales	3420
Scotland	2700
Northern Ireland	2470

* Calculated on the basis of population numbers in each region.

priority groups, those with special needs and individuals who cannot find a GDP, are catered for. In addition, oral health promotion and the collection of epidemiological data are undertaken by the CDS. There have been cutbacks in the funding of the CDS such that it is not possible for the service to be the 'safety net' for all patients.

The government is currently reviewing the structure of the way dental services are organised. However, as GDPs are independent contractors change may be a slow process. Many general dental practitioners are trying to build up the numbers of private patients in an effort to reduce their commitment to the National Health Service.

10.11 CONCLUSION

Dental ill health is very expensive to treat but it is one of the few diseases where the preventive messages are straightforward and if implemented offer a tangible health gain. The nursing profession is in an ideal position to offer advice to parents and their children and thereby reduce the unnecessary suffering caused by dental ill health.

REFERENCES

BDA Advisory Service (1997) *Into General Practice*. British Dental Association, London.

Berkovitz, B.K.B., Holland, G.R. & Moxham, B.J. (1977) *Colour Atlas and Textbook of Oral Anatomy*. Wolfe Medical Publications, London.

Blinkhorn, A.S. (1993) Dental health promotion for the United Kingdom in the year 2000. *Community Dental Health*, **10**, 65–70.

Blinkhorn, A.S. & Mackie, I.C. (1992). *Practical Treatment Planning in Paediatric Dentistry*. Quintessence Publishing Company, London.

Blinkhorn, A.S. & Mackie, I.C. (1996) My child's just knocked out a front tooth. *British Medical Journal*, **312**, 512.

Blinkhorn, A.S., Brown, M.D., Attwood, D. & Downer, M.C. (1981) The effect of fluoridation on the dental health of urban Scottish schoolchildren. *Journal of Epidemiology and Community Health*, **35**, 98–101.

Blinkhorn, A.S., Holloway, P.J. & Davies, T.G.H. (1983) The combined effects of a fluoride dentifrice and fluoride mouthwash on the incidence of dental caries. *Community Dentistry & Oral Epidemiology*, **11**, 7–11.

Blinkhorn, A.S., Holloway, P.J. & Wilson, N.H.F. (1994) Future of preventive dentistry. *British Medical Journal*, **309**, 1302–3.

COMA. (1991) *Dietary Reference Values for Food Energy and Nutrients in the United Kingdom*. HMSO, London.

Davies, R.M. & Ellwood, R.P. (1995) The use of fluoride toothpaste in an oral health strategy for the North West of England. In: *Achieving the Targets for Oral Health*, Eden Bianchi Press, Manchester.

Downer, M.C. (1994a) The 1993 national survey of children's dental health: a commentary on the preliminary report. *British Dental Journal*, **176**, 209–14.

Downer, M.C. (1994b) Caries prevalence in the United Kingdom. *International Dental Journal*, **44**, 367–70.

Edgar, W.M. & O'Mullane, D.M. (eds) (1990) *Saliva and Dental Health*. British Dental Journal Publications, London.

Hägg, U. & Taranger, J. (1986) Timing of Tooth Emergence. A prospective longitudinal study of Swedish urban children from birth to 18 years. *Swedish Dental Journal*, **10**, 195–206.

Hardwick, J.L. (1969) The incidence and distribution of caries throughout the ages in relation to the Englishman's diet. *British Dental Journal*, **108**, 9–17.

Hinds, K. & Gregory, J.R. (1995) National Diet and Nutrition Survey: Children Aged $1\frac{1}{2}$–$4\frac{1}{2}$ years. Vol. 2: Report of the Dental Survey. HMSO, London.

Holloway, P.J. & Joyston-Bechal, S. (1994) How should we use dietary fluoride supplements? *British Dental Journal*, **177**, 319–20.

Kay, E.J. & Blinkhorn, A.S. (1987) Factors influencing the extraction of teeth by general dental practitioners. *Journal of Community Dental Health*, **4**, 3–9.

Konig, K.G. (1993) Role of fluoride toothpastes in a caries preventive strategy. *Caries Research*, **27**, (suppl 1), 23–8.

Knox, E.G. (1985) Fluoridation of Water and Cancer: a Review of the Epidemiological Evidence. Report of a Working Party. HMSO, London.

Levine, R. (1996) *Scientific Basis of Dental Health Education*. Health Education Authority, London.

Löe, H. and Brown, L.J. (eds) (1993) Classification and epidemiology of periodontal diseases. *Periodontology 2000*, vol. 2. Munksgaard, Copenhagen.

Loesche, W.J. (1986) Role of *streptococcus mutans* in human dental decay. *Microbiological Review*, **50**, 353–80.

Mackie, I.C. (1995) Children's dental health and medicines that contain sugar. *British Medical Journal*, **311**, 141–2.

Melberg, J.R. (1991) Fluoride dentifrices: current status and prospects. *International Dental Journal*, **41**, 9–16.

Murray, J.J. (1993) General anaesthesia and children's dental health: present trends and future needs. *Anaesthesia and Pain Control in Dentistry*, **2**, 209–16.

O'Brien, M. (1994) *Children's Dental Health in the UK, 1993.* HMSO, London.

Pearce, E.I.F. (1991) Salivary inorganic and physical factors in the aetiology of dental caries, and their role in prediction. In: *Dental Caries, Markers of High and Low Risk Groups and Individuals*, (ed. N.W. Johnson). Cambridge University Press, Cambridge.

Rugg-Gunn, A.J. (1988) Diet and dental caries. In: *The Prevention of Dental Disease*, (ed. J.J. Murray), 2nd edn. Oxford Medical Publications, Oxford.

Rugg-Gunn, A.J. & Edgar, W.M. (1985) Sweeteners and dental health. *Community Dental Health*, **2**, 213–23.

Rugg-Gunn, A.J., Hackett, A.F., Appleton, D.R., Jenkins, G.N. & Eastoe, J.E. (1984) Relationship between dietary habits and caries increment assessed over two years in 405 English adolescent children. *Archives of Oral Biology*, **29**, 983–92.

Seward, M.H. (1972) Treatment of teething in infants. *British Dental Journal*, **132**, 33–6.

Shaw, W.C., O'Brien, K.D., Richmond, S. & Brook, P. (1991) Quality control in orthodontics: risk/benefit considerations. *British Dental Journal*, **170**, 33–7.

Simonsen, R.J. (1993) Why not sealants? *Journal Public Health Dentistry*, **53**, 211.

Sreebny, L.M. (1982) Sugar availability, sugar consumption and dental caries. *Community Dentistry and Oral Epidemiology*, **10**, 1–7.

Stamm, J.W., Stewart, P.W., Bohannan, H.M., Disney, J.A., Graves, R.C. & Abernathy, J.R. (1991) Risk assessment for oral diseases. *Advances in Dental Research*, **5**, 4–17.

Stephan, R.M. (1940) Changes in hydrogen ion concentration on tooth surfaces and in carious lesions. *Journal American Dental Association*, **27**, 718–23.

Stephen, K.W. & Campbell, D. (1978) Caries reduction and cost benefit after 3 years of sucking fluoride tablets daily at school. *British Dental Journal*, **144**, 202–6.

Stewart, R.E., Witkop, C.J. & Bixler, D. (1982) The dentition. In: *Paediatric Dentistry, Scientific Foundations and Clinical Practice*, (eds R.E. Stewart, T.K. Barber, K.C. Troutman & S.H.Y. Wei). C.V. Mosby Company, St Louis.

Sullivan, P.G. (1994) Craniofacial growth. In: *Orthodontics and Occlusal Management*, (ed. W.C. Shaw), Wright, Butterworth-Heinemann Ltd, Oxford.

Ten Cate, A.R. (ed.) (1980) *Oral Histology: Development, Structure and Function.* C.V. Mosby Company, St Louis.

Thylstrup, A. and Fejerskov, O. (1994) Clinical and pathological features of dental caries. In: *Textbook of Clinical Cariology*, (eds A. Thylstrup & O. Fejerskov), Munksgaard, Copenhagen.

Todd, J.E. & Lader, D. (1991) *Adult Dental Health, 1988, UK.* HMSO, London.

Whelton, H. & O'Mullane, D.M. (1997) Public health aspects of oral diseases and disorders, dental caries. In: *Community Oral Health*, (ed. C.M. Pine). Wright, Butterworth-Heinemann, Oxford.

Winter, G.B. (1980) Problems involved with the use of comforters. *International Dental Journal*, **30**, 28–38.

World Health Organization (1994) Fluorides and oral health. *Technical Report Services*, **846**, WHO, Geneva.

Part 3

Common Problems in Childhood

11

Immunisation and Prevention: An Up-To-Date Perspective

Sean Magennis

11.1 INTRODUCTION

It is every child's right to be immunised. All health care professionals are responsible for ensuring that the children they care for are granted this right. Members of the primary health care team must share the vision of the eradication of infectious disease through the medium of immunisation. The realisation of this vision demands a high level of skill, knowledge and commitment from the team. Only teams fulfilling these requirements will be in a position to support parents in making informed decisions on behalf of their children. This chapter considers background and current evidence surrounding this issue.

11.2 HISTORICAL BACKGROUND

Primitive societies used talismans to ward off disease. The expression 'hair of the dog' owes its derivation not to the cure for the Sunday morning hangover, but to attempts by primitive healers to prevent dog-bite victims from developing rabies by inoculating the offending bite with the hair of the rabid dog.

Plague was replaced by smallpox as the most dreaded disease in England in the mid seventeenth century, although smallpox epidemics had been described by Gregory of Tours as early as AD 581. It is known that the ancient Chinese healers in AD 1000 were grinding up smallpox pustule scales, and blowing them up the nostrils of their patients to try to prevent them catching the disease. In 1714 Dr John Woodward published in 'Philosophical Transactions' details of the work of two Greeks, Pylarini and Timoni, who were inoculating patients with smallpox pus by applying it on a needle and scratching the skin. Finally, in 1796, Edward Jenner demonstrated that inoculating patients with cowpox material afforded them protection against smallpox. At that time, smallpox affected most of the population and had a 10% mortality rate.

In the nineteenth century, vaccination became so well established that Parliament passed several Acts making vaccination compulsory, and defaulting parents punishable by fines. By the end of the twentieth century so successful was smallpox vaccination that the World Health Organization declared smallpox eradicated from the world in 1980.

Although vaccinating children is one of the safest and most cost effective of all preventive measures, resistance to the concept is almost as old as the idea itself. Indeed, opposition to compulsory vaccination in the UK was so strong that legislation enforcing compulsory vaccination was repealed in 1948. Compulsion, however, continues in the USA, where children may not enter school unless they have completed their vaccination programme.

If we are to be equally successful in eradicating diseases like poliomyelitis and measles, the partnerships between the members of the primary health care team, the patients and their parents will have to function in an atmosphere of security, trust and mutual respect.

As compulsion is unlikely to be politically acceptable in the UK for the foreseeable future, the government introduced an alternative vehicle to drive up immunisation rates. General practitioners have always relied for part of their income on being paid for providing certain services to their patients. Payment for vaccinations has been made in the past on the basis of a single fee for each vaccination carried out by the practice. This payment was made irrespective of which member of the practice actually administered the vaccine. No payment was made if, for example, a health visitor or community physician administered the vaccine. Since the inauguration of the 'New GP Contract' in 1990, instead of being paid for individual vaccines, the GP has been set targets to achieve in order to trigger any payments for childhood vaccinations. A higher rate target fee is payable if the practice attains a level of 90% vaccination of eligible children, and a lower fee if only 70% of eligible children are vaccinated. If less than a 70% rate is achieved then no fee is payable. Reaching the higher rate target will generate an income of approximately £2235 per annum per GP, whereas reaching the lower rate will only generate £745 per annum per GP (Ingram 1995). The success of this inducement is a clear illustration of how established management techniques can help the achievement of health service objectives.

11.3 PARENTAL PERSPECTIVE

Health professionals must not underestimate how daunting it is for a parent to bring a fit, healthy, happy child along for a vaccination. Even the better informed and motivated parents cannot help but experience pangs of uncertainty that vaccinating a child for long-term statistical gain might bring about some immediate harm to their loved one. Many parents will never have heard of anyone who has had diphtheria, tetanus, polio or even whooping cough. It is easy to rationalise that if these diseases are so rare, it might be safe to avoid vaccination. In the late 1970s a major setback occurred following adverse publicity claiming a link between pertussis (whooping cough) immunisation and brain damage in children (Kulenkampff *et al.* 1974). This led to a substantial fall in uptake of the vaccine and a corresponding rise in the number of children contracting the disease and developing its complications (Office of Health Economics 1984). Other parents believe that alternative strategies of avoiding diseases will adequately protect their children. Avoiding contact with ill children and the use of homeopathic medicines are often cited as reasons for non-vaccination, although the Faculty of Homeopathy advises that children should be immunised in accordance with current guidelines. Previous history of measles or rubella is another disincentive in some parents' minds, despite the problem that these conditions are difficult to diagnose in children. Parents may believe that eczema and asthma are contraindications, or that premature babies should have their immunisations delayed. Some parents may even cite selective extracts from the literature to support their case for non-vaccination (Moskowitz 1984).

To counteract these understandable fears and concerns, the members of the primary health care team must be armed with the latest knowledge of the subject and present a united approach to the issue, based on the best available evidence. Nothing undermines the team's credibility more than dissent between different team members on the correct approach to a vaccination issue. Without training, update courses and regular communication between members, the team are doomed to fail some of their patients.

The MMR debate

In 1998, in an article published in the *Lancet*, Dr Andrew Wakefield and his team suggested a possible link between the MMR vaccine and the development of inflammatory bowel disease (IBD) and autism (Wakefield *et al.* 1998). They theorised that children genetically susceptible to autism may have their intestinal function damaged by the vaccine, resulting in IBD and autism. Wakefield's advice was to vaccinate children with separate vaccines until further research was carried out. The paper was widely reported and misreported in the media.

Expert review (DoH 1998) and subsequent published work (Peltola *et al.* 1998) reported no evidence of such a link. The government's Chief Medical Officer, on the basis of this expert review, recommended that:

'children should receive MMR vaccine at appropriate times, and should not be given separate component vaccines, since there is no evidence that doing this has any benefit and it may even be harmful'. (DoH 1998)

Despite this advice confidence in the MMR vaccine has fallen. Although the full impact of Wakefield *et al.*'s paper on subsequent MMR vaccination uptake has yet to be seen, there has been an increase in parental refusal to consent to MMR in Lanarkshire, Scotland from April to July 1998 (*CDR Weekly* 1998). While some parents continue to refuse to give consent for MMR, others delay the decision, which in itself may carry risks. Others are opting for single vaccines injected separately for each of measles, mumps and rubella. Single vaccines have not been available in Britain since shortly after the publication of Wakefield's paper but parents have travelled abroad to obtain them.

Notwithstanding the small but growing number of legal claims on behalf of parents who believe their children have been damaged by vaccines, the need for health professionals to have the most up to date information and to advise parents of the government's recommendations regarding MMR vaccination is vital.

11.4 IMPLICATIONS FOR PRIMARY HEALTH CARE TEAMS

Unfortunately, the management structures of the primary health care team may actually interfere with effective co-operation. Responsibility for encouraging, providing, facilitating and paying for the necessary training may fall on the team members themselves, the GP in the case of practice nurses, and the Community Healthcare Trust in the case of district nurses and health visitors. It is therefore vital to ensure a consistent quality and content wherever the training occurs. Employers have a duty to provide the time and money to achieve these standards. Teams function best when well led. Leaders of the team may be chosen for specific tasks, utilising the skills of the members most appropriately. Appointing someone to lead the vaccination team will mean choosing the person with the best knowledge and skills whose attitude will help the team function as an efficient unit. The team will require a member whose 'selling' skills will enable them to overcome the resistance of reluctant parents by carefully listening to and addressing their concerns sensitively and knowledgeably.

Why immunise?

A knowledge of the clinical features of the diseases against which immunisation is effective is indispensable for all involved health service staff. It serves to enhance motivation, and will be expected by parents seeking advice. A résumé of their salient features follows.

Diphtheria
Diphtheria is a notifiable infectious disease caused by the *Corynebacterium diphtheriae*. It affects the upper respiratory tract and is associated with the formation of a grey membrane, which may obstruct the airway. Its incubation period is two to five days and patients may remain infectious for up to four weeks. Although the bacterium is sensitive to antibiotics, it produces a potentially lethal toxin, which attacks the heart and nervous system. Its complications are paralysis, myocardial damage and in 10% of patients, death. Prior to the introduction of the vaccine, there were 46,281 cases and 2480 deaths in 1940. In 1994 there was one death.

There has been an epidemic of diphtheria in the former Soviet Union since 1991, which resulted in 1700 deaths in 1995 (DoH 1996). A recent study (Maple *et al.* 1995) highlighted the worrying fact that 38% of blood donors in the UK were found to be susceptible to diphtheria. A reinforcing dose of low dose diphtheria vaccine is now recommended for school leavers.

Tetanus
Tetanus (lockjaw) is a notifiable disease caused by the toxoid of *Clostridium tetani*. It is characterised by muscle spasm, rigidity and convulsions. It may cause death from sudden cardiac arrest. It is usually contracted from soil contaminated with tetanus spores. The incubation period is two to sixty days although it is most commonly seven to ten days (Adams *et al.* 1969). It is not spread from person to person. In the West, it is now most common in elderly people. Fifty three per cent of cases in the UK are aged over 65 years and 75% aged over 45 years. The World Health Organization (1992) reported that 50% of neo-natal

deaths and 25% of infant deaths in developing countries, are due to tetanus.

Pertussis

Pertussis (whooping cough) is a notifiable disease caused by the bacterium *Bordetella pertussis*. It has an incubation period of seven to ten days and is spread by droplet infection. Patients are infectious from day 7 until day 21 after infection. Initially the disease may present with fever, malaise, anorexia and non-specific upper respiratory symptoms. After this catarrhal stage the cough may become paroxysmal, with prolonged bouts followed by the distinctive 'whoop'. Complications are commonest in infants under six months and include pneumonia, vomiting, convulsions, brain damage and death. It is difficult to diagnose early and treatment with antibiotics is only effective in the catarrhal stage. However, it is recommended that treatment is given even in the paroxysmal stage, in order to reduce infectivity to others. After the adverse publicity in the 1970s uptake of vaccination fell to 30%. As a result, major epidemics with over 100,000 cases occurred in England and Wales until 1983. Uptake improved to 94% by 1992, when notifications dropped back to 1873, the lowest level ever recorded. By 1990 the total deaths from pertussis had fallen to six, all in infants under four months of age. The immunisation schedule was accelerated in 1990 and the death rate fell further to only five, in the four year period to 1995, averaging just over one per annum (DoH 1996).

Polio

Polio is a notifiable disease caused by a virus of which there are three types, I, II, and III. The last three polio epidemics in the UK were due to type I. The virus is spread by the faecal/oral route. The incubation period is 3 to 21 days, and cases may be infectious for more than six weeks. Typically the illness begins with sore throat, anorexia and occasionally nausea, vomiting and diarrhoea. However, the virus multiplies in nerve cells and this may lead to the complications of meningitis, paralysis and death from respiratory muscle paralysis or brain stem damage. In 1955 4000 cases of paralytic polio were notified in England and Wales, compared with 28 cases in the 10 year period between 1994–95. Indigenous wild polio virus seems to have been eradicated from England and Wales (Joce *et al.* 1992).

Haemophilus influenzae

Haemophilus influenzae was originally, but incorrectly, thought to be the cause of flu epidemics when first discovered in 1892. This bacillus has been found to cause many illnesses, among the most serious are: meningitis, septicaemia, epiglottitis, septic arthritis, osteomyelitis, pneumonia and pericarditis. Haemophilus meningitis is a notifiable disease. Before the introduction of the routine vaccination in 1992, one in every 600 children in the UK developed some form of invasive haemophilus disease by their fifth birthday. Meningitis was the most common; 1 in 10 children with meningitis suffered neurological damage and 1 in 20 children who contracted it died. Notification of haemophilus meningitis has fallen from 484 cases in 1992 to 60 in 1995. It would appear that the introduction of the vaccine in the UK has been as successful as it was in the USA in reducing the numbers of children suffering from haemophilus infections (Hargreaves *et al.* 1996).

Measles

Measles is still a dreaded disease in many developing countries. It was estimated as late as 1987 to kill at least 2 million children annually. It has been a notifiable disease in England and Wales since 1940. Immunisation has more than halved the death rate. Measles is due to a paramyxovirus, has an incubation period of about 10 days and a further delay of about four days before the rash appears. It is highly contagious from about day 10 till day 18. Its diagnosis causes some difficulty but may be aided by the simple formula of:

- rash for three days;
- fever for at least one day; and
- one or more of the following: cough, conjunctivitis, coryza.

The identification of Koplik's spots (appear like grains of salt on irregular bright red spots on the buccal mucosa) the day before the rash appears, may also assist diagnosis. The Department of Health recommends that saliva samples are taken from all notified cases of measles mumps and rubella, to allow confirmation of diagnosis (Brown *et al.* 1994). Although often a mild disease, complications of measles can be life threatening, and range from severe conjunctivitis, enteritis and stomatitis, to pneumonia, encephalitis and death. One in 15 cases results in complications, and one in 1000 may develop encephalitis. Of these 15% may die, and up to 40% suffer permanent brain damage. Subacute sclerosing panencephalitis (SSPE) is a rare (one in a million) but serious long-term complication (Miller *et al.* 1992). It leads to a slow inevitable disintegration of the brain, followed by decerebrate rigidity then death.

Mumps

Mumps is a notifiable disease, it is also due to a paramyxovirus and has an incubation period of 14 to 21 days. Spread is by infected saliva and cases are infectious from several days before the parotid swelling to several days after its appearance. It classically causes swelling of one or both parotids, but may affect other salivary glands, the testes, ovaries and pancreas. Despite popular belief, there is no evidence that it causes sterility, although atrophy of testis, epididymis and prostate can occur (Rima 1994). Rarely fatal, mumps can cause deafness and otitis, and is a common cause of viral meningitis and sometimes encephalitis. Before the introduction of the vaccine mumps was responsible for 1200 hospital admissions each year in England and Wales.

Rubella

Rubella is a mild exanthematous notifiable disease due to a togavirus. The incidence rises from age one to four and peaks between five and nine years. It is rare below the age of one. The incubation period is 14 to 21 days and cases are infectious from seven days before the rash until five days after the rash, but highest on the day before and first day of symptoms. The rash usually begins on the face and spreads to the trunk then limbs. It is pink and maculopapular and the lesions are initially discrete but later tend to coalesce. Typically, sub-occipital and post-auricular lymph nodes are enlarged. Arthralgia of multiple joints can occur in adults. Complications are rare but include thrombocytopenia, encephalitis and Guillain-Barre syndrome. Rubella is most difficult to diagnose accurately as it may be impossible to distinguish it from other viral exanthemata; therefore only serological confirmation should be accepted as indicative of infection.

Maternal rubella causes fetal damage in 90% of cases if it occurs in the first 10 weeks of pregnancy. This falls to 34% by 12 weeks, 17% by 16 weeks and is rare after 18 weeks (Miller *et al.* 1982). Deafness is most common, but mental retardation, cataracts, cardiovascular defects, microcephaly and growth retardation occur. When it was realised that immunising pre-pubertal girls and non-immune women would never eradicate rubella, in 1988 rubella was added to the vaccination schedule for children. To prevent the re-emergence of further epidemics of measles and rubella, a two-dose schedule of MMR vaccine was introduced in October 1996.

Tuberculosis

Tuberculosis is a notifiable disease caused by a mycobacterium. In humans the organism is usually spread by droplet infection, and rarely by drinking contaminated milk. Primary tuberculosis may present with cough, haemoptysis, fever, anorexia and failure to thrive in children. Complications include bronchopneumonia, pleural effusions, collapsed lung and disseminated disease (miliary TB). Non-respiratory sites affected by tuberculosis include lymph nodes (scrofula – believed at one time to be cured by the touch of the monarch), kidney, bladder, ovaries, testes and bones and joints. Rarely it may cause meningitis. Gastrointestinal tuberculosis is often due to consumption of infected milk. In the West, post-primary disease is commoner than primary disease and involves a reactivation of a dormant infection, or occasionally a new exogenous infection. These patients may present with fever, weight loss, malaise, night sweats, anorexia in addition to their respiratory symptoms as in the primary disease.

It is estimated that one third of the population of the world is infected with the organism, resulting in 8 million cases of disease and 3 million deaths per annum. The incidence and mortality in the UK has been gradually declining for almost 200 years but since 1987 there has been an increase. As a result of the long period of declining incidence the debate has resurfaced as to whether it is justifiable to continue vaccination of the population as a whole rather than vaccinating targeted high risk groups. Other European countries, for example, Sweden, have discontinued their BCG (Bacille Calmette-Guérin) vaccination regimen (Fine & Rodrigues 1990). The rate of decline had slowed in the 1960s mainly as a result of immigration from the Indian subcontinent. The incidence in the white population of the UK was 4.7 in 100,000 in 1988, whereas in the Indian immigrant population it was 134.6 in 100,000. Four hundred deaths per year are attributed to tuberculosis in England and Wales and men have double the incidence and mortality of women.

Guidelines for practice

Table 11.1 represents the immunisation schedule for babies and children in the UK.

11.5 MEDICO-LEGAL ISSUES

Consent

Consent may be written, verbal or implied. For informed consent to be given, patients or their parents or guardian must be informed of the possibility of common minor reactions and even rare serious reactions. They should of course be advised of the expected benefits of the procedure. Written consent is the ideal for medico-legal reasons. Verbal consent is acceptable, but unless witnessed may be hard to prove. Implied consent is assumed for example when a parent brings a child to an immunisation appointment. The use of protocols, which include the signing of written consent forms for each immunisation, can help to verify a high and consistent level of care. It must be remembered that children are entitled to give or refuse consent once they are old enough to understand the benefits and potential adverse effects (Shield & Baum 1994). It is good practice to encourage children to involve a parent in their decision. The spirit of the famous Gillick case has been challenged by subsequent decisions by the Court of Appeal, where children's refusal to consent to treat-

ment has been deemed irrational and, as such, evidence of their lack of competence to refuse consent (Devereux *et al.* 1993). Clinicians must consider each child individually and in case of doubt as to the child's competence to give or refuse consent, seek legal advice. As one might expect, recording of initial consent is associated with high rates of completed courses of vaccination (Pearson *et al.* 1993).

Prescribing

Under current regulations doctors retain the responsibility for the prescription of vaccines. The Department of Health has decreed that doctors may delegate the responsibility for immunisation to nurses providing the following conditions are fulfilled:

(1) The nurse is willing to be professionally accountable for this work as defined in the UKCC guidance on the 'Scope of Professional Practice'.
(2) The nurse has received training and is competent in all aspects of immunisation, including the contraindications to specific vaccines.
(3) Adequate training has been given in the recognition and treatment of anaphylaxis.

Legally doctors are obliged to issue a prescription for any vaccine before it is administered. Both the Royal College of Nursing and the General Medical Services Committee of the British Medical Association have recently called for the Department of Health to issue an Executive Letter to give nurses more legal protection until the law can be changed (Waters 1997). The nurse prescribing pilots have recently been evaluated and the latest white papers on primary care propose the extension of the scheme (Bradley *et al.*

Table 11.1 Immunisation schedule.

Age	Vaccines
2 months	Diph/Tet/Pertussis Polio Hib
3 months	Diph/Tet/Pertussis Polio Hib
4 months	Diph/Tet/Pertussis Polio Hib
12–15 months	Measles/Mumps/Rubella
3–5 years	Diph/Tet Polio Measles/Mumps/Rubella
10–14 years	BCG
13–18 years	Diph/Tet (with low dose diphtheria, i.e. Td)

1997). As with the administration of any drugs the following are a must:

- identify that the vaccine is the correct one;
- note that the expiry date has not been passed;
- record the date, the vaccines given and their batch numbers;
- record the site of each vaccine;
- ensure only correctly stored vaccines are used.

11.6 CONTRAINDICATIONS

Acute illness

If a child has an acute illness with fever or systemic upset it is wise to consider postponing vaccination until recovery.

Severe reaction

If a patient has a severe local or general reaction to a previous dose, then immunisation with the same vaccine should not proceed without specialist advice. The following are severe:

- Local: an extensive area of redness and swelling, which becomes indurated and involves most of the antero-lateral surface of the thigh or a major part of the circumference of the upper arm.
- General: fever of 39.5°C or above within 48 hours of vaccination; anaphylaxis; bronchospasm; laryngeal oedema; generalised collapse. Prolonged unresponsiveness; prolonged inconsolable or high-pitched screaming for more than four hours; convulsions or encephalopathy occurring within 72 hours.

Pertussis

There are no additional contraindications. Where a neurological problem exists which is still evolving, immunisation should be deferred until it is stable. If in doubt seek a specialist opinion.

Diphtheria and tetanus

No additional contraindications.

Haemophilus influenzae type b (Hib)

No additional contraindications, but its safety in pregnant women has not been established.

The live vaccines

The live vaccines are polio (oral polio virus i.e. OPV), MMR and BCG. Contraindications to live vaccines include:

- Children receiving high dose steroids, that is 2 mg/kg per day for more than one week or 1 mg/kg per day for one month should postpone vaccination with live vaccines until three months after the treatment has been stopped.
- Children with untreated malignancy or on treatment with chemotherapy or radiotherapy should not have live vaccines until six months after such treatment has ended.

Polio (oral polio virus i.e. OPV)

In addition to the above general contraindications to vaccination and those peculiar to live vaccines, children with diarrhoea or vomiting, and women in the first four months of pregnancy should have vaccination postponed. Oral polio virus (OPV) should not be given to the siblings or other household contacts of immunocompromised children, who should be given inactivated polio vaccine (IPV). Extreme hypersensitivity reactions to penicillin, neomycin, polymyxin or streptomycin (although rare) are contraindications to OPV.

Measles/mumps/rubella (MMR)

In addition to the above general contraindications to vaccination and those peculiar to live vaccines children with allergies to neomycin or kanamycin should not be given MMR. Children who have received another live vaccine (excluding polio), should delay MMR for three weeks, and children who have an injection of immunoglobulin should delay MMR for three months.

BCG (Bacille Calmette-Guérin)

In addition to the general contraindications to vaccination and those peculiar to live vaccines, BCG should not be given to any HIV (human immunodeficiency virus) positive individuals. It should also be withheld from patients with a positive tuberculin protein skin test and pregnant women.

11.7 ADVERSE REACTIONS

Mild redness and soreness at the injection site, and slight pyrexia and irritability may occur in approximately 15% of vaccinated babies. In 1995 of 14 million doses of vaccine distributed in the UK there were 152 reported reactions classified as serious. The risk of serious illness following natural infection greatly exceeds this.

The National Childhood Encephalopathy Study (DHSS 1981) failed to demonstrate statistically any increased risk of brain damage and encephalopathy after pertussis vaccination, despite three years of case finding and follow up. The American Academy of Pediatrics, the US National Vaccine Advisory Committee and the US Advisory Committee on Immunization Practices similarly found no proven link between the two.

Some specific adverse reactions are known to occur in addition to the general reactions outlined above and these are shown in Table 11.2.

Good injection technique can minimise the risk of local reactions. Parents should be advised of the need to have paracetamol available and how to manage fever.

Anaphylaxis

In addition to the reactions outlined so far and in Table 11.2, any patient receiving any vaccine must be considered at risk of developing an anaphylactic reaction to it. These reactions are extremely rare but may be fatal (see Figure 11.1). During the 1994 Measles Rubella Campaign approximately 8 million

Table 11.2 Specific adverse reactions to immunisation.

Vaccination	Adverse reaction
Diphtheria	Neurological reactions occasionally reported.
Tetanus	Rarely peripheral neuropathy.
Pertussis	Increased risk of febrile convulsions if given after child is six months old, especially with the third dose. No increased risk if given before six months old.
Polio (OPV)	Vaccine associated poliomyelitis has been reported in recipients and contacts at a rate of one per million doses of vaccine. If all contacts were immune this could be halved.
Haemophilus influenzae type b (Hib)	No additional risks.
Measles/mumps/rubella (MMR)	Febrile convulsions in 1 in 1000 in days 6–11 post vaccine. Thrombocytopaenia in 1 in 24,000. Rarely arthralgia or arthritis.
Bacille Calmette-Guérin (BCG)	Vertigo and dizziness occasionally. Large ulcers and abscesses at injection site. Keloid formation at injection site. Lymphadenitis rarely. Rarely dissemination of the organism.

- Flushing
- Urticaria
- Angioedema
- Hoarseness/stridor
- Rhinorrhoea
- Wheezing
- Abdominal pain
- Nausea and vomiting
- Metallic taste
- Tachycardia
- Hypotension
- Respiratory arrest
- Cardiac arrest

Figure 11.1 Features of anaphylaxis.

children were vaccinated. Eighty one cases of ana-phylaxis were reported. Available data suggests all made a full recovery. However all staff engaged in immunisation should be fully conversant with the diagnosis and management of anaphylaxis. It is important to be able to distinguish the condition from simple faints and convulsions. The presence of a strong carotid pulse is highly suggestive that collapse is due to a faint or convulsion.

Management of anaphylaxis

(1) Call for help and an ambulance immediately.
(2) Place child in recovery position.
(3) Maintain airway.
(4) Give intramuscular adrenaline (see Table 11.3 for dosages).
(5) Begin cardiopulmonary resuscitation if necessary.
(6) Give IV hydrocortisone.
(7) Consider nebulised salbutamol.
(8) Send to hospital for assessment.

Table 11.3 Recommended dose of adrenaline 1 in 1000 (1 mg/ml).

Age	Dose*
Under 1	0.05 ml
1–2	0.1 ml
2	0.2 ml
3–4	0.3 ml
5	0.4 ml
6–10	0.5 ml

* By intramuscular or subcutaneous injection in all cases.

11.8 SPECIAL SITUATIONS

Some children, for example from abroad may present with an unknown immunisation history. Assume children are unimmunised unless there is concrete evidence to the contrary. Such children should have the full primary course of three doses of diphtheria/tetanus/pertussis, polio and Hib, with boosters of diphtheria/tetanus and polio at five and then ten years later. Only children less than one year old need three doses of Hib. Those between one and four years require a single dose and it is unnecessary after the fourth birthday. Children above the age of one year require two doses of measles/mumps/rubella at least three months apart. Children aged over ten years should have tetanus and low dose diphtheria (Td), with MMR and OPV. Boosting should be with Td and OPV at five, then ten years later.

Splenectomy increases the risk from bacterial infections especially for the first two years. In addition to the routine schedule patients are advised to have pneumococcal vaccine (if aged over two years), Hib (irrespective of age), influenza and meningococcal (A and C) vaccine. Patients on haemodialysis should be screened for evidence of immunity to hepatitis B and given a course of three doses of hepatitis B vaccine if not immune. Annual monitoring for immunity should be carried out and if anti-HBs antibodies fall below 10 miu/ml reimmunisation is required.

Chronic renal disease and renal transplant increase infection risk and should be considered for Hib, pneumococcal and annual influenza vaccines.

Technique

Polio vaccine is given orally, BCG intradermally and diph/tet/pertussis, Hib and MMR given either intramuscularly or by deep subcutaneous injection. BCG is normally given over the insertion of the left deltoid muscle in the upper arm. Stretch the skin between thumb and finger and with the other hand insert the needle (26G) with its bevel upwards about 2 mm into the superficial layers of the dermis, almost parallel with the surface. Raise a tense bleb of about 7 mm diameter which blanches. The absence of resistance to injection suggests that the needle is too deep. In this case withdraw and reinsert. Intramuscular injections should be given into the antero-lateral thigh, using a 25G or 23G needle.

It is not necessary to use alcohol swabs to clean the skin. Dirty skin may be washed with soap. If any disinfectants are used the skin must be allowed to dry as they can inactivate live vaccines.

Storage

- All the vaccines referred to in this chapter should be stored in a refrigerator at a temperature between 2 and 8 degrees Celsius.
- Maximum and minimum temperatures should be recorded daily.
- Air should be allowed to circulate around vaccines which should not be stored in the refrigerator door.
- Stock should be rotated to facilitate the use of oldest vaccines first.
- Food should not be stored in the same refrigerator as vaccines.
- Vaccines are now delivered to centres by a commercial company in refrigerated vans to maintain the cold chain.

11.9 CONCLUSION

An overview of the present situation has been given, for the future the World Health organization objectives for the millennium include the eradication of polio, neo-natal tetanus, measles and congenital rubella. Developments may add chickenpox, rotavirus, meningococcal and Respiratory Syncytial Virus vaccines to our therapeutic armoury. Even small advances such as the recent availability of combined Hib/diph/tet/pertusssis vaccines are of significant benefit to children and their parents. One injection replaces two which will be welcomed by patient, parent and clinician. There is already evidence that the accelerated schedule of vaccination has reduced the incidence of post-vaccination febrile convulsions fourfold (Farrington *et al.* 1995).

REFERENCES

Adam, E.B., Laurence, DR and Smith, J.W.G. (1969) *Tetanus*. Blackwell Scientific, Oxford.

Bradley, C.P., Ross, J.T. and Blenkinsopp, A. (1997) Developing prescribing in primary care. *British Medical Journal*, **314**, 744–7.

Brown, D., Ramsay, M., Richards, A. and Miller, E. (1994) Salivary diagnosis of measles: a study of notified cases in the UK, 1991–1993. *British Medical Journal*, **308**, 1015–1017.

Community Disease Report (1998) *CDR Weekly*, **8**, 317–20.

Department of Health (1996) *Immunisation against Infectious Disease*. HMSO, London.

Department of Health (1998) *Measles, measles mumps rubella (MMR) vaccine, Crohn's disease and autism*. London: 27 March 1988. (PL/CMO/98/2). Cardiff: Welsh Office, 27 March 1998. (CMO(98)7).

Devereux, J.A., Jones, D.P.H. and Dickson, D.L. (1993) Can children withhold consent to treatment. *British Medical Journal*, **306**, 1459–61.

DHSS (1981) *Whooping cough*. Reports from the Committee on Safety of Medicines and the Joint Committee on Vaccination and Immunisation. HMSO, London.

Farrington, P., Pugh, S., Colville, A., Flower, A., Nash, J. Morgan-Capner, P. *et al.* (1995) A new method for active surveillance of adverse events from Diphtheria/Tetanus/Pertussis and MMR Vaccines. *Lancet*, **345**, 567–69.

Fenner, F., Anderson, D.A., Arita, I., Jezek, Z. & Ladnyi, I.D. (1980) *Smallpox and its Eradication*. World Health Organization, 1980, Geneva.

Fine, P.E.M. and Rodrigues, L.C. (1990) Mycobacterial disease. *Lancet*, **335**, 1016–19.

Fisher, P. (1990) Enough nonsense on immunisation. *British Homeopathy Journal*, **79**, 198–200.

Hargreaves, R.M., Slack, M.P.E., Howard, A.J., Anderson, E. & Ramsay, M.E. (1996) Changing patterns of *Haemophilus influenza* disease in England and Wales after introduction of Hib vaccination programme. *British Medical Journal*, **312**, 160–61.

Ingram, M. (1995) *Managing Immunisation in General Practice*. Radcliffe Medical Press, Oxford.

Joce, R., Wood, D., Brown, D. & Begg, N. (1992) Paralytic poliomyelitis in England and Wales 1985–1991. *British Medical Journal*, **305**, 79–82.

Kulenkampff, M., Schqartzman, J.S. & Wilson, J. (1974) Neurological complications of inoculations. *Archives of Disease in Childhood*, **49**, 46–9.

Maple, P.A., Efstratiou, A., George, R.C., Andrews, N.J. & Sesardic, D. (1995) Diptheria immunity in United Kingdom blood donors. *Lancet*, **345**, 963–5.

Miller, C., Farrington, C.P. & Harbert, K. (1992) The epidemiology of subacute sclerosing panencephalitis in England and Wales 1970 to 1989. *International Journal of Epidemiology*, **21**, 998–1006.

Miller, E., Craddock-Watson, J.E. & Pollok, T.M. (1982) Consequences of confirmed maternal rubella at different stages of pregnancy. *Lancet*, **ii**, 781–4.

Moskowitz, R. (1984) The case against immunisation. *The Homeopath*, **4**, 4.

Office of Home Economics (1984) *Childhood Vaccination: Current Controversies*. Office of Health Economics, London.

Pearson, M., Makowiecka, K., Gregg, J., Woollard, J., Rogers, M. & West, C. (1993) Primary immunisations in Liverpool. I: Who withholds consent? *Archives of Disease in Childhood*, **69**, 110–114.

Peltola, H., Palja, A., Leinikki, P., Valle, M., Davidkin, I. & Paunio, M. (1998) No evidence for measles, mumps, and rubella vaccine-associated inflammatory bowel disease or autism in a 14-year prospective study. *Lancet*, **351**, 1327–8.

Rima, B.K. (1994) Mumps virus. *Encyclopedia of Virology*, (ed. R.G. Webster & A. Granoff), Academic Press, London.

Shield, J.P.H. & Baum, J.D. (1994) Children's consent to treatment: listen to the children – they will have to live with the decision. *British Medical Journal*, **308**, 1182–83.

Wakefield, A.J., Murch, S.H., Linnell, A.A.J., Casson, D.M., *et al.* (1998) Ileal-lymphoid-nodular hyperplasia, non-specific colitis and pervasive developmental disorder in children. *Lancet*, **351**, 637–41.

Waters, A. (1997) CPS refuses to protect nurses from prosecution. *General Practitioner*, 7 March, p. 3.

Whitman, C., Belgharbi, L., Gasse, F., Torel, C., Mattei, V. & Zoffman, H. (1992) Progress towards the global elimination of neonatal tetanus. *World Health Statistics Quarterley*, 45, 248–56.

12

Managing Infections: How to Help Parents
Jane Willock

12.1 INTRODUCTION

With the implementation of national immunisation schemes, many life-threatening childhood infections, such as poliomyelitis, tetanus, diphtheria, measles and pertussis are becoming less common. In addition, improvements in treatment and antibiotic therapy have reduced the complications of diseases, such as scarlet fever, for which there is no immunisation. This chapter will consider evidence concerning childhood infections, including intestinal parasites, skin and hair problems and guidelines for practice.

12.2 CURRENT CONTEXT

Table 12.1 shows the incidence of notifiable diseases in 1994, associated with very few deaths. However, in Britain today some infections such as tuberculosis are again on the increase.

Tuberculosis most commonly affects the lungs; 394 cases of respiratory tuberculosis were reported in children under the age of 20 years in 1994 (OPCS 1996). Tuberculosis can also affect bones, intestines, kidneys and other parts of the body; 221 non-respiratory cases were reported in children under 20 years in 1994 (OPCS, 1996). National data have shown that between 1988 and 1992 the notification rate of tuberculosis in the poorest 30% of the population in England and Wales increased, particularly in the younger age groups, but no increase was observed in the remainder of the population. In 1992, 29% of notified cases occurred in the 10% of the population with the highest deprivation index. Overcrowding was demonstrated to be the factor most strongly related to the incidence of tuberculosis, followed by the proportion of ethnic minority residents in a district (Bhatti et al. 1995). Evidence from the USA and Africa suggests that there has been an increase in the incidence of tuberculosis in people infected with human immunodeficiency virus (HIV); this is not yet evident in the UK. However, if the number of people infected with HIV rises, the risk of exposure of tuberculosis and the increase in the number of infections in children is expected to rise (OPCS 1995).

Smoking and secondary inhalation of cigarette smoke has been significantly associated with the frequency of tonsillitis (Hinton et al. 1993), otitis media (Etzel et al. 1992; Ey at al. 1995), and respiratory tract infections (OPCS 1995). Cigarette smoke decreases the beat of the cilia lining the mucous membranes of the respiratory tract and middle ear. This leads to stagnation of the respiratory and ear secretions, increasing susceptibility to respiratory and ear infections (Agius et al. 1995). A pronounced socio-economic gradient in smoking is evident in adults, with unskilled manual groups having the highest consumption (Bunting 1997).

Breast feeding provides some protection for the infant from infections such as gastrointestinal illness, respiratory illness, and otitis media by providing a nutritionally balanced diet, antimicrobial and anti-inflammatory agents and some antibodies (Duncan et al. 1993; Beaudry et al. 1995; Henschel & Inch, 1996). This is discussed in more depth in Chapter 7.

Table 12.1 Incidence of notifiable diseases in England and Wales in 1994 (all ages) 1994 Communicable Disease Statistics, Office for National Statistics © Crown Copyright 1999.

Disease	Number of cases	Number of deaths
Measles	16375	1
Rubella	6326	0
Scarlet fever	6193	1
Whooping cough	3964	3
Mumps	2494	0
H. influenzae meningitis	52	1
Diphtheria	9	2
Acute poliomyelitis	0	0
Respiratory tuberculosis	Approx. 80 per million population	Approx. 8 per million population

(Office for National Statistics 1996)

Housing conditions may also contribute to infection. The number of households accepted as homeless rose from 53,000 in 1978 to 145,800 in 1990. Over 80% of these households had dependent children or a member who was pregnant (OPCS 1995). Hygiene may be a problem for poor and homeless families due to lack of hot water, lack of laundry facilities and insufficient clothing and bedding to enable frequent changing. Damp, cold accommodation increases the prevalence of respiratory tract infections, and overcrowding increases the spread of most infections. Babies and children in bed and breakfast accommodation are more susceptible to gastrointestinal and respiratory infections, and have higher rates of malnutrition than babies and children in stable accommodation (Lowry 1991). It should also be remembered that for disadvantaged families a nutritious diet may be much harder to achieve (see Chapter 9).

12.3 CHILDHOOD INFECTIONS

The common cold

The common cold is an everyday problem for children and their parents. Symptoms are nasal discharge caused by damage to capillary cells by the cold virus, nasal congestion, sneezing, watery eyes, sore throat, tickly cough caused by excess fluid draining down the throat, and mild fever (Gleeson 1993; Sinclair 1996). The child may also develop sinusitis and a headache. The nasal discharge is usually colourless and watery, a coloured discharge may indicate infection.

Infants with nasal congestion have problems feeding as it is difficult to breathe through the mouth and suck at the same time. Children in their first year at school tend to catch frequent colds when they mix with many other children. Children with respiratory tract infections generally find breathing easier if they are sitting up, or propped up on three or four pillows when in bed; infants can be nursed in a 'sitta chair' and the head end of the cot can be raised slightly during sleep times (placing a pillow under the covers to stop the infant sliding down under the covers).

Vasoconstrictors work by constricting the blood vessels in the nasal mucosa and therefore reducing the mucosal thickness and secretions. Examples of vasoconstrictors are ephedrine and pseudoephedrine. Topical vasoconstrictors can cause rebound congestion which may be worse than before the medication was used, they should therefore not be used more than twice a day or for longer than a week. Most topical vasoconstrictors are not recommended for infants under three months, and it is recommended that the pharmacist's advice is sought before administering vasoconstrictors to children under two years (Sinclair 1996). The contents of inhalation capsules should be applied according to the instructions and not applied directly to the baby's face (Blake 1993).

Care of infants and children with colds

Mild fever and discomfort may be relieved with paracetamol. Care should be taken to check the ingredients of cold remedies to prevent inadvertently giving a double dose of paracetamol.

Topical decongestants, such as Karvol, used in the evening help the child to sleep at night. Propping the child up on extra pillows may also help to relieve congestion. Children should be taught to blow their noses closing one side of the nose and blowing one nostril at a time to prevent infected mucous spreading into the Eustachian tubes and causing an ear infection. Tissues and handkerchiefs used for nose blowing should not be used to wipe the eyes as they may transfer infection into the eyes and cause conjunctivitis (Gleeson 1993).

The child should be given extra fluids preferably of a sugar-free kind, to compensate for the nasal discharge. Infants may find it easier to take feeds if the milk is given slowly with a feeder beaker or a teaspoon, as they may find sucking a bottle difficult and tiring.

Eye infections

'Sticky eyes' and conjunctivitis

Conjunctivitis is one of the most common infections in the neo-natal period and can affect up to one in four babies (Krohn *et al.* 1993). Usually there is no infection and cooled, boiled water or sterile saline can be used to soften and remove exudate from the eye lashes and around the eyes. If pus is present swabs should be taken for culture to confirm a diagnosis. These should be put into standard and chlamidial transport medium, and a medical diagnosis should be sought.

Conjunctivitis may be caused after birth by staphylococcal, streptococcal or pseudomonal organisms, or during delivery by *Neisseria gonorrhoeae* or *Chlamydia trachomatis* from the birth canal of an infected mother. There were 268 reported cases of opthalmia neonatorum in England and Wales in 1994 (OPCS 1996). Gonococcal infection is now quite rare in industrialised countries.

Ordinary bacterial infections such as those caused by *Staphylococcus* can be treated with chloramphenicol eye drops or ointment. Parents should be taught the correct technique for cleaning the eyes and instilling eye drops or applying eye ointment. The baby's eyes should first be cleaned to remove exudate, the drops or ointment applied making sure that liquid from one eye does not enter the other eye. Separate bottles of eye drops or tubes of ointment should be used for each eye to prevent any cross infection occurring. Excess medication can be gently removed from the edges of the eyelids with sterile cotton wool approximately one minute after installation (Delahoussaye 1994).

Ear infections

External otitis

External otitis refers to inflammation of the external auditory meatus with accompanying discharge. Excessive wetness (swimming, inadequate drying of ears after bathing, high atmospheric humidity), dryness (previous infection, dry skin conditions, insufficient cerumen), and trauma (e.g. foreign bodies) make the skin of the ear canal vulnerable to infection from normal skin flora and introduced infection.

The predominant symptom is severe ear pain, especially when the pinna is handled. The external auditory meatus is red and swollen, and may be almost closed. There may be a small amount of offensive discharge. Lymph nodes around the ear may be enlarged and painful. Conductive hearing loss may occur as a result of oedema of the skin and tympanic membrane, serous or purulent secretions, and in chronic external otitis, skin thickening due to longstanding chronic infection. External otitis may be caused by bacterial, viral and fungal infections. *Candida* and *Staphylococcus* are the most common infectious agents.

Acute otitis media

One of the most common infections in early childhood, it is estimated that 76% of children will have had at least one episode of otitis media by the age of two years (Hunsberger & Feenan 1994). The child will have a fever, pain, and a red, bulging tympanic membrane. The tympanic membrane may perforate and a purulent discharge from the ear may be seen. Infants may also present with irritability, crying and vomiting, loss of appetite, loose stools, and general malaise.

The infective agent may be bacterial or viral, most commonly *Streptococcus pneumonae* and *Haemophilus influenzae* (Levine 1991; Mair 1996). Otitis media may also be caused by obstruction of the Eustachian tube by enlarged adenoids (Levine 1991). Paracetamol should be administered to relieve pain and fever. Nasal decongestants may be effective. A medical diagnosis should be sought and antibiotic therapy may be commenced.

Complications include otitis media with effusion, conductive deafness, mastoiditis, perforation of the tympanic membrane, chronic otitis media and facial palsy (Levine 1991).

Otitis media with effusion (glue ear)

At least 50% of all pre-school children have at least one episode of otitis media with effusion (OME). Conductive hearing loss is extremely common. Severe persistent OME (affecting about 7% of children) may result in significant language delay, behaviour disturbance and occasionally disturbance in balance (Hall 1996).

Deafness is caused by fluid in the middle ear. This may be unrecognised until the child is screened for hearing impairment (Levine 1991). Parents' worries should be taken seriously, as it has been reported that one case in three of otitis media with effusion is diagnosed when parents report vague symptoms in their child such as tugging at the ears, and suspected hearing impairment (Alho *et al.* 1995).

The average length of otitis media with effusion is 1–2 months, and some children are more prone to this condition than others. In most cases the condition spontaneously resolves and hearing improves. In children prone to OME examination of the ears about every six months should detect children in need of intervention. In these cases surgical treatment, in the form of grommets to drain the middle ear, is often recommended although the efficiency of this procedure is questionable. (Effective Health Care 1992; Hogan *et al.* 1997).

Tonsillitis

Tonsillitis is often associated with ear infections and hearing problems. The tonsils, although part of the immune system, may harbour organisms that lead to recurrent infections. If frequent, this can lead to disrupted schooling due to prolonged periods of illness and surgical removal of the tonsils may be necessary.

The child may complain of a sore or painful throat, high temperature and reduced appetite. If the palatine tonsils become very oedematous they may meet in the midline, obstructing the entry of air and food. Enlargement of the adenoids may block the space behind the posterior nares, making nose breathing impossible, this will result in mouth breathing, dry mouth, impaired sense of taste and smell, and speech impairment (Clarke 1995). The child with tonsillitis may also complain of abdominal pain due to mesenteric adenitis (Levine 1991). Infections are mainly caused by streptococcal strains.

Tonsillitis is usually treated with antibiotics and symptomatic relief for painful throat and pyrexia provided by cool drinks and paracetamol (Mair 1996). The criteria for the removal of the tonsils is controversial as the tonsils protect the respiratory and alimentary tracts from infection. This is especially important for young children who are more susceptible to upper respiratory tract infections (Clarke 1995). The mortality rate associated with a combined tonsillectomy and adenoidectomy ranges from 0.004 to 0.006%, and the risk of local haemorrhage associated with surgical intervention requiring treatment ranges from 0.49–4.00%. It is not recommended for children with a submucous cleft palate to undergo adenoidectomy as this can result in speech impairment (Berman 1995).

The complications of tonsillitis include otitis media, chronic tonsillitis, peritonsillar abscess, airway obstruction and post-streptococcal allergic disorders such as acute nephritis and rheumatic fever (Levine 1991).

Meningococcal meningitis

Amongst the childhood diseases meningitis causes most anxiety in parents and recent media attention to small local outbreaks has added to the atmosphere of panic.

The infective agent in meningitis is *Neisseria meningitidis*. It is probably spread through respiratory droplets. Colonisation of the upper respiratory tract is usually asymptomatic and can last for weeks or months (Estabrook 1996). The child may initially experience headache (possibly with photophobia), followed by neck stiffness, malaise, fever and petechial reddish-purple rapidly spreading rash which does not blanch on applying pressure (Disabato & Wulf 1994).

Meningitis is fatal in about 85% of cases (Fielder 1995) and any child suspected of contracting the disease should be referred to a hospital immediately for emergency treatment.

Chickenpox

Chickenpox is one of the commonest of the childhood diseases and most children will develop chickenpox at some time, usually in the pre-school and early school years.

The varicella zoster virus causes chickenpox and it is spread by droplet from respiratory secretions and to a lesser extent contact from skin lesions (not crusts) and contaminated objects. The incubation period for chickenpox is two to three weeks, usually 13 to 17 days, and the child will probably be infectious one day before the eruption of the lesions to six days after the first crop of vesicles, when crusts have formed. Usually once a child has had chickenpox he or she is immune to further infection, but second infections have been reported.

The child has a mild pyrexia, malaise and anorexia in the first 24 hours then in the acute phase of the disease the very itchy rash begins as a macula rash, rapidly becoming papula, then becoming vesicular. All three stages may be present at the same time. The rash spreads from the body to the face and upper limbs.

Secondary bacterial infections, such as pneumonia, abscesses or cellulitis, may develop as complications to chickenpox. Other complications include encephalitis, varicella pneumonia, haemorrhages in the vesicles and petechiae on the skin, chronic or transient thrombocytopenia, and Reye's syndrome if aspirin is administered.

Management of chickenpox involves:

- application of calamine lotion and diphenhydramine hydrochloride to relieve itching;
- keeping the skin clean to prevent secondary infection;
- administering paracetamol to make the child more comfortable;
- keeping nails short; use scratch mittens for babies;
- teaching older children to apply pressure to itchy area rather than scratching;
- strict isolation at home.

Where the child is at risk of complications strict isolation in hospital away from other high risk patients is required. For children at risk of complications, for example those who are immunosuppressed, on steroid therapy or immunosuppressive therapy, Varicella Zoster Immunoglobulin (VZIG) within three days of exposure is indicated. An anti-viral agent (such as acyclovir) is recommended for high risk patients.

Infectious mononucleosis (glandular fever)

Glandular fever can be particulary debilitating and is more common in older children. It is caused by the Epstein-Barr virus and is probably transmitted by saliva. It has an incubation period of 30 to 50 days and the infectious period may be as long as six months.

The child will have a fever, lasting up to 14 days, headache and malaise, followed by a sore throat and lymphadenopathy especially in cervical glands. A thick white exudate may be present on enlarged tonsils, and petechiae on the soft palate. There may some splenomegaly and hepatomegaly. Complications can include hepatitis, pneumonia, meningitis and myelitis.

Symptomatic treatment of fever, sore throat and malaise is recommended (Rudd 1991).

For a summary table of other childhood diseases see Appendix 12.1. Also see Chapter 11, which describes childhood diseases for which immunisation is available.

12.4 INTESTINAL PARASITES

Any child or adult can become infested with intestinal parasites and it should not be associated with squalor or poor standards of hygiene. Table 12.2 outlines some common intestinal parasites.

Prevention of infection by intestinal parasites in children is difficult; for example a child may hold hands with a child with threadworm eggs under his or her nails. Sucking fingers also increases the likelihood of infestation. However, advice can be given to prevent spread within a family:

- keep children's nails short and take particular care where threadworms are present;
- infected children should wear close fitting pants at nighttime, to prevent scratching;
- take extra care over hand washing, especially after visits to the toilet.

Factors such as overcrowding, poor sanitation and environmental sources need to be taken into account when planning the most realistic approach to treat-

Table 12.2 Common intestinal parasites.

Parasite	Source	Features	Diagnosis	Specific management
Giardia lamblia Flagellate protozoan	Ingestion of food or water contaminated by the cysts of the parasite (Porter *et al.* 1988, 1990).	Endemic in most countries, high prevalence in young malnourished children. Trophozoite form may adhere to small intestinal mucosa disrupting structure and reducing absorptive function. May be asymptomatic, however young children may have failure to thrive, anorexia, diarrhoea, vomiting. Older children may complain of abdominal pain, also may have loose stools or constipation. Stools – malodorous, greasy, may be watery.	Stool microscopy, jejunal juice microscopy or intestinal biopsy.	Most infections resolve spontaneously, but many last for months or years. Metronidazole.
Threadworm (Enterobius vermicularis)	Household dust.	Perianal and vulval pruritus – this may lead to sleep problems, irritability and bedwetting in young children.	'Tape test' – sticky tape pressed against the perianal area will reveal threadworms on microscopic examination. Mobile thread-like worms are easily seen between buttocks of sleeping child.	Difficult to eradicate, treatment only necessary if symptomatic. Whole family should be treated. Mebendazole – children over 2 years: 100 mg as single dose, may be repeated 2–3 weeks later if re-infection is suspected. Not recommended for children under 2 years. Piperazine – dose and administration vary with age of child and preparation. Hygiene measures to prevent re-infection.
Roundworm (Ascaris lumbricoides)	Ingestion of eggs from hands that have been in contact with contaminated dust, soil and contaminated inadequately washed raw fruit or vegetables.	Rare gut symptoms include pain, obstruction, appendicitis, and rarely intestinal perforation and peritonitis. Pneumonitis and eosinophilia during larval stage if infestation is heavy.	Positive stool culture for ova and parasites.	Mebendazole – children over 2 years: 100 mg twice daily for 3 days. Piperazine treats adult phase – may be given as a single dose. Improvements in hygiene.

Toxocara canis and catis	Dog and cat excreta. Strongly associated with puppy ownership and pica (the habit of eating dirt).	Many cases are asymptomatic. General malaise, cough irritability and dizziness. Eosinophilia, hepatomegaly, bronchospasm. May lead to sight impairment or complete loss of vision (an estimated 100 to 200 cases of toxocara eye disease are diagnosed each year) or epilepsy if larvae encapsulate in the eye or the brain. (Elliott, 1995)	Eosinophilia. Serological diagnosis by enzyme linked immunosorbent assay (ELISA) test (Rée et al. 1984).	Diethylcarbamide corticosteroids. Regular de-worming of pets.
Tapeworm (Taenia saginata – beef tapeworm, Taenia solium – pork tapeworm)	Ingestion of tapeworm larvae from inadequately cooked pork or beef, or from hands after handling raw pork or beef.	Adult lengthens in small intestine by generating segments. Larvae may form cysts and calcify in the tissues such as brain or eye.	Positive stool culture for ova and parasites.	Adult tapeworms may be killed by niclosamide – age specific dose.

(Hull & Johnston 1993; Feroli 1994; Powell 1995; Joint Formulary Committee 1998) ment and prevention of recurrence of intestinal parasites. Parents and children need to be given information about taking medication, hand washing and personal hygiene to prevent re-infestation. Families living in poverty may need practical assistance to ensure that they are able to follow advice.

12.5 GUIDELINES FOR PRACTICE

Caring for a sick child at home

Gastroenteritis

Diarrhoea in children under two years is very common. Rehydration, using a solution of rehydration sachets made up according to manufacturer's instructions, should be advised. Parents should be made aware that they should not make up rehydration solution too concentrated as it may lead to sodium overload. Babies become dehydrated very quickly and may need to be admitted to hospital for rehydration.

Toddlers may have diarrhoea due to changing diet from baby food to more adult food; this is normal and parents should not worry as long as the child is happy and thriving. However, if the child is drawing his knees up with coliky abdominal pain and passing bloody or red currant jelly-like stools, intussusception should be considered, this is an emergency and the child should be immediately referred to a paediatrician. In children aged 5–16 years episodes of diarrhoea are fairly common, usually viral in origin and self limiting. At this age sensitivity to gluten may be diagnosed, coeliac disease may be unrecognised until the child starts infant or junior school and failure to thrive compared with peers becomes apparent. Appendicitis in this age group may present with a mild change in bowel habit and vague abdominal pain in the first 12 to 24 hours (Kerrigan 1996).

Children who have diarrhoea and are not dehydrated, and children who had mild to moderate dehydration but have been rehydrated can take age-appropriate diets (Provisional Committee on Quality Improvement, Sub-Committee on Acute Gastroenteritis 1996). The duration of diarrhoea in milk fed infants has been shown to be reduced when a low-lactose milk feed is given rather than normal cows' milk (Wall *et al.* 1994). Antidiarrhoeal agents are not very effective in childhood and can be harmful, therefore parents are best advised to avoid them (Davies & Jenkins 1992).

Fever

High temperature can make children feel uncomfortable, irritable, and can precipitate a febrile convulsion. Febrile convulsions affect about 3% of children and are one of the most common neurological conditions in childhood. They mainly occur in children aged between six months and three years, affecting children under 18 months most frequently. Boys are twice as susceptible as girls, and there appears to be a genetic predisposition. A sudden rise in temperature to above 38.8°C is usually the main precipitating factor, and in 25% of affected children convulsions recur with subsequent fevers. There appears to be little risk of neurological damage following a febrile convulsion (Fielder 1995).

There are two types of febrile convulsion, simple and complex. Simple febrile convulsions last from 10 to 15 minutes and are generalised. Complex febrile convulsions last longer and have focal features (Fielder 1995). It is important to reassure parents that these convulsions are not a form of epilepsy. Parents should be taught how to measure their child's temperature and how to maintain it within normal limits. Research has shown that tepid sponging of children does not significantly reduce their temperature and can cause shivering and agitation (Herder 1994). The most effective way to reduce a child's temperature is to administer paracetamol, give the child a warm (36°C) shallow bath then dress in light underwear (vest and nappy) in a comfortably warm room (Kinmonth *et al.* 1992).

Parents can be taught how to care for children with febrile convulsions. The child should be protected from injury; sharp or hard objects should be removed if they are near the child. The child should not be restrained, if secured in a pram or pushchair he/she should be taken out and placed on the floor, parents should not try to restrain the child or place anything in the mouth. After the convulsion, the child should be placed on his or her side (to prevent the tongue obstructing the airway) in the cot, and someone should stay with the child until consciousness is regained. If prescribed, parents can be taught how to administer rectal drugs such as paracetamol or diazepam.

Hydration and nutrition during minor illness

When caring for a child with a fever, parents should be advised to encourage intake of cool fluids to replace body fluids lost in sweating. A good rough guide would be 1.5–2 litres of fluid per day for a child over 12 months, this is essential if the child is sweating a lot. Children with a sore throat may not be able to tolerate acidic fruit drinks, but may find more relief with milky drinks. If an infant is breast fed, this should not be discontinued. Parents should be reassured that the child will come to no harm from not eating for two or three days as long as there is sufficient fluid intake. These children can be supplemented with high calorie drinks such as milk shakes, and normal diet can be reintroduced gradually.

12.6 SKIN AND HAIR PROBLEMS

Common non-infectious skin problems

Napkin dermatitis (nappy rash)

Napkin dermatitis is the most common form of non-allergic, irritant, contact dermatitis in infancy, occurring in approximately 50% of young children. The peak age of incidence is between 9 and 12 months and the incidence is reported as higher in bottle fed than breast fed infants (Campbell & Glasper 1995).

Napkin dermatitis is characterised by the appearance of a red rash on the waist, buttocks and thighs, often sparing the crevices of the groin and perineum (Ryan 1993). It is caused by the prolonged contact of the skin with urine and faeces, resulting in the breakdown of urine to form ammonia and other irritant products harmful to tender skin (Ryan 1993). Residues of detergent in towelling nappies may also have an irritant effect and the use of waterproof pants helps to create an ideal environment for napkin dermatitis to develop (Jethwa 1994). The use of disposable nappies does reduce (but not eliminate) its incidence (Carter & Dearmun 1995).

Seborrhoeic dermatitis

Seborrhoeic dermatitis is a chronic inflammatory reaction of the skin that occurs most commonly on the scalp (cradle cap) but may involve the eyelids, external ear canal, nasolabial folds and inguinal region (Campbell & Glasper 1995). It appears as thick, scaly, oily lesions that may or may not be mildly pruritic. The cause of seborrhoeic dermatitis is unknown, although it is more common in early infancy when sebum production is increased. Incidence is not associated with a positive family history.

Infectious skin problems

Candida albicans ('thrush')

Candida albicans or 'thrush' is a fungal infection which presents in the mouth as white discrete patches surrounded by erythema, or in the nappy area as an erythematous rash with numerous sharply marginated satellite lesions which may involve the insides of the thighs and the abdomen (Nicol & Hill 1994). These lesions are characteristic and diagnosis can be made on this observation alone (Randall & Soefer 1983). Often the mouth and the nappy area are affected at the same time. Oral Candida can cause pain and discomfort and therefore impair feeding. Candida nappy rash does not improve when commercial barrier creams are used.

Cold sores

Cold sores occur as a result of herpes simplex virus infection. Transmission is by contact from hands and objects such as towels and flannels. From initial contact with the virus to appearance of the infection takes approximately 2–20 days. Once infected the virus remains latent and can be reactivated by several factors such as fever, emotional upset, exposure to sunlight, trauma, menstruation and immunodepression (Nicol & Hill 1994).

Cold sores comprise grouped burning and itching vesicles surrounded by an area of inflammation, usually on or near junctions with mucosal tissues (lips, nose, genitals, buttocks). Vesicles become dry, forming a crust, followed by shedding of the crust and spontaneous healing in 8–10 days. Cold sores may be accompanied by regional lymphadenopathy.

Scarring can occur if secondary infection is introduced. In severe cases stomatitis may inhibit intake of food and drink due to pain, which can be temporarily relieved with anaesthetic mouthwashes. Salty, fizzy and fruity drinks are most irritating and should be avoided, bland and milky drinks are tolerated best (Nicol & Hill 1994). Cold sores may be aggravated by corticosteroids and can be fatal in immunosuppressed children.

Stye (hordeolum)

A stye is caused by a staphylococcal infection of the glands on the margins of the eyelid producing a small abscess. It is usually contracted by hand to eye contact by children rubbing their eyes. Frequent infections may be associated with visual impairment due to children rubbing their eyes when their vision is not clear. The stye itself has no detrimental effect on vision (Nicol & Hill 1994).

The stye causes pain, redness and periauricular lymph node enlargement. The surrounding eyelid becomes tender and swollen. Superficial abscesses spontaneously come to a head, rupture and heal within one to two days.

Headlice (pediculosis capitis)

Headlice are most likely in the pre-school and early school age probably due to the close group activity at this age. It is thought to be more common in white people than any other group due to the makeup of the hair shaft (Colson 1995). Transmission is by direct hair to hair contact, especially short, clean hair. Infection from such things as combs, hats and clothing is debatable (Sutkowski 1989)

The headlouse usually lives its entire life on the head of the child it infests. The eggs ('nits') are silvery, greyish or white in colour and are attached to the hair shaft near the scalp by a cement-like substance. They are most easily seen behind the ears and at the nape of the neck. The egg hatches within a week and the hatched nymph matures into an adult louse which may be seen as a black speck which moves and jumps on the scalp (Feroli 1994). Within 7 to 10 days it punctures the scalp and sucks blood. After a week the child may develop an allergic response with intense itching and scratching may introduce secondary infection. The allergic reaction subsides after prolonged exposure.

Paronychia

Paronychia is a *Staphylococcus aureus* infection at the margins of the nails especially in neo-nates. It appears as redness around the nail margins, which may have exudate and flaking skin, and is spread by washing in an unclean bowl especially or by wearing unclean mittens. Multiple paronychiae indicate systemic infection and should be treated as an emergency with systemic flucloxacillin, as septicaemia can rapidly lead to death.

Furunculosis (boils)

The usual agent of infection producing boils is a pathogenic *Staphylococcus*. The bacteria invade the sebaceous glands and hair follicles, usually at the sites of disruption in the skin, for example scratches or grazes. The skin becomes red around a hair follicle followed by the growth of a pustule with tenderness, heat, and swelling due to odema. The centre becomes yellow with pus and eventually drains purulent material. Healing occurs in one or two weeks. The most commonly affected sites are the back of the neck, the axillas, the buttocks and the thighs. Boils are most common in diabetic patients and patients with a compromised immune status. A systemic effect may be malaise if severe. Boils tend to heal with scar formation (Nicol & Hill 1994).

Carbuncles are similar to furuncles but affect adjacent hair follicles and drain through multiple openings. They may enlarge through multiple openings, enlarging to the size of an egg or an orange and are very painful. When they drain they leave a large ulcerated area which may take several weeks to granulate and usually leaves a scar.

Cellulitis

Cellulitis can be caused by infection with *Streptococcus*, *Staphylococcus* or *Haemophilus influenzae* and results in inflammation of skin and subcutaneous tissues with intense redness, swelling, and firm infiltration (a firm area under the skin). Infection usually occurs at or near the site of a wound or skin trauma; anywhere, but most commonly fingertips, periorbital cheeks, and over large joints. Facial cellulitis may occur with dental disease (Hanna 1991); otitis media may be associated with facial cellulitis. Lymphangitis 'streaking' is frequently seen, and involvement of regional lymph nodes is common. It may progress to abscess formation and can be very painful due to intense pressure in tissues.

If systemic symptoms are present the child may need admitting to hospital for parenteral antibiotics (Hooton 1995). Systemic effects include: fever, malaise, lethargy.

Shingles

Once infection with primary varicella (chickenpox) is resolved, the virus often persists in a dormant form which later may result in shingles. Initial neuralgic pain (usually mild in children), hyperaesthesia or itching is followed by the appearance of crops of vesicles on the skin tracing the course of a nerve, usually the posterior root ganglion or posterior horn of the spinal cord. Chickenpox may follow exposure to shingles. In children with depressed immunity, shingles can be fatal.

Impetigo

Impetigo is very contagious and spreads rapidly in environments such as nurseries, occuring most frequently in children under 10 years of age. It is most common in middle to late summer. It is caused by *Staphylococcus aureus* and *Streptococcus pyogenes* and is spread by contact, especially through using shared towels. Impetigo may also be transmitted by insect bites. It is particularly infectious among those living in crowded conditions with poor sanitary facilities.

The face, hands and scalp are most frequently involved; an initial small patch of redness enlarges rapidly into a spreading vesicle, which bursts and forms a scab (Colson 1995). It tends to spread peripherally in sharply modulated irregular outlines. Regional lymph nodes may also be involved. Pruritis is common.

Scarring occurs if lesions develop secondary infection and, rarely, post-streptococcal glomerulonephritis if nephritogenic strains of streptococci are involved (Nicol & Hill 1994).

Ringworm

Ringworm results from infection with the *Microsporium canis* fungus. In children it most commonly affects the scalp; in adults it is more commonly seen in the groin and as a fungal disease of the nails. Children typically have one or more scaly patches of hair loss where the hair in the affected areas is broken off just above the skin surface, producing an irregular stubble. Ringworm of the trunk or limbs is usually associated with scalp ringworm. The lesions are roughly circular with a red scaly edge and central clearing.

Scabies

The infective agent in scabies is the mite *Sacroptes scabiei*. It may be difficult to indentify the source of infection as the incubation period may be up to two months; transmission is by close contact. Most commonly scabies is found in creases of the skin and between fingers and toes, although it can occur anywhere on the body. Characteristic burrows can be seen as fine grey lines 5–10 mm long, although they can be obscured by excoriation due to scratching (Colson 1995). Itching tends to start at night as the warmth of the bed increases the irritation (Feroli 1994). Irritation is severe and secondary bacterial infection may be introduced due to scratching.

Verruca (warts)

Infection with the human papilloma virus causes verrucas. The source of infection is contact, probably through an abrasion or cut. Verrucas are auto-innoculable. They appear as small benign tumours, usually with a well defined margin, and have grey or brown papules with a roughened texture. They can occur anywhere but usually on exposed areas such as fingers, hands, face and soles of the feet. They may be single or multiple and are asymptomatic. Verrucas are common in children and tend to disappear spontaneously.

Variants of verruca include the:

- Common wart (infection with verruca vulgaris) – skin coloured to brown, rough surface epithelial growth, may be single or multiple, most frequently on backs and palms of hands and fingers and around nails.
- Juvenile wart (verruca plana juvenilis) – skin coloured to brown, slightly raised smooth lesion. Multiple lesions commonly located on face and backs of hands.
- Plantar wart (verruca plantaris) – located on plantar surface of feet, practically flat due to pressure, may be surrounded by a collar of hyperkeratosis.

Repeated irritation of warts may cause them to enlarge (Hooton 1995).

Tinea pedis (athlete's foot)

The infectious agent in athlete's foot is a fungus and transmission is by contact with infected surfaces. Infection manifests as scaling in the web spaces between the toes, occasionally extending to the dorsal surfaces of the feet sometimes with itchy vesicles. Athlete's foot is uncommon in childhood.

The spread of many skin infections can be largely prevented by washing with soap and water, frequent changes of clothes, bedding and towels. However, for families living in adverse circumstances such as poverty, this may be an unachievable goal. Table 12.3 outlines specific management and treatment of the skin and hair problems described above.

Table 12.3 Specific management of common skin and hair infections and infestations.

Condition	Specific management/treatment
Napkin dermatitis	Prevention is best achieved through regular nappy changes, careful washing of the nappy area with mild soap and water and application of a water repellent barrier cream (Jethwa 1994). If towelling nappies are used they must be soaked and washed in appropriate solutions to remove ammonia. Once nappy rash is present such hygiene practices are even more essential in order to keep the skin clean and dry. Avoidance of the occlusive environment of the nappy and exposing the skin to light and air aids drying and healing, but in practice may be only possible for short periods. Mild forms may be treated with a standard nappy rash cream. Severe forms may require an antibacterial and/or antifungal preparation (Jethwa 1994). Medical advice should be sought if the condition does not settle or recurs frequently.
Seborrhoeic dermatitis	Regular shampooing of the infants hair and careful hygiene may prevent cradle cap (Campbell and Glasper 1995). Once present treatment is aimed at removing the crusts. Daily shampooing with a mild shampoo or soap. Leaving the shampoo until the crusts have softened then thoroughly rinsing before removing the loosened crusts with a fine tooth comb or soft facial brush is advised (Campbell and Glasper 1995).
Candida albicans ('thrush')	Treatment for oral candida is with the use of an oral liquid or gel fungicide. It often results from inadequate sterilisation of feeding equipment, parents should be taught how to wash and sterilise feeding equipment. It also may occur during antibiotic treatment when the body's natural flora is reduced, or in sick or immunosuppressed children. Candida nappy rash is treated using an antifungal cream or ointment which should be continued for a few days after the rash has disappeared or the infection may reoccur (Denyer and Turnbull 1996).
Cold sores	Avoid secondary infection by keeping area clean, and avoid touching with fingers. Topical antiviral cream (acyclovir) is effective in preventing recurrence. Oral antiviral may be needed if severe recurrence. Hospitalisation and IV antivirals needed for immunosuppressed children.
Stye (Hordeolum)	If infection does not resolve in two days, warm compresses may be applied every couple of hours and a topical ophthalmic antibiotic may be needed.
Headlice (Pediculosis capitis)	Infestation may be prevented by twice daily combing of the hair from roots to tips, and daily washing with normal shampoo. Parents should be advised to inspect their child's hair at least weekly for eggs, especially at the hair roots. The 'wet combing' method of removing lice is recommended. The hair is combed with a fine tooth comb after washing with ordinary shampoo. Using a conditioner makes the hair more slippery and the lice can be detached more easily. This should be repeated every three to four days over a two week period (Scowen 1996). Lotions and shampoos containing malathion or pyrethroids can be bought over the counter, preparations containing carbaryl are now under the prescription only category. Alcohol-based lotions are not recommended for people with eczema, sensitive skin or asthma (Scowen 1996). Insecticidal shampoos may lead to the development of resistant strains of headlice if used frequently as a preventative measure, for this reason, parents should be advised to use lotions only if infestation is suspected, carefully following the instructions. It has been recommended that the type of insecticide used is rotated every two or three years to reduce the chance of resistance occurring (Ward 1992). After treatment, the hair should be combed with a fine toothed comb starting at the roots to remove the eggs. Dipping the comb in vinegar may help to loosen tightly attached eggs. All family members and other close contacts should also be treated at the same time. The school authorities should be notified so that contacts can be traced and treated (Colson 1995). A louse repellent product containing piperonal, a natural substance found in plants, is available from chemists. This does not kill headlice, but deters them from infesting hair (Maunder1993).

Continued on next page

Table 12.3 *Contd.*

Condition	Specific management/treatment
Furunculosis (boils)	The painful boil should be protected from trauma by a dressing. Penicillin or a broad spectrum antibiotic may be used. If the boils are recurrent, treatment may be continued for two months after the last boil has cleared up (Colson 1995). Incision and drainage of severe lesions followed by wound irrigation with antibiotics; drain may be needed if extensive.
Cellulitis	Oral or parenteral antibiotics. Rest and immobilisation of affected area, minimal activity for affected child. Hot moist compresses to area.
Shingles	Symptomatic management, analgesics for pain, mild sedation may be helpful, local moist compresses and drying lotions. The ophthalmic variety of shingles may need systemic corticotrophin (ACTH) and/or corticosteroids. Acyclovir in immunosuppressed children. Isolate from other children if in hospital, keep away from school.
Impetigo	Topical antibiotics may be used after gently releasing the crusts with saline (Colson 1995). Education in meticulous hand washing, avoid sharing flannels and towels. Systemic administration of oral or parenteral antibiotics if lesions are severe or extensive (Hooton 1995). Good handwashing techniques and isolation of the child's face flannel, towels, drinking cups, bed linen, etc.
Ringworm	Oral griseofulvin for 4–6 weeks. Topical anti-fungal agents are not effective (Burns 1991).
Scabies	The child should be washed and dried well. The prescribed cream or lotion such as benzyl benzoate is applied all over the body except for the face and scalp, paying special attention to skin creases and crevices and between fingers and toes, this is left on for 24 hours. A second application is applied without washing off the first application. This is also left on for a day. The treatment can then be washed off. This one treatment should be sufficient if the instructions are followed. All family members should be treated for scabies even if they show no signs as the long incubation period makes it impossible to tell whether they have been infected (Denyer and Turnbull 1996).
Verruca (warts)	Local destructive therapy individualised according to location, type and number. Surgical removal, electro-cautery, curetage, cryotherapy (liquid nitrogen), caustic solutions, X-ray treatment, hypnotherapy. Plantar warts – apply caustic solution to wart, wear foam insole with hole cut in to relieve pressure on wart. Soak for 20 min after 2–3 days, dry and apply more caustic solution. Repeat until wart comes out. Destructive removal techniques may leave scars which cause pain when walking. Verrucas are common in children and tend to disappear spontaneously.
Athlete's foot (Tinea pedis)	Treatment with a topical imidazole such as clotrimazole (Burns 1991).

12.7 SUMMARY

This chapter has provided an overview of many of the common infections in childhood and their treatment. It is intended as a reference for community nurses primarily so that they are better prepared to help parents and their children through these difficult and distressing periods. It is in this way as a support and educator of parents and families that nurses in the community can have a significant impact on the wellbeing of children.

REFERENCES

Agius, A.M., Wake, M., Pahor, A.L. & Smallman, L.A. (1995) Smoking and middle ear ciliary beat frequency in otitis media with effusion. *Acta Otolaryngology*, 115, 44–9.

Alho, O-P., Oja, H., Koivu, M. & Sorri, M. (1995) Otitis media with effusion in infancy: how frequent is it? how docs it develop? *Archives of Otolaryngology, Head, Neck Surgery*, 121, 432–6.

Bandolier (1996) Verrucas and games. September, 3 (9), 3.

Bass, D.M. (1996) Rotavirus and other agents of viral gastro-enteritis. In: *Nelson Textbook of Pediatrics* (eds R.E. Behrman, R.M. Kliegman, A.M. Arvin). WB Saunders Company, Philadelphia.

Beaudry, M., Dufour, R. & Marcoux, S. (1995) Relation between infant feeding and infections during the first six months of life. *Journal of Pediatrics*, 126, 191–7.

Berman, S. (1995) Otitis media in children. *New England Journal of Medicine*, 332 (23), 1560–5.

Bhatti, N., Law, M.R., Halliday, R. & Moore-Gillon, J. (1995) Increasing incidence of tuberculosis in England and Wales: a study of the likely causes. *British Medical Journal*, 310, 967–9.

Blake, K.D. (1993) Dangers of common cold treatments in children. *Lancet*, 341, 640.

Bunting, J. (1997) Morbidity and health related behaviour of adults – a review. In: *Health Inequalities* (eds F. Drever & M. Whitehead) Office for National Statistics, HMSO, London.

Burns, A. (1991) Skin disorders. In: *Jolly's Diseases of Children* (ed. M. Levine). Blackwell, Oxford.

Campbell, S. and Glasper, E.A. (eds) (1995) *Whaley and Wong's Children's Nursing*, Mosby, London.

Carter, B. & Dearmun, A.K. (eds) (1995) *Child Health Care Nursing*, Blackwell Science, Oxford.

Chiesa, C., Pacifico, L., Nanni, F. & Orefici, G. (1994) Recurrent attacks of scarlet fever. *Archives of Paediatric and Adolescent Medicine*. 148, 656–9.

Clarke, F. (1995) The child with disturbance of oxygen and carbon dioxide exchange. In: *Whaley and Wong's Children's Nursing* (eds S. Campbell & E.A. Glasper). Mosby, London.

Colson, J. (1995) Nursing support and care: meeting the needs of the child and family with altered integumentary function. In: *Child Health Care Nursing: Concepts, Theory and Practice* (eds B. Carter & A.K. Dearmun) (ch. 23). Blackwell Science, Oxford.

Davies, A., Jenkins, H.R. (1992) Management of gastro-enteritis in early childhood, *Drugs*, 44 (1), 57–64.

Delahoussaye, C.P. (1994) Families with neonates. In: *Family Centred Nursing Care of Children* (eds C.L. Betz, M. Hunsberger & S. Wright), 2nd edn, Ch. 4. WB Saunders Company, Philadelphia.

Denyer, J., Turnbull, R. (1996) The skin. In: *Children's Nursing* (eds L. McQuaid, S. Huband & E. Parker). Churchill Livingstone, Edinburgh.

Disabato, J., Wulf, J. (1994) Altered neurologic function. In: *Family Centred Nursing Care of Children* (eds C.L. Betz, M. Hunsberger & S. Wright), 2nd edn, Ch. 40. WB Saunders Company, Philadelphia.

Duncan, B., Ey, J., Holberg, C.J., Wright, A.L., Martinez, F.D. & Taussig, L.M. (1993) Exclusive breast feeding for at least four months protects against otitis media. *Pediatrics*, 91 (5), 867–72.

Effective Health Care (1992) The treatment of persistent glue ear in children: are surgical interventions effective in combating disability from glue ear? November, No. 4.

Elliott, R. (1995) Toxocara canis: health risks and prevention. *Health Visitor*, 68 (8), 324–6.

Estabrook, M. (1996) Meningococcal infections. In: *Nelson Textbook of Pediatrics* (eds R.E. Behrman, R.M. Kliegman & A.M. Arvin). WB Saunders Company, Philadelphia.

Etzel, R.A., Pattishall, E.N., Haley, N.J., Fletcher, R.H., Henderson, F.W. (1992) Passive smoking and middle ear effusion among children in day care. *Pediatrics*, 90 (2, pt 1), 228–32.

Ey, J.L., Holberg, C.J., Aldous, M.B., Wright, A.L., Martinez, F.D., Taussig, L.M. & Group Health Medical Associates (1995) Passive smoke exposure and otitis media in the first year of life. *Pediatrics*, 95 (5), 670–77.

Feroli, K.L. (1994) Infectious disease. In: *Family Centered Nursing Care of Children* (eds C.L. Betz, M. Hunsberger & S. Wright), 2nd edn. WB Saunders Company, Philadelphia.

Fielder, A. (1995) The child with cerebral dysfunction. In: *Whaley and Wong's Children's Nursing* (eds S. Campbell & E.A. Glasper). Mosby, London.

Gadomski, A. & Horton, L. (1992) The need for rational therapeutics in the use of cough and cold medicine in infants. *Pediatrics*, 89 (4, pt 2), 774–6.

Gleeson, S. (1993) Back to school: common infections and infestations (Part 2). *Professional Care of Mother and Child*, Oct, 3 (9), 261–7.

Gow, D. (1995) Health problems of early childhood. In: *Whaley and Wong's Children's Nursing* (eds S. Campbell & E.A. Glasper), Mosby, London.

Hall, D.M.B. (ed.) (1996) *Health for All Children*, 3rd edn. Oxford University Press, Oxford.

Hammerschlag, M.R. (1996) Chlamidia. In: *Nelson Textbook of Pediatrics* (eds R.E. Behrman, R.M. Kliegman & A.M. Arvin). WB Saunders Company, Philadelphia.

Hanna, C.B. Jr (1991) Cefadroxil in the management of facial cellulitis of odontogenic origin. *Oral Surgery, Oral Medicine, Oral Pathology*, 71 (4), 496–8.

Henschel, D., Inch, S. (1996) *Breast Feeding: a Guide for Midwives*. Books for Midwives, England.

Herder, S. (1994) Sponge baths for fever: a waste of nursing time. *American Journal of Nursing*, **94** (10), 55.

Hinton, A.E., Herdman, R.C.D., Martin-Hirsch, D. & Saeed, S.R. (1993) Parental cigarette smoking and tonsillectomy in children. *Clinical Otolaryngology*, **18**, 178–80.

Hogan, S.C., Stratford, K.J., Moore, D.R. (1997) Duration and recurrence of otitis media with effusion in children from birth to 3 years: prospective study using monthly otoscopy and tympanometry, *British Medical Journal*, **314**, 350–3.

Hooton, M. (1995) Health problems of middle childhood. In: *Whaley and Wong's Children's Nursing* (eds S. Campbell & E.A. Glasper). Mosby, London.

Hull, D. & Johnston, D.I. (1993) *Essential Paediatrics*, 3rd edn. Churchill Livingstone, Edinburgh.

Hunsberger, M., Feenan, L. (1994) Altered respiratory function. In: *Family Centered Nursing Care of Children* (eds C.L. Betz, M. Hunsberger & S. Wright), 2nd edn. WB Saunders Company, Philadelphia.

Jethwa, K. (1994) Nappy rash: a pharmaceutical approach. *Professional Care of Mother and Child*, Oct., **4** (7), 219–20.

Joint Formulary Committee (1998) *British National Formulary*, **35** (March 1998) Section 5.5. British Medical Association, London; The Pharmaceutical Press, Oxford.

Kerrigan, P. (1996) Management of diarrhoea by the primary health care team, *Professional Care of Mother and Child*, **6** (2), 37–8.

Kinmonth, A-L., Fulton, Y. & Campbell, M.J. (1992) Management of feverish children at home. *British Medical Journal*, **305**, 1134–6.

Krohn, M.A., Hillier, S.L., Bell, T.A., Kronmal, R.A., Grayston, J.T. *et al.* (1993) The bacterial etiology of conjunctivitis in early infancy. *American Journal of Epidemiology*, **138** (5), 326–32.

Levine, M. (1991) Disorders of the ear, nose and throat. In: *Jolly's Diseases of Children* (ed. M. Levine). Blackwell, Oxford.

Lowry, S. (1991) *Housing and Health*. British Medical Association, London.

Mair, E.J. (1996) Hearing and vision. In: *Children's Nursing* (eds L. McQuaid, S. Huband & E. Parker). Churchill Livingstone, Edinburgh.

Maunder, J.W. (1993) An update on headlice. *Health Visitor*, **66** (9), 317–8.

McIntosh, K. (1996) Respiratory syncitial virus. In: *Nelson Textbook of Pediatrics* (eds R.E. Behrman, R.M. Kliegman & A.M. Arvin). WB Saunders Company, Philadelphia.

Nicol, N.H. & Hill, M.J. (1994) Altered skin integrity. In: *Family Centered Nursing Care of Children* (eds C.L. Betz, M. Hunsberger & S. Wright), 2nd edn, Ch. 38. WB Saunders Company, Philadelphia.

Office of Population Censuses and Surveys (1991) *General Household Survey: Cigarette Smoking 1972 to 1990*. OPCS Monitor SS 91/3. HMSO, London.

Office of Population Censuses and Surveys (1995) *The Health of Our Children: Decennial Supplement* (ed. Beverley Botting). HMSO, London.

Office for National Statistics (ONS) (1996) *1994 Communicable Disease Statistics*. HMSO, London.

Porter, J.D., Ragazzoni, H.P., Buckanon, J.D., Waskin, H.A., Juranek, D.D. & Parkin, W.E. (1988) *Giardia* transmission in a swimming pool. *American Journal of Public Health*, **78** (6), 659–62.

Porter, J.D.H., Gafney, C., Heymann, D. & Parkin, W. (1990) Food outbreak of *Giardia Lamblia*, *American Journal of Public Health*, **80** (10), 1259–60.

Powell, C. (1995) Health problems of early childhood (ch 16), in: S. Campbell & E.A. Glasper (eds) *Whaley and Wong's Children's Nursing*. Mosby, London.

Provisional Committee on Quality Improvement, Sub-Committee on Acute Gastroenteritis (1996) Practice parameter: the management of acute gastroenteritis in young children. *Pediatrics*, **97** (3), 424–31.

Randall, J.L., Soefer, E.F. (1983) Care of the infant and child. In: *Family Medicine: Principles and Practice* (ed. R.B. Taylor), 2nd edn, Ch. 39. Springer Verlag, New York.

Rée, G.H., Voller, A. & Rowland, H.A.K. (1984) Toxocariasis in the British Isles 1982–1983. *British Medical Journal*, **288**, 628–9.

Rudd, P. (1991) Immunisation and infectious diseases. In: *Jolly's Diseases of Children* (ed. M. Levine). Blackwell, Oxford.

Ryan, T. (1993) Wrong assumptions in the nappy area. *Professional Care of Mother and Child*, **3** (3), 4–6.

Scowen, P. (1996) Head lice: a problem for 1 in 10 primary school children. *Professional Care of Mother and Child*, **6** (5), 139–40.

Sinclair, A. (1996) Nasal decongestants. *Professional Care of Mother and Child*, **6** (1), 9–11.

Sutkowski, K. (1989) Tackling headlice. *Health Visitor*, **62** (3), 96–7.

Walker-Smith, J.A. (1992) Advances in the management of gastroenteritis in children. *British Journal of Hospital Medicine*, **48** (9), 582–5.

Wall, C.R., Webster, J., Quirk, P., Robb, T.A., Cleghorn, G.J. & Davidson, G.P. *et al.* (1994) The nutritional management of acute diarrhoea in young infants: effect of carbohydrate ingested. *Journal of Pediatric Gastroenterology and Nutrition*, **19** (2), 170–74.

Ward, K. (1992) The management of skin infestations. *Nursing Standard*, **6** (23), 28–30.

White, A., Freeth, S. & O'Brien, M. (1992) *Infant Feeding 1990*. Office of Population Censuses and Surveys, HMSO, London.

APPENDIX 12.1: CHILDHOOD DISEASES

Infection and epidemiology	Features	Complications	Specific management
Bronchiolitis *Infective agent* – mainly respiratory syncytial virus in infants under 1 year. *Transmission* – droplets from respiratory tract conveyed in air, on hands or on objects. *Incubation* – about 4 days. *Infectious period* – 5 to 12 days after appearance of symptoms, can be more than 3 weeks.	Children over 1 year and adults may have cold-like symptoms. Infants under a year, especially 2nd to 7th month of life, become more severely ill. *Prodromal* – infants display cold-like symptoms, cough usually starts after 1–3 days with sneezing and low grade fever. Soon after the cough has developed, the child begins to wheeze audibly. In mild infections symptoms may not progress further. *Acute phase* – if illness progresses, cough and wheezing increase with air hunger, chest hyperexpansion, and intercostal and subcostal recession. Respiratory rate may increase to more than 70 breaths per minute with central cyanosis, listlessness and apnoeic spells.	Dehydration. In severe cases brain damage due to oxygen starvation, death (2% mortality in hospitalised infants). Recurrent pulmonary infections due to chronic lung damage.	Symptomatic treatment, most infants seem to breathe better when propped up at an angle of 10 to 30 degrees or sat in a 'sitta' chair. Small amounts of fluids should be offered frequently. If the infant is unable to take fluids, exhibits any signs of dehydration or respiratory distress, they should be immediately referred for a hospital opinion. (McIntosh 1996)
Erythema infectiosum (slapped cheek disease, fifth disease) *Infectious agent* – human parvovirus B19. *Transmission* – unknown, possibly respiratory secretions and blood. *Incubation* – usually 1 to 4 days, occasionally as long as 20 days. *Infectious period* – not known, but before the onset of symptoms in children.	Rash appears in three stages: *Stage 1* – erythema on face especially cheeks, with circumoral pallor, this disappears by 1–4 days. *Stage 2* – about 1 day after the rash appears on the face maculopapular red spots appear symmetrically distributed on upper and lower limbs, rash progresses from proximal to distal surfaces, this rash may last a week or more. *Stage 3* – after rash has subsided, it may reappear if the skin is irritated or traumatised due to heat, cold, sun or friction. In children with aplastic blood disorders rash is usually absent and prodromal illness includes headache, fever, myalgia, lethargy, nausea, vomiting and abdominal pain.	Self limiting arthritis and arthralgia. May result in fetal death if mother is infected during pregnancy, but there is no evidence of congenital abnormalities. Children with immune deficiency or haemolytic disease may have an aplastic crisis.	Isolation is not necessary, no special care needed. Avoid contact with pregnant women and immunocompromised children.

Continued on next page

APPENDIX 12.1: *Contd*

Infection and epidemiology	Features	Complications	Specific management
Exanthema subitum (roseola infantum, sixth disease) *Infectious agent* – human herpes virus type 6. *Transmission* – unknown, the infection is virtually limited to children between the ages of six months and two years. *Incubation* – unknown. *Infectious period* – unknown.	Persistent high fever for 3 to 4 days in child who appears well. Sudden drop in temperature to normal with appearance of discrete rose pink macular or maculopapular rash, this appears first on the trunk then spreads to the neck, face and extremities. The rash is non-purpuric and fades on pressure. It lasts 1 to 2 days. Other symptoms are lymphadenopathy around the neck and behind ears, cough and coryza.	Febrile convulsions.	Antipyretics for fever, anticonvulsants for children with a history of febrile convulsions.
Influenza *Infectious agent* – influenza viruses. *Transmission* – droplet infection from the respiratory tract. *Incubation* – 1 to 3 days.	Sudden onset of fever often associated with chills and rigors, headache, cough and myalgia. May develop conjunctivitis and tonsillitis. May be associated with vomiting and diarrhoea.	Pneumonia and apnoea in early infancy.	Symptomatic treatment of pyrexia, headache, sore throat. (Rudd 1991)
Rotavirus gastroenteritis *Infectious agent* – rotaviruses. *Transmission* – contact with infected material via faecal-oral route. *Incubation* – less than 48 hours.	Mild to moderate fever and vomiting followed by the onset of frequent watery stools. Gross blood is absent in the stools. Vomiting and fever usually cease during the second day of illness, but diarrhoea often continues for 5–7 days. Diarrhoea may lead to severe dehydration.	Severe dehydration especially in infants.	Oral rehydration solutions should be used initially to rehydrate the child, if dehydrated, over 6 to 8 hours. Thereafter normal feeding can be recommenced, supplemented by oral rehydration solutions to make up for fluid losses in stools. Prolonged use of clear fluids has not been shown to be beneficial and may actually prolong the duration of the diarrhoea. Breast feeding should be continued even during rehydration. Some infants may benefit from lactose-free infant formula for several days. (Bass 1996)

Scarlet fever

Infectious agent – group A β-haemolytic streptococci.

Transmission – direct contact or droplet from nasopharyngeal secretions, indirect contact with contaminated articles, ingestion of contaminated food and milk.

Incubation – mainly 2–4 days, can be 1 to 7 days.

Infectious period – during incubation period and clinical illness, approximately 10 days, also during first 2 weeks of carrier phase and may persist for months.

Second and third attacks of scarlet fever have been reported (Chiesa *et al.* 1994).

Prodromal stage – sudden high fever, very rapid pulse, vomiting, headache, shivering, abdominal pain.

Enanthema – enlarged, oedematous tonsils covered with patches of exudate, may resemble membrane in diphtheria in severe cases; oedematous, bright red pharynx; tongue becomes coated and papillae swollen and red (white strawberry tongue); by fourth or fifth day white coat sloughs off leaving prominent papillae (red strawberry tongue); palate covered with erythematous punctate lesions.

Exanthema – rash appears within 12 hours after prodromal signs; red pinhead sized punctate lesions rapidly becoming generalised but absent on face; face becomes flushed with striking circumoral pallor; rash on body is more intense in folds of joints, axilla, groin. By the end of the first week skin sloughs off, like fine sandpaper on torso and in sheets on palms and soles. This may take three weeks or longer.

Otitis media, peritonsillar abscesses, sinusitis. Rarely carditis and polyarthritis.

Isolation until 24 hours after treatment has been initiated, bed rest during febrile stage, antipyretics and analgesics. Antiseptic mouthwash or lozenges, encourage fluids especially during the febrile stage, and soft bland foods when the child is able to eat, avoid irritating fluids such as citrus juices, or rough foods.

Treatment of choice is a full course of penicillin (or erythromycin if child is sensitive to penicillin) fever should subside 24 hours after starting treatment. Carriers should have antibiotic therapy (carriers are diagnosed by nose and throat cultures).

(Randall & Soefer 1983; Feroli 1994; Colson 1995; Gow 1995)

13

Managing Atopic Eczema: Evidence and Issues

Barbara Elliott

13.1 INTRODUCTION

A range of non-infectious skin problems can affect young children. Some are minor and generally of short duration such as seborrhoeic dermatitis (cradle cap) and napkin dermatitis (see Chapter 12). Other skin diseases such as atopic eczema, epidermolysis bullosa and psoriasis may be far more serious in terms of their effect on the child and family. The main focus of this chapter will be on the evidence pertaining to atopic eczema and its management. Atopic eczema is a very common skin condition in young children and many of the issues are relevant to other skin conditions and/or other atopic diseases.

13.2 CLARIFICATION OF TERMS

Atopic dermatitis is described as:

'an inherited skin condition of varying morphology associated with numerous pharmacologic and immunologic abnormalities and a tendency to produce specific IgE (reagins) in response to common environmental antigens.'
(Krafchik 1988, p. 695)

Traditionally the term eczema has been used to describe the infantile form of atopic dermatitis or when the inflammation of the skin is the result of internal events. Dermatitis is used more often to describe inflammation caused by external factors. However the two terms are used interchangeably in the literature (Burton 1992).

13.3 INCIDENCE OF ATOPIC DISEASES

Atopic eczema is a relatively common disease particularly in childhood and its incidence appears to be increasing. It was estimated that atopic eczema affected approximately 10% of the population (Taylor et al. 1984) and that the incidence in childhood was approximately 5% (David 1983). More recent studies have indicated a higher incidence. Neame et al. (1993) found that 14% of children under five years of age suffered from the disease and it has been suggested that the lifetime prevalence of atopic eczema in children aged 3–11 years is 20% (Kay et al. 1994). The majority of sufferers develop the disease in the first year of life (David 1983; Atherton 1994; Kay et al. 1994).

The incidence of the other major atopic disease, for example asthma, also appears to be increasing (Burney et al. 1990; Strachan et al. 1994). National Asthma Campaign (1993a) estimate that one in ten children suffer from asthma. Increased air pollution due to road traffic has been suggested as a possible cause for the increase (Read 1991) as well as tobacco smoke (National Asthma Campaign 1993b). It is likely that the situation is more complicated and other factors may be implicated. Children who already have eczema appear to have at least a three fold increased risk of developing asthma (Atherton 1994).

Management of asthma by nurses in the community is described in Kenrick and Luker (1995) and Bryar and Bytheway (1996).

13.4 RECOGNITION OF ATOPIC ECZEMA

Physical appearance

The word eczema is derived from the Greek language and literally means 'to boil over'. This is a very apt description of the presentation of the disease, which appears initially as red itchy skin and develops rapidly into a rash of pustules which eventually break down and leak serous fluid or 'boil over'. The hair is dry and there may be signs of lymphadenopathy.

In infancy the eczematous lesions frequently appear first on the cheeks (Krafchik 1988, Atherton 1994), other areas may also be involved. In childhood the anticubital and popliteal areas are most affected with the neck and flexures of the wrists and ankles also involved. It is also common for the disease to affect the hands (Atherton 1994). As the child reaches puberty the face again becomes involved with the neck and body (Krafchik 1988).

The most regular visible characteristic of the rash is erythema and when atopic eczema worsens the first visible sign is increased redness (Atherton 1994). Children with eczema often have dry scaly skins even in areas where other features of the disease are not apparent. Other family members who do not suffer from eczema may also have this dry skin known as ichthyosis. Eczema may cause altered pigmentation in affected skin due to its effects on the melanocytes. This causes a temporary loss of pigmentation which may last for several months.

If eczema becomes a chronic condition lichenification is a major feature, the lesions becoming thickened with a leather-like appearance and an increase in normal skin markings. In dark skinned children this lichenification causes the skin to appear darker which may cause them and their parents distress (Atherton 1994). Despite the severity of some

children's eczema and the distressing appearance of their skin this disease rarely results in permanent scarring.

Symptoms

Atopic eczema is characterised by a chronic pruritic inflammation of the skin. Many cases are mild but in some the disease is severe, disfiguring and disabling. The majority of children with atopic eczema fall between these two extremes.

The most distressing symptom of atopic eczema is pruritis (David 1983; Krafchik 1988) and the desire to scratch may be overwhelming (Frank 1987). Children with severe eczema may lapse into a trance-like state, scratching frantically, apparently oblivious of their surroundings. The irritation is often so severe that the pain of torn, bleeding skin is preferable to the itching. The damage done to the skin may be considerable, and the bleeding and exudation stains clothes and bedding and may cause such materials to stick to the child's skin.

Continuous scratching can lead to other complications such as lichenification, excoriation and the introduction of infection (Buckley 1984). Broken skin is readily infected by commensal organisms or other pathogens introduced by dirty finger nails or other objects used by children to scratch. Small babies may find it easier to rub themselves against objects rather than use their finger nails, and older children become adept at finding new ways to relieve their itching. Scratching may cause temporary hair loss particularly noticeable on the eyebrows and in the scalp.

The child who is itchy is also usually irritable, and parents and carers are frequently irritated themselves by a child whose behaviour is erratic and uncontrollable and whose constant scratching is deemed to be antisocial and annoying (David 1983). Psychological irritability also increases the itchiness of the skin although the mechanisms for this are unknown (Atherton 1994). Sufferers may be able to ignore their skin whilst absorbed in an interesting activity, but once their brain is unoccupied or 'irritated' by other factors the itchiness of their skin becomes more apparent. This creates a vicious cycle which parents and carers need to break through distraction and activity.

Linked with the itchiness and irritability of children with atopic eczema is their inability to sleep. Children may find it difficult to get to sleep and/or may wake several times in the night scratching and screaming.

Regularly disrupted nights constitute the greatest single burden for the family, many parents not having had a full night's sleep for years (David 1985).

Diagnosis

The symptoms of different skin diseases may be similar and a clear diagnosis may initially be difficult. Doctors may refer to all infantile rashes as eczema (Atherton 1994), which can be very confusing for parents. It should be remembered that a diagnosis of eczema does not always mean that the child has atopic eczema.

For years there has been a lack of a precise definition of atopic eczema (David 1985). In 1994 a working party of 16 doctors was established to develop a minimum list of reliable discriminators for atopic dermatitis (Williams *et al.* 1994b). Their study suggested that cases of atopic dermatitis could be distinguished from other inflammatory skin diseases by six features. These are:

(1) history of flexural involvement;
(2) onset under the age of two years;
(3) history of an itchy rash;
(4) personal history of asthma;
(5) history of a dry skin;
(6) visible flexural dermatitis.

Visible flexural dermatitis is a key feature in diagnosing atopic eczema (Williams *et al.* 1995) and it is the only physical sign considered to be a useful indicator of the disease, historical features being far more important (Williams *et al.* 1994b). This is important for community nurses, as they are often in the best position to obtain an accurate history of a child's skin problems.

13.5 CAUSES OF ATOPIC ECZEMA

The actual cause of atopic eczema is unknown. It is thought to have multi-factorial causation.

Genetic predisposition

The atopic diseases, atopic eczema, asthma, urticaria, allergic rhinitis and allergic conjunctivitis, are fre-quently familial. Van Bever (1992) found that 66% of patients with atopic eczema had a family history of the disease. A family history of other atopic diseases such as asthma has also been found to be a strong predictor of the disease (Hide & Guyer 1981; Fergusson *et al.* 1982). The actual nature of the genetic predisposition remains uncertain and it would appear that environmental factors determine whether the genetic trait manifests itself.

Allergy

Allergy to specific antigens is generally accepted as one of the factors involved in the pathogenesis of atopic eczema. Some experts believe that allergy to a wide variety of stimuli is the cause of atopic eczema (Atherton 1994). Others believe that the relative importance of allergy varies in different sufferers (David 1989).

The identification of allergic triggers is problematic. Tests are available to detect the number of IgE antibodies to particular antigens both in the blood and in the skin. However such tests can be expensive and difficult to interpret (David 1991a). There is no currently available test for the identification of foods that can provoke atopic eczema and, possibly because of this, there has developed a wide range of unconventional allergy tests offered by private clinics (Atherton 1994). The results of these tests are generally considered to be spurious (David 1985; Atherton, 1994).

Early feeding practices

The fact that the majority of cases of atopic eczema develop early in life has led to much interest in the effects of early infant feeding upon the incidence of this disease. The relationship between early feeding practices and the incidence of allergic diseases has been researched and debated for over 50 years. The quality and design of studies varies markedly and the evidence remains inconclusive. The Department of Health (1994) requested that further investigation be made of dietary factors which initiate atopic disorders in early childhood.

Families with a history of atopic disease need clear advice from community nurses regarding the best way to feed their children in order to minimise the risk of disease developing.

13.6 FEEDING ADVICE

Despite the controversies the current advice regarding infant feeding for **genetically predisposed infants** is as follows:

- Exclusive breast feeding for the first few months of life will reduce the risk of atopic eczema. Where the genetic risk is high this may be halved by exclusive breast feeding (Atherton 1994).
- Breast feeding probably does not have a protective effect but rather prevents the introduction of harmful cows' milk proteins in formula feeds. For this reason breast feeding must be exclusive with no 'top up' feeds of formula milk.
- Food antigens from a mother's diet are transmitted in minute amounts to her baby via breast milk (Cant *et al.* 1985). This may cause sensitisation in babies who are exclusively breast fed. Restricting maternal diets has been found to reduce both the incidence of atopic eczema (Chandra *et al.* 1989) and the severity of existing atopic eczema (Lake *et al.* 1981; Cant *et al.* 1986). Maternal diets excluding egg and cows' milk may be considered for breast fed babies at extremely high risk of developing atopic eczema, but should be carefully monitored by a dietician to ensure adequate nutrition is maintained for both mother and baby (Atherton 1994).
- Cows' milk does increase the risk of a wide range of allergic responses in babies with a family history of atopy (Lucas *et al.* 1990) and therefore should be avoided until the age of at least one year, including any milk formulae derived from cows' milk or weaning foods containing cows' milk protein (Atherton 1994).
- Soya based formulae do not appear to reduce the risk of atopic eczema (Halpern *et al.* 1973; Kjellman & Johansson 1979) and should not be recommended as an alternative to breast feeding.
- Goats' milk should not be used in children under six months and probably not in the first year (DHSS 1980).
- If breast feeding is not possible, casein hydrolysate formula is the best alternative (Chandra *et al.* 1989; Sampson *et al.* 1991). Due to its high cost, it should only be given on the advice of a doctor (Atherton 1994).

- Weaning should not commence before four months and no later than seven months, vegetables and fruits being introduced first (Atherton 1994). Foods should be introduced gradually and individually. Egg should not be introduced until at least two years. The introduction of nuts and nut products should be delayed in children from atopic families, especially if they already have eczema or asthma as they are at increased risk of developing nut allergy (Tariq *et al.* 1996).

Critical reviews of some of the research evidence linking early infant feeding and the incidence of allergy, and recommendations for future research can be found in Cant (1986) and Obeid (1996) and more details regarding infant diets can be found in Atherton (1994).

Other factors

There are many substances in the environment which are thought to contribute to the incidence and aggravation of atopic eczema. Of these the most common offenders are: house dust mites, pollens, moulds and animal fur. Considerable research has focused on whether such environmental antigens are the cause of atopic eczema.

House dust mites have been considered to be an aetiological factor in the incidence of atopic eczema for some time (Beck & Korsgaard 1989). The increased numbers of house dust mites found in well heated and well insulated houses with fitted carpets has been suggested as a reason for the marked increase in atopic eczema in children from social classes I and II (Williams *et al.* 1994a).

The general consensus of opinion would now seem to be that contact with environmental antigens is a major contributory cause of atopic eczema, but the relative importance of such contact remains unclear (Atherton 1994).

13.7 COURSE AND SEVERITY

In general, the condition of a child's skin deteriorates over a few years and then gradually improves until it is no longer a problem. How long this takes varies, but it is suggested that for 50% of children with eczema at one year the disease is no longer a problem by the age of five years (Atherton 1994).

The course and the severity of the disease are influenced by many factors. The complex interaction of these factors means that the disease fluctuates dramatically both from child to child and within the same child at different times. The relative importance of these factors varies between children.

Allergy

Once atopic eczema is apparent allergic reactions can aggravate the disease. Parents will become aware of particular foods and environmental allergens which cause deterioration in their child's skin condition. Careful history taking is therefore essential in identifying possible allergens particularly in view of the inadequacies of laboratory tests.

Irritants

The skin of individuals with atopic eczema appears to be particularly sensitive to a great variety of chemical and physical irritants which cause deterioration in the disease state. Soaps, detergents, antiseptics, solvents, salt, preservatives and some fruit and vegetables can all have an irritant effect on eczematous skin (Atherton 1994). Certain fibres, particularly pure wool, and smoke are also frequently irritants.

Climatic factors

The influence of climate, particularly sunlight and humidity, on the skin of sufferers of atopic eczema has been studied (Rajka 1989; George *et al.* 1991; Turner *et al.* 1991). Climates with low humidity tend to dry the skin and therefore cause deterioration. Cold winter winds may be particularly harmful. Possibly the most detrimental climatic factor is sudden changes of temperature and humidity (Atherton 1994).

Psychological factors

There exists a large amount of anecdotal literature supporting the relationship between emotional stress and conflict and dermatological disorders. The role of stress in atopic eczema has been noted (Faulstich & Williamson 1985; Gil *et al.* 1987). It would appear that there is a link between stress and family environment

and the severity of atopic eczema in a child, but it cannot be assumed that the relationship is causal.

In the past it has been suggested that the psychological make up of sufferers was largely responsible for the incidence and evolution of atopic eczema (Sneddon 1980; Medansky 1980), but now it is recognised that personality traits of children and adults with atopic eczema are both a cause and result of their disease (Atherton 1994). It has been suggested that children with chronic physical disorders have twice the risk of developing psychosocial maladjustment than healthy children (Pless & Nolan 1991). In particular children with atopic eczema have been found to have a significantly greater number of behaviour symptoms with an excess of clinginess and dependency, fearfulness and sleep difficulty than healthy controls (Daud *et al.* 1993).

13.8 LIVING WITH ATOPIC ECZEMA

The worst aspects of skin diseases are their effects on activities and feelings (Jowett & Ryan 1985; Kurwa & Finlay 1995). Whilst it is advocated that the activities of children with atopic eczema should not be restricted (Atherton 1994), many parents report that their children with this disease are not always able to pursue normal childhood activities, either due to the pain of excoriated, sore skin or the reactions of others (Elliott 1994). Balancing their child's need for opportunities to develop and socialise normally with their desire to protect them and avoid deterioration of the child's skin is a very real issue for parents of children with eczema. Atherton (1994) recommends that children with atopic eczema should not be treated as different, as it is this, rather than the condition itself, which will lead to permanent damage.

The skin is the largest and most visible organ in the body. Perception of good health depends on its appearance as well as its function, and any disease or treatment which affects a child's skin is bound to have social consequences both for the child and his or her parents. It is frequently assumed that skin disorders are infectious and contagious, and they carry connotations of dirtiness and poor hygiene practices. A large number of eczema sufferers experience unpleasant remarks and ridicule from others and the most common setting for such incidents is school (Jowett & Ryan 1985). Coming to terms with such reactions is a significant feature of living with a skin disease.

Parents also report suffering because of the misconceptions of others regarding skin diseases, and they have been accused of abusing and neglecting their children (Elliott 1994). The stress of social encounters and having to deal with hurtful comments may make mothers reluctant to take their eczematous children out.

Parents may have concerns regarding their child's irritable behaviour and these may be compounded by fears that their child is exploiting the condition in order to get his or her own way (Elliott 1994). This fear would seem justified, as it is claimed that children with eczema are quick to appreciate its manipulative value (Atherton 1994). Parents may find it difficult to discipline their child if doing so results in a bout of furious scratching which causes lasting skin damage.

Living with, and caring for, a child with atopic eczema can be emotionally demanding for parents. Feelings such as anger, both at the disease and at the child, guilt, helplessness, frustration, despair and depression have all been described (Elliott 1994). Sleep problems and consequent tiredness may exacerbate parents' emotions. An increase in marital problems in families with children with chronic illness has been found (Donnelly *et al.* 1987) although there is no clear evidence of an increase in divorce (Cadman *et al.* 1991). The demands of caring for a child with atopic eczema may put a strain on marital relationships, particularly when parents spend little time alone together without their children (Elliott 1994). Siblings may also suffer from having a child with atopic eczema in the family. They may resent the special attention often demanded by the child and required when giving treatments. Parents need to be aware of this and alert to any developing jealousies in order to compensate their other children.

Caring for a child with atopic eczema involves work which is in addition to normal childcare. Usual activities involved in caring for children such as bathing, dressing, feeding and entertaining may become onerous tasks. Preventing their child from scratching is one of the prime objectives for parents, and this involves keeping their child occupied and preventing boredom, a difficult task when the child is irritable and has a short concentration span. The overwhelming desire to scratch can make undressing

and nappy changing very difficult, and bleeding and exudation may cause clothes to stick to the child's skin, adding to the trauma for both child and carer.

Avoidance of allergens brings additional work for carers. If diet is implicated in the child's disease the effort involved in shopping, preparing food and meal times may be increased. Minimising contact with house dust mites involves extra cleaning, dusting and washing (Nocoon 1991). The disease itself generates more 'dirt' in terms of bleeding, exudation and exfoliation, combined with greasy creams and ointments. The result is often the need for daily changes of bedding and clothing, and a strict routine of damp dusting and vacuuming (Elliott 1994). The irritant effect of certain chemicals and fibres means that parents have a limited number of cleaning products available to them which may increase the burden of work. Families may be entitled to claim for a Disability Living Allowance, and the National Eczema Society provides one-off payments to help with special purchases such as clothing and bedding. The experiences of mothers caring for a child with atopic eczema are discussed in more depth by Elliott and Luker (1996).

13.9 GUIDELINES FOR PRACTICE

Management of atopic eczema

The multifactorial causation of atopic eczema means that treatment often involves several different approaches and often has to be conducted on a 'trial and error' basis over several months (Atherton 1994). There is no proven cure for the disease, the aim of treatment is to control the symptoms and prevent deterioration of the skin. The fluctuating nature of the disease means that once an ideal treatment is found for an individual, there is no guarantee that this will remain useful (Atherton 1994). This can be immensely frustrating for parents who desperately want to see their child relieved of the condition.

There is a degree of dissatisfaction with the medical management of atopic eczema both from within the medical profession (David 1985) and the parents of children with the disease (Elliott 1994). This situation, coupled with the fact that rashes are so common in young children means that parents are often bombarded with well meaning advice from family, friends, the media, and total strangers. Studies have indicated that there may be serious risk to the health of children with atopic dermatitis subjected to lay or unsupervised treatment (Webber *et al.* 1989).

Parents carry a major responsibility for the success or failure of treatments, which have to be given on a regular basis and often require considerable time and effort. Failure of parents to comply with prescribed treatment is a common cause of apparent failure of treatment (Fischer 1996). Reasons for non-compliance, such as lack of understanding, fear of steroids, and time and cost are amenable to help from nurses. As care and treatment are mainly given at home, community nurses are in an excellent position to offer much needed support and advice to parents and help alleviate some of their distress and frustration. Where nurses are involved with such parents the benefits have been described in the literature (Broberg *et al.* 1990; Spowart 1993; Bridgman 1994, 1995b; Venables 1995).

Nursing assessment

Careful assessment and history taking is a vital role for community nurses involved with children with skin problems. This may form the basis for diagnosis and an essential source of information regarding possible causative and aggravating factors.

Interventions

The main aims of care are to:
(1) hydrate the skin;
(2) reduce inflammation;
(3) break the cycle of pruritis and scratching;
(4) prevent, identify and treat infection;
(5) support the child and family.

Hydrate the Skin
Emollients in the form of ointments, creams, bath oils and aerosols are an essential part of skin care. They moisturise dry skin and reduce the desire to scratch. Mild eczema may be controlled with emollients alone (Watts 1996).

Daily tepid baths with a suitable emollient and soap substitute such as aqueous cream are recommended to return moisture to the skin and keep it clean (Atherton 1994). Baths may also be used to relieve

intense itching. As for any children baths should be fun and an opportunity to play. However it should be remembered that emollients will make the bath very slippy and a bath mat should always be used.

Skin should always be patted dry and more emollient applied. Emollients should be applied at regular intervals throughout the day, whenever the skin feels dry and to relieve itching, preferably every 1–2 hours (Atherton 1994). The advice of 'thinly and often' rather than 'thickly and rarely' is useful in avoiding problems of clothes and furnishings becoming greasy and washing machines damaged (Atherton 1994). Care should be taken to prevent emollients becoming contaminated with microorganisms. This is a particular risk with large pots into which fingers are regularly dipped. The lid should be kept on when not in use and hands washed before application.

Occasionally, a child's skin may become intolerant of preparations that have been used successfully in the past, or the skin may be sensitive to additives and preservatives contained in the preparation. An alternative can usually be found and a comprehensive list of emollients is given in Atherton (1994, pp. 99, 101 and 103).

Reduce inflammation
In combination with emollients the most commonly used and effective standard treatment for atopic eczema is topical steroids (David 1991b). They are used for their anti-inflammatory and immunosuppressive effects. The use of oral steroids is rarely justified and they are only used for extremely severe atopic eczema and for very short periods.

Parents may express concern about side effects of steroids such as growth suppression and atrophy of the skin, and fear of such side effects is a common reason for parents not giving prescribed treatment (Elliott 1994; Fischer 1996). Topical steroids are grouped according to their potency from group 1, low potency, to group 5, very high potency. A list of the common steroid preparations and their potencies is given in Atherton (1994, pp 111). The potential for harmful side effects relates not only to the potency of the preparation but also to the area of skin to which the preparation is applied, the amount applied and the age and size of the child.

In general the least potent preparation that will maintain efficacy should be used and parents can be assured that group 1 preparations virtually never cause side effects and group 2 preparations are unlikely to (Atherton 1994). No dermatologist would now use group 4 or 5 preparations undiluted for eczema in children for more than a few days (Atherton 1994). Nothing stronger than hydrocortisone (group 1) should ever be used on babies (Atherton 1994) or on the face. There are no validated guidelines as to the safe daily dosage of topical steroids (David 1991b) and reactions tend to be very individual. Any side effects will take time to develop, and careful monitoring of a child's skin and height may be necessary if prolonged use of steroids is prescribed. Parents can generally be reassured that correct and careful use of topical steroids will not harm their child, and, if used correctly, they can do much to alleviate suffering.

The amount of steroid preparation applied needs to be carefully measured. Parents should be informed by their doctor or pharmacist how to measure out the correct dose, either using a ruler or, more commonly, the finger tip measure (Watts 1996). To be absorbed most effectively steroid preparations should be applied at least 30 minutes after an emollient.

The effectiveness of topical steroids can be enhanced with application of wet wrap bandages. This technique also causes a cooling effect of the skin and often a rapid improvement of skin inflammation and may be used with emollients alone. There are different protocols for the application of wet wraps described in the literature (Atherton 1994; Turnbull & Atherton 1994; Bridgman 1995a, 1995b; Watts 1996). This type of bandaging has been well evaluated and can be a very effective treatment for exacerbation of eczema, reducing the number of disturbed nights and disruption of daily activities and preventing admission to hospital for some children (Mallon et al. 1994).

Other types of bandaging using coal tar or ichthamol paste medicated bandages may be helpful in reducing irritation, inflammation and lichenification (Watts 1996).

Break the cycle of pruritus and scratching

One of the most important considerations in the management of atopic eczema must be the removal of causative and aggravating factors (Burton 1990). Some factors such as woollen clothes may be relatively easy to avoid, but others such as pets may be more difficult. Any avoidance strategies must balance the benefits to the skin with the disadvantages to the child and family. Special diets may be particularly disrupting to family life and should not be undertaken

lightly. Restricted diets should also be carefully monitored by a dietician to ensure that adequate nutrition for a growing child is maintained.

Antihistamines may be used for their sedative effect, particularly at nighttime. They appear to reduce the pruritus of atopic eczema and thus are helpful for children who find they cannot get to sleep or wake often in the night (Atherton 1994). They may cause some drowsiness the next day, which is particularly problematic in school children, and they should not be used during the day except in special circumstances.

In recent years doctors have examined the use of behaviour therapy to stop patients with atopic eczema scratching. Bridgett and Staughton (1996) describe a successful combined approach to treatment, where conventional treatments with emollients and steroids are used in conjunction with habit reversal where new behaviours are taught to combat scratching.

Prevent, identify and treat infection

Eczematous skin provides an attractive environment for microorganisms, and frequent scratching can be a source of infection. Keeping fingernails short and filed daily with an emery board will help reduce the risk of the child introducing infection when scratching, as will daily bathing and washing with a soap substitute. Antiseptic solutions may be used in the bath to help reduce skin bacteria.

The skin of patients with atopic eczema is frequently colonised with *Staphylococcus aureus* (Dhar *et al.* 1992). Exacerbation of eczema due to infection with this organism is common and physical signs of infection are not always reliable (David & Cambridge 1986). Nurses should be alert to this possibility when a child's condition deteriorates unexpectedly and take swabs for bacterial and/or viral culture as necessary.

Viral infections by herpes simplex are also common although the reasons for this are not clear (Goodyear *et al.* 1996). The resulting eczema herpeticum can be very severe and occasionally life threatening (Ewing *et al.* 1989). The virus is frequently contracted from a close family member with a cold sore, and children with atopic eczema should avoid physical contact with anyone with a cold sore which should also be kept covered. There is often confusion regarding immunisations and children with atopic eczema. However none of the vaccinations routinely offered to children in the UK are any more hazardous to children with atopic eczema than to other children

(Atherton 1994). The routine immunisations should all be given at the recommended time, and there is no strong evidence that immunisations can cause atopic eczema (Atherton 1994). The only vaccines that are still grown in eggs are influenza and yellow fever, and therefore these should not be given to anyone who is allergic to egg. If a child is being treated with oral steroids vaccinations with live viruses should not be given.

Support the child and family

The management of atopic eczema should not be confined to the application of skin creams, a holistic approach should be adopted to encompass all aspects of life (Spowart 1993). Indeed, it has been suggested that quality of life be taken into account when evaluating treatment as objective clinical assessment alone cannot provide a complete picture (Kurwa & Finlay 1995).

The long-term nature of the problems of eczema sufferers means that it is essential for nurses to establish a stable therapeutic relationship with the child and parents, and gain their confidence and co-operation in order to achieve compliance and treatment success (Watts 1996). The amount of effort needed to carry out treatment successfully should not be underestimated, and this should be matched by support from health professionals (Watts 1996).

Enabling parents and children to develop effective ways of coping with the disease is an important role for the nurse. This may involve educating others about the disease and treatment regimens. Children with atopic eczema should be targeted for extra health visitor visits, as their mothers may be reluctant to take their children to clinics for fear of adverse comments, and the usual advice given to parents may be inappropriate.

Parents may well request advice regarding new and/or unconventional treatments. Probably the most publicised new treatment for atopic eczema is the use of Chinese herbs. This treatment has been found to have a beneficial effect on children with extensive and severe atopic eczema (Sheehan et al. 1991). There is concern about the hepatotoxity of such treatments (David 1991b) and patients should be carefully monitored. The herbs should only be prescribed by qualified doctors trained in traditional Chinese medicine. A drug company now manufactures a formulation of Chinese herbs as granules, but this drug is not licensed for use in this country.

Phototherapy has also been used with success to treat older children with atopic eczema which did not respond to more conventional treatment. The most successful is oral PUVA (a combination of UVA phototherapy and oral psoralem) which, despite concerns about long-term hazards such as skin cancer and cataract formation, is considered justified in a small number of older children with disabling atopic eczema (Sheehan et al. 1993). More recently narrowband UVB phototherapy has been used with success in children with atopic eczema (Collins & Ferguson 1995).

Treatment of atopic eczema with evening primrose oil has received considerable attention, but results of clinical trials were not conclusive (Bamford et al. 1985). Despite this Atherton (1994) suggests that a small number of children may benefit from such treatment, and recommends a three-month trial in any child with extensive eczema that has not responded to the usual external treatments.

National Eczema Society

The National Eczema Society provides information, advice and support for sufferers of eczema. It is also a useful resource for professionals working with patients with this disease. Books and leaflets are produced aimed at different professionals and there is one specifically for community health care nurses (Spowart & Muir 1994). Research is also funded and in 1993 a course 'Eczema Care in the Community' was developed to meet the needs of primary care and community staff for further information and training. This course has been well evaluated and continues to run across the UK (Hay 1996).

Just as a final note; psoriasis and epidermolysis bullosa are relatively rare in young children and these are discussed in detail in books concerned with the care of sick children such as Carter and Dearmun (1995).

13.10 CONCLUSION

This chapter has paid particular attention to the management of atopic eczema. Management has included not only common treatments but also avoidance strategies for families whose children are particularly at risk of developing this disease. With the increasing prevalence of atopic diseases and the continued emphasis on managing children's treatment at home, it is essential that community nurses have the skills and knowledge to care for these children effectively.

REFERENCES

Atherton, D.J. (1994) *Eczema in Childhood The Facts.* Oxford Medical Publications, Oxford.

Bamford, J.T., Gibson, R.W. & Renier, C.M. (1985) Atopic eczema unresponsive to evening primrose oil. *Journal of American Accademy of Dermatology,* **13** (6), 959–65.

Beck, H.I. & Korsgaard, J. (1989) Atopic dermatitis and house dust mites. *British Journal of Dermatology,* **120** (2), 245–51.

Bridgett, P.N. & Staughton, R. (1996) *Atopic Skin Disease. A Manual for Practitioners.* Wrightson Biomedical Publishing, Petersfield.

Bridgman, A. (1994) Management of atopic eczema in the community. *Health Visitor,* **67** (7), 226–7.

Bridgman, A. (1995a) The use of wet wrap dressings for eczema. *Paediatric Nursing,* **7** (2), 24–7.

Bridgman, A. (1995b) *A Guide to Wet Wraps.* Seton Healthcare Group plc, Oldham.

Broberg, A., Kalimo, K., Lindbald, B. & Swanbeck, G. (1990) Parental education in the treatment of childhood atopic eczema. *Acta Dermato-Venereologica (Stockh),* **70** (6), 495–9.

Bryar, R. & Bytheway, B. (1996) *Changing Primary Health Care, The Teamcare Valleys Experience.* Blackwell Science, Oxford.

Buckley, R.H. (1984) Allergic eczema. In: V.C. Kelley (ed.) *Practice in Pediatrics.* Hayes and Row, Philadelphia.

Burney, P.G.J., Chinn, S. & Roner, R.J. (1990) Has the prevalence of asthma increased in childhood? Evidence from the national study of health and growth 1973–1986, *British Medical Journal,* **300**, 1306–10.

Burton, J.L. (1990) *Essentials of Dermatology.* 3rd edn. Churchill Livingstone, Edinburgh.

Burton, J.L. (1992) Eczema, lichenification, prurigo and erythroderma. In: *Textbook of Dematology.* (eds R.H. Champion, J.L. Burton & F.J.G. Ebing). 5th edn. Blackwell Science, Oxford.

Cadman, D., Rosenbaum, P., Boyle, M. & Offord, D.R. (1991) Children with chronic illness: family and parent demographics and psychosocial adjustment. *Pediatrics,* **87** (6), 884–9

Cant, A., Marsden, R.A. & Kilshaw, P.J. (1985) Egg and cow's milk hypersensitivity in exclusively breast fed infants with eczema and the detection of egg protein in breast milk. *British Medical Journal,* **291**, 932–5.

Cant, A.J., Bailes, J.A., Marsden, R.A. & Hewitt, D. (1986) Effect of maternal dietary exclusion on breast fed infants with eczema: two controlled studies. *British Medical Journal,* **293** (6541), 231–3.

Carter, B. & Dearmun, A.K. (eds) (1995) *Child Health Care Nursing: Concepts, Theory and Practice.* Blackwell Science, Oxford.

Chandra, R.K., Puri, S. & Hamed, A. (1989) Influence of maternal diet and use of formula feeds on development of atopic eczema in high risk infants. *British Medical Journal,* **299**, 228–30.

Collins, P. & Ferguson, J. (1995) Narrowband UVB air-conditioned phototherapy for atopic eczema in children. Correspondence *British Journal of Dermatology,* **133**, 653–67.

David, T.J. (1983) The investigation and treatment of severe eczema in childhood. *International Medicine Supplement,* (6), 17–25.

David, T.J. (1985) The overworked and fraudulent diagnosis of food allergy and food intolerance in children. *Journal of the Royal Society of Medicine,* suppl 5, **78**, 21–31.

David, T.J. (1989) Dietary treatment of atopic eczema. *Archives of Disease in Childhood,* **64**, 1506–9.

David, T.J. (1991a) Conventional allergy tests. *Annals of Allergy,* pp. 281–2.

David, T.J. (1991b) Recent developments in the treatment of childhood atopic eczema. *Journal of the Royal College of Physicians of London,* **25** (2), 95–101.

David, T.J. & Cambridge, G.C. (1986) Bacterial infection and atopic eczema. *Archives of Disease in Childhood,* **61** (1), 20–3.

Daud, L.R., Garralda, M.E. & David, T.J. (1993) Psychosocial adjustment in preschool children with atopic eczema. *Archives of Disease in Childhood,* **69** (6), 670–6.

Department of Health and Social Security (1980) *Artificial Feeds for the Young Infant.* HMSO, London.

Department of Health (1994) Weaning and the Weaning Diet. *Report on Health and Social Subjects* 45, HMSO, London.

Dhar, S., Kanwar, A.J., Kaur, S., Sharma, P. & Ganguly, N.K. (1992) Role of bacterial flora in the pathogenesis and management of atopic dermatitis. *Indian Journal of Medical Research Section A – Infectious Diseases,* **95**, 234–8.

Donnelly, J.E., Donnelly, W.J. & Thong Y.H. (1987) Parental perceptions and attitudes towards asthma and its treatment: a controlled study. *Social Science and Medicine,* **24**, 431–7.

Elliott, B.E. (1994) *The effects of having a child with severe atopic eczema as described by the written accounts of mothers.* unpublished M.Sc thesis, University of Manchester, Manchester.

Elliott, B.E. & Luker, K. (1996) The experiences of mothers caring for a child with severe atopic eczema. *Journal of Clinical Nursing*, **6**, 241–7

Ewing, C.I., Roper, H.P., David, T.J. & Haeney, M.R. (1989) Death from eczema herpeticum in a child with severe eczema, mental retardation and cataracts. *Journal of the Royal Society of Medicine*, **82** (3), 169–70.

Faulstich, M.E. & Williamson, D.A. (1985) An overview of atopic dermatitis: towards a bio-behavioural integration. *Journal of Psychosomatic Research*, **29**, 647–54.

Fergusson, D.M., Horwood, L.J. & Shannon, F.T. (1982) Risk factors in childhood eczema. *Journal of Epidemiology and Community Health*, **36**, 118–22.

Fischer, G. (1996) Compliance problems in paediatric atopic eczema. *Australian Journal of Dermatology*, **37**, s10–s13.

Frank, G. (1987) Scratching the surface. *Nursing Times*, **83** (39), 66–8.

Gil, K.M., Keefe, F.J., Sampson, H.A., McCaskill, C.C., Rodin, J. and Crisson, J.E. (1987) The relation of stress and family environment to atopic dermatitis symptoms in children. *Journal of Psychosomatic Research*, **31** (6), 673–84.

George, S., Bilsland, D., Johnson, B.E. & Ferguson, J. (1991) Narrowband UVB (TL-01) air conditioned therapy for chronic severe adult atopic eczema. *Annals of Allergy*, p. 17.

Goodyear, H.M., McLeish, P., Randall, S., Buchan, A., Skinner, G., Winter, M. *et al.* (1996) Immunological studies of herpes simplex virus infection in children with atopic eczema. *British Journal of Dermatology*, **134**, 85–93.

Halpern, S.R., Sellars, W.A., Johnson, R.B., Anderson, D.W., Saperstein, S. & Reisch, J.S. (1973) Development of childhood allergy in infants fed breast, soy or cow milk. *Journal of Allergy and Clinical Immunology*, **52**, 139–51.

Hay, C. (1996) National Eczema Society. *Primary Health Care*, **6** (11), 22–3.

Hide, D.W. & Guyer, B.M. (1981) Clinical manifestations of allergy related to breast and cow's milk feeding. *Archives of Diseases in Childhood*, **56**, 172–5.

Jowett, S. & Ryan, T. (1985) Skin disease and handicap; an analysis of the impact of skin conditions. *Social Science and Medicine*, **20**, 425–9.

Kay, J., Gawkrodger, D.J., Mortimer, M.J. & Jaron, A.G. (1994) The prevalence of childhood atopic eczema in a general population. *Journal of the American Academy of Dermatology*, **30** (1), 35–9.

Kenrick, M., Luker, K.A. (1995) *Clinical Nursing Practice in the Community*. Blackwell Science, Oxford.

Kjellman, N.I.M. & Johansson, S.G.O. (1979) Soy versus cows' milk in infants with bi-parental history of atopic disease: development of atopic disease and immunoglobulins from birth to four years of age. *Clinical Allergy*, **9**, 347–58.

Krafchik, B.R. (1988) Eczematous dermatitis. In: *Paediatric Dermatology*, (eds R.C. Hansen & L.A. Schachner) Churchill Livingstone. New York

Kurwa, H.A. & Finlay, A.Y. (1995) Dermatology inpatient management greatly improves life quality. *British Journal of Dermatology*, **133**, 575–8.

Lake, A.M., Kleinman, R.E. & Walker, W.A. (1981) Enteric alimentation in specialised gastrointestinal problems: an alternative to total parenteral nutrition. *Advances in Pediatrics*, **28**, 319–39.

Lucas, A., Brooke, O.G., Morley, R., Cole, T.J. & Bamford, M.F. (1990) Early diet of preterm infants and development of allergic or atopic disease: randomised prospective study. *British Medical Journal*, **300**, 837–40.

Medansky, R.S. (1980) Dermatopsychosomatics: an overview. *Psychosomatics*, **21**, 195–200.

Mallon, E., Powell, S. & Bridgman, A. (1994) Wet wrap dressings for the treatment of atopic eczema in the community. *Journal of Dermatological Treatment*, **5**, 97–9.

National Asthma Campaign (1993a) *Asthma at School 4*, National Asthma Campaign, London.

National Asthma Campaign (1993b) *Asthma and the Environment: Air Pollution II*, National Asthma Campaign, London.

Neame, R.L., Berth-Jones, J. & Graham-Brown, R.A.C. (1993) A population based prevalence study of atopic dermatitis in the UK. *Journal of Investigative Dermatology*, **100**, 543.

Nocoon, A. (1991) Social and emotional impact of childhood asthma (editorial). *Archives of Disease in Childhood*, **66** (4), 458–60

Obeid, A. (1996) Infant feeding and allergy: a critical review. *Paediatric Nursing*, **8** (6), 17–22.

Pless, I.B. & Nolan, T. (1991) Revision, replication and neglect: research on maladjustment in chronic illness. *Journal of Child Psychology and Psychiatry*, **32** (2), 347–65.

Rajka, G. (1989) *Essential Aspects of Atopic Dermatitis*, Berlin, Springer Verlag.

Read, C. (1991) *Air Pollution and Child Health*, London, Greenpeace.

Sampson, H.A., Bernhisel-Broadbent, J., Yang, E. & Scanlon, S.M. (1991) Safety of casein hydrolysate formula in children with cow milk allergy. *Journal of Pediatrics*, **118** (4), pt 1, 520–5.

Sheehan, M.P., Atherton, D.J., & Hui Lo, D. (1991) A controlled trial of Chinese medicinal plants in widespread non-exudative atopic eczema. *Annals of Allergy*, p. 17.

Sheehan, M.P., Atherton, D.J., Norris, P. & Hawk, S. (1993) Oral psoralem photochemotherapy in severe childhood atopic eczema an update. *British Journal of Dermatology*, **129** (4), 431–6.

Sneddon, J. (1980) The psychiatrist and the dermatologist – which ticket of admission? *Practitioner*, **224**, 97–100.

Spowart, K. (1993) Management of eczema in children. *Paediatric Nursing*, **5** (8), 9–12.

Spowart, K. & Muir, M. (1994) *A Practical Guide to the Management of Eczema. Community Healthcare Nurses.* National Eczema Society, London.

Strachan, D.P., Anderson, H.R., Limb, E.S., O'Neill, A. & Wells, N. (1994) A national survey of asthma prevalence, severity and treatment in Great Britain, *Archives of Disease in Childhood*, **70**, 174–8.

Tariq, S.M., Stevens, M., Matthews, S., Ridout, S., Twisleton, R. & Hide D.W. (1996) Cohort study of peanut and treenut sensitisation by age of 4 years. *British Medical Journal*, **313** (7056), 514–17.

Taylor, B., Wadsworth, J., Wadsworth, M. & Peckham, C. (1984) Changes in the reported prevalence of childhood eczema since the 1939–45 war. *Lancet*, ii, 1255–7.

Turnbull, R. & Atherton, D.J. (1994) The use of wet wraps in childhood atopic eczema. *Paediatric Nursing*, **6** (2), 22–6.

Turner, M.A., Devlin, J. & David, T.J. (1991) Holidays and atopic eczema, *Archives of Disease in Childhood*, **66**, 212–15.

Venables, J. (1995) Dermatology nursing in practice: management of children with atopic eczema in the community. *Dermatology in Practice*, Oct, pp. s1–4.

Van Bever, H.P. (1992). Recent advances in the pathogenesis of atopic dermatitis. *European Journal of Paediatrics*, **151**, 870–73.

Watts, J. (1996) Atopic eczema practical management. *Primary Health Care*, **6** (11), 17–21.

Webber, S.A., Graham-Brown, R.A. Hutchinson, P.E. & Burns, D.A. (1989) Dietary manipulation in childhood atopic dermatitis. *British Journal of Dermatology*, **12** (1), 91–98.

Williams, H.C., Strachan, D.P. & Hay, R.J. (1994a) Childhood eczema: disease of the advantaged? *British Medical Journal*, **308** (6937), 1132–5.

Williams, H.C., Burney, P.G.J., Hay, R.J., Archer, C.B., Shipley, M.J., Hunter, J.J.A. *et al.* (1994b) The UK Working Party's Diagnostic Criteria for Atopic Dermatitis. I. Derivation of a minimum set of discriminators for atopic dermatitis. *British Journal of Dermatology*, **131**, 383–96.

Williams, H.C., Forsdyke, H., Boodoo, G., Hay, R.J. & Burney, P.G.J. (1995) A protocol for recording the sign of flexural dermatitis in children,. British Journal of Dermatology, **133**, 941–9.

14

Sleep Disorders in the Pre-school Child: How the Health Professionals Can Help

Pam Pritchard

14.1 INTRODUCTION

Children's sleep, or the lack of it, seems to be a major preoccupation for many parents. All parenting issues seem intensely important, but this one seems even more charged with a wide range of emotions. Sleep – or the lack of it – in both the parent and child can undermine the coping abilities of even the most confident parent; it can precipitate family discord, and upset both the marital relationship and that of the parent and child.

This chapter is written from a practical perspective and outlines current accepted practice underpinned by evidence from some of the classic literature on this subject.

14.2 THE SCALE OF THE PROBLEM

Frequent night waking occurs in approximately 20% of one to two year olds, 14% of three year olds and 8% of four year olds (Richman *et al.* 1975; Jenkins *et al.* 1980). There are no sex differences in the rates of sleep disturbance in young children, and no social class difference (Richman *et al.* 1982). However, there is considerable persistence of the problem. Forty six per cent of children with sleeping problems as babies still have sleep problems at the age of five years

(Butler & Golding 1986). The more severe the difficulty, the greater the likelihood of persistence of the problem. About a third of children with sleep problems also show other behavioural difficulties, which may, in part, be due to a chronic lack of sleep.

Some parents become very distressed at being awakened frequently during the night, whereas others may feel that this is expected, and are less concerned. Some parents enjoy having their child share their bed, others feel this is not an area of negotiation. As each parent feels differently about what is expected and reasonable for their child, equally there is no universal advice that will suit all parents. Each child and family is individual, as each has separate and differing needs. There is no single 'right' way of responding, parents need to decide what is appropriate for them and their child.

Sleep difficulties may be part of a larger behavioural problem. Toddlers with strong wills and persistence may be seen as being out of control by their parents who may find setting limits difficult both during the day and at night time. The interaction between parent and child is a critical issue and parental responses to the sleep difficulty can nevertheless increase or decrease the problem. No child needs to be a 'poor sleeper'; a new sleep pattern can be learned, as all other behaviours are learned, by a parent giving the child cues, routine and consistency.

Consequently, it is important that both parents participate in trying to solve a sleep difficulty. Fathers are often overlooked by health professionals, but may be equally involved in the care of their child. Often it is in the evening and at night that are times when the family is together, and excluding one parent from discussion could undermine parents working together. Parental confidence is a key aspect of success in managing sleep problems, so joint decision making between the professional and parents is critical for advice to be successful. It is easy for health visitors to meet mothers, but it requires perhaps a special effort, a separate appointment at a mutually convenient time, to meet both parents together.

Sleep patterns

The first years of life are a time of rapid change, and there is a wide variation in the amount of sleep children need, and in their waking and sleeping patterns. Newborn babies sleep on average about 16 hours a day, this is made up of frequent, brief, periods of waking with little diurnal pattern, interrupting an otherwise unbroken sleep. Over the first three months the total hours of sleep do not decline significantly but the pattern consolidates into fewer, more prolonged episodes of waking and a greater concentration of

sleep at night. At this stage about 70% of babies do not wake at night (Flower & Tufnell 1994).

By the end of the first year, the total hours of sleep will have fallen to about 10, and some 10% of children will be waking every night, or several nights a week. There appears to be an association between wakefulness in babies and breast feeding (Eaton Evans & Dugdale 1988), also with complications in pregnancy and delivery (Blurton Jones *et al.* 1978).

Between one and three years, children's sleep may become more disrupted, which may be related to certain developmental factors. Going to sleep requires a surrender of the external world for an internal one, which may seem frightening and lonely, and this may explain the need for the 'transitional objects' that bridge the gap. Teddies, blankets and cuddlies can become essential as comforters, and particularly important at a stressful time.

Most children in the first three years of life have a daytime nap or naps, though by four to five years old this has been outgrown and a slightly earlier bedtime is commonplace.

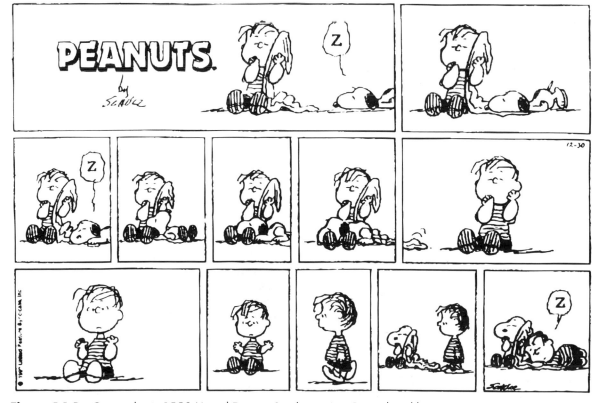

Figure 14.1   Copyright © 1990 United Feature Syndicate, Inc. Reproduced by permission.

Types of sleep problems

The commonest sleep difficulties in young children are night waking and difficulties in settling at bedtime; these patterns may co-exist. There are a number of variations on the theme, but often the child may refuse to go to bed, then wake frequently throughout the night, again settle with difficulty, or end up sleeping with the exhausted parents.

14.3 ASSESSMENT

A detailed assessment of the child's sleep pattern and the parents' interaction and coping mechanisms is essential before an effective treatment plan can be offered. Health professionals can be impatient to intervene and offer advice, often little information is gathered, and consequently non-specific 'blanket' advice is given which is usually ineffective. A careful, planned assessment and a detailed understanding of the situation are vital to an effective management approach.

History of the problem

The history should identify when the problem started, and how long it has been continuing. Some children have never slept well, and have been seen to be difficult since birth. Others may have been disrupted by a specific event, teething, illness or an emotional upset. It is important to listen to the 'story', to gain an insight into the worries and concerns of the parents and truly to understand, not only their level of stress, but also their coping mechanisms. It is also essential to discover whether parents feel their child is waking because of hunger, thirst, discomfort, and so on. A strategy for change has to come from the parents' frame of reference, not that of the professional.

Settling routine

It is helpful to know where the child is settled to sleep in the evening, and how the child is settled to sleep by the parent. For example, perhaps the child lies on the settee sucking a bottle, or lies in the parents' bed with mother beside the child stroking his or her head. The time that this usually occurs, and length of time it takes the child to settle to sleep, together with the routine that the parents follow, is essential information.

Night waking

The frequency of the waking and the duration that the child is awake is information that will help you to understand what is happening in the middle of the night. What the child does on waking, and how the parents respond provide an interactive picture. It may give information as to why the behaviour is maintained.

Daytime naps

Children who have sleep problems often compensate by having a nap or series of naps in the day, perhaps being lulled to sleep by the movement of the pram or car. Whether these are excessive or age-appropriate, and whether the timing of the nap is possibly interfering with a preferred evening settling time, need to be determined.

Sleep diary

Asking parents to complete a sleep diary can provide an accurate record of the child's sleep pattern and involves all of the above. It avoids distorted memories, and helps parents think through their involvement with their child's night time behaviour. Often the diary can clarify issues for parents as well as for professionals.

Parents who do not complete a diary are unlikely to carry through an agreed plan of action. So the way in which parents are able to comply with this task can aid assessment of parental motivation. Without a diary it is impossible to formulate an accurate sleeping 'plan'. So 'no diary no treatment plan' is a good rule to remember.

Usually, a week of recording is ample, or four or five nights may be enough. Obviously, when a treatment plan is implemented, the diary can be helpful to record the change in the child's sleeping pattern. This supplies feedback to parents and professionals and monitors progress.

By the end of the assessment, it is important to know what aims and goals the parents want to see. It is important to be sure that they want the situation to change. Some parents are happy to live with a wakeful child that (to us) seems impossible. Do not assume that this is a problem. Equally, a parent may be upset because their child wakes once a night, but they may find it impossible to go back to sleep, once awakened. Again do not be dismissive of a difficulty that may be very stressful for a parent.

14.4 SLEEP PATTERNS HYPOTHESES

Sleeping patterns have been demonstrated by a recent videotaped study of young children's night time behaviour (Minde *et al.* 1993). It showed that *all* children in the sample woke regularly during the night. The 'poor' sleepers were those who were unable or unwilling to go back to sleep, and cried, or called out to a parent. The 'control' children went back to sleep after a period of approximately 10 minutes, without disturbing anyone, and self-settled by hugging a toy or by sucking their thumb.

In order to go to sleep adults (and children) develop their own individual method of settling to sleep (you may get into bed a particular way, snuggle down, turn on your left side and put your hand under the pillow, etc.). During sleep the brain continues to be active in certain ways and, during the night, cycles of sleep occur, moving from light sleep to deep sleep and back again, the light stages are when we dream and the deep stages are when it is most difficult to wake up.

In the lighter stages of sleep it is possible to be aware of a loud noise (lorry changing gear or dog barking) but, in order to slip back to a deeper level of sleep, we often repeat the settling routine that we used to go to sleep in the evening. For a child if this settling routine involves an external object such as drinking from a bottle or being cuddled by his or her mother, the child will be unable to settle to sleep again without this, so he or she will consequently wake and cry for this to happen.

Also, if infants are settled to sleep by their mother, say, lying beside them, their last memory before sleep will be of their mother's presence. When they wakes or are disturbed, they will consequently fully expect their mother still to be there. They will panic, and become upset. Consequently, in order to solve a

problem of night waking it is essential to explore fully the existing settling routine. The child will need to be taught the skill of settling himself or herself to sleep, rather than relying upon external attention. For example an alternative settler perhaps a dummy instead of a bottle could then be offered to the child, so the child could self-settle, by putting the dummy in.

If, for instance, a mother lies with her child as part of a settling routine, this can continue but the mother should, for example, kiss the child and leave the room, leaving the child to go to sleep *independently*. Again an alternative settler can be negotiated, a doll that the child is particularly fond of instead of the mother, a soft toy, or special blanket is equally suitable. With an older child, the child could choose a new toy 'instead' of Mummy so that there is partnership in the proposed change.

14.5 MANAGING CHANGE

The message for many years has been that a child needs to learn a set routine of getting ready for bed and falling asleep. A regular, set sequence of wash, change, drink, cuddle and so on, enables the child to be calm and learn what is expected. The consistency of this approach will give security to the child who will follow the 'cues' and learn to go to sleep by the new routine.

Ferber (1986) suggests that this works well, that a child's sleep associations need not include the parents, and the child can develop his or her own way to get to sleep. Obviously the child may not be keen on the new routine. He or she will cry because the old routine was familiar, and learning anew is strange and difficult. Ferber suggests that visits from a parent are made to show they are 'still there', but are progressively less frequent so the child learns to accept a longer and longer separation, and eventually settles without feeling deserted.

White (1978), author of *The First Three Years of Life*, suggests a 'cry-it-out' approach is still very effective, and does no harm to a child's emotional well being. He suggests that, for a healthy normal child, this will be successful if used consistently between seven to ten days.

After a bedtime routine, the parent leaves the room and allows the child to cry until he or she falls asleep. No maximum amount of time for crying is set. The parent responds to the first cry to make sure that there is nothing 'wrong', such as an illness. The prediction is that with each incident, the length of crying will decrease, until the child goes to sleep.

Leach (1989), recommends checking the child at consistent five minute intervals, whereas Brazelton (1984) recommends that, after going to the child several times, a parent simply calls out reassuringly to the child without going into the room. He also stresses the importance of encouraging attachment to a 'lovey' as an important part of the settling routine.

There are a number of variations on the theme, Douglas and Richman (1984), in their definitive work with children with sleep disturbances, suggest a 'checking' routine similar to that of Leach of returning to the child every five minutes. They also suggest a careful assessment and 'diary' and a soothing, settling routine at bedtime.

This management advice has remained a standard since that date, but reconciling the contradictory views on the timing of returning and checking of the child is difficult. Evidence is conflicting, as some studies suggest that a frequent response produces more crying, others finding the opposite.

What follows is a synthesis from the author's own practice outlining two different strategies for managing change:

Strategy A

A fixed checking time of 15 minutes for a baby 6–24 months and 20 minutes for children of two years and older (Pritchard & Appleton 1988). Thinking from a child's perspective, it seems to give the wrong message to 'pop' into the room every five minutes, when the message given by the parent should be that of restfulness, quiet and sleep. Also, the unpredictable intervals of 5, 10, 15 minutes suggested by progressively lengthening the time interval might provoke anxiety in the child, and hence increase crying. The 15/20 minute rule allows for the escalation of the child's distress, then allows the child to relax and begin to calm. The timing could give the child a sense of security by its repetition.

The message to the child is that it is sleep time, so a firmness of approach, with no undue sympathy or contact is advocated. Often the child responds, as he

or she picks up on the firmness of manner and knows that in this case, the parent means to carry it through. Consistency of approach is essential, so, once begun, this should be continued every night, so the child learns very quickly (usually in about four nights).

Parents do have very different temperaments and tolerance for crying, so it is essential that both partners are committed to working together and supporting each other through this method. It is helpful, perhaps, to emphasise the rapid improvement in the child's settling (and night waking), if they can persevere.

Some parents find their child's crying extremely difficult to cope with. They become upset themselves, or feel the child becomes 'hysterical', or in such a state that it is emotionally damaging to the child. Carefully talking through the meaning of the crying may help parents see it more objectively. It is important that parents do not feel the crying reflects the child's being hungry, thirsty or in pain. So helping parents exclude these possibilities one by one, can help them to reach a considered decision. Some parents will describe the crying as being 'like a tantrum' and with this, you can think together what the child is demanding, which is, of course to come out of the cot! When it is put in this way, most parents feel better equipped to cope with the child's distress, and less anxious about hearing a child cry. Parents may need reassurance that a child who is well loved and cared for during the day will not be damaged or feel rejected if parents set firm limits about nighttime behaviour.

It is helpful for the professional to provide extra support for parents at this time. The offer of a home visit from a health visitor on the morning following the implementation of the new routine, to discuss any difficulties the parents may have encountered, can be reassuring. Many small aspects of management that are worrying parents can then be ironed out. Parents can be encouraged to stay on track, and further visits arranged to suit the family. These may be daily or weekly depending on anxiety or progress. However, no matter how everybody tries, or how logical the agreed plan is, there are some parents who simply find a rigid routine too stressful and impossible to implement.

Strategy B

A 'graded steps' approach may help to lessen the crying and be more acceptable to parents (Douglas &

Richman 1984). The overall aim, for the child to learn to settle to sleep unaided, remains the same. However, the settling routine is broken down into small stages, the child learning to accept one stage with little protest before moving on to the next.

The starting point is moving slightly away from the present settling routine. For example, if a parent is lying beside the child, the parent leaves a gap between them, then moves to the edge of the bed, then sits in a chair by the bed and so on, until the parent reaches the door. The process of gradual separation involves the parent having less physical contact and being less responsive (not talking and so on) to the child. The parent should reassure the child only by being there not by interaction. This too can be difficult to achieve, some children resist separating from their parents, or insist their parent interacts with them (sitting on the parent's face or pulling parent's hair and such like).

The routine in practice can be difficult to implement. Parents need to be committed and disciplined, to be clear as to what stage they have reached, and to continue to move forward. Similarly, when the child wakes in the night, the parent resettles the child by repeating the 'settling' routine.

If the child becomes ill, however, it is easy for the routine to break down and parents may have to start all over again.

This graded steps approach is much slower than the more direct approach and, again, support from the professional is helpful when planning each stage of withdrawal. It could be, however, a method of choice for a child with special needs. In these cases, the problems of settling and waking at night are the same as with any other child. Clear routines are essential together with a consistency of approach. The management of change may be slower, but this is determined by the child's level of ability and developmental delay.

Managing night waking

If a child has learned that when he or she cries a parent will go to him or her and offer a drink or engage in play and so on, the child is likely to continue to do this as the end result is pleasurable. It becomes a habit. The aim is for the child to settle back to sleep independently, the same strategy being followed as in the settling routine.

For a young child it is important that he or she is reassured, no food or drink is offered, there is no play or going downstairs, or into the parents' bed. If the child needs to be changed, this should be done with minimal attention (Pritchard & Appleton 1988). With an older child, that perhaps comes downstairs or goes into the parents' bed, it involves the parents being committed to returning the child to its own bed, each time. A calm, firm approach is advocated, again giving the child minimal attention (Douglas 1989).

Some children can be very persistent. In one instance a child (aged three years) came downstairs 76 times (hence the joy of keeping a record chart!). The parents succeeded at the 77th time, the child remained in bed, and did not come out of her bed *at all* on successive nights.

If parents find this physically exhausting, a baby gate could be placed across the child's bedroom door. It is important that this restrains the child, and is, in itself, safe, that is the child cannot climb over it. This is particularly helpful for those children who are between 18 months and three years who sleep in a bed. Parents may be anxious that the child may fall, or play in other bedrooms/bathroom if they have free access.

Managing extreme tantrum behaviour

It is important that during assessment you discover what the child is likely to do in its persistence to get its own way. If parents report that the child 'becomes hysterical' you will need to know what is meant by this, for instance does the child vomit, hold his or her breath, or headbang? And so on. If this is likely, if for example the child usually resorts to this behaviour if thwarted during the day, it is helpful to discuss a management procedure or some coping mechanism that the parents can follow during the night. It is much better to prepare for this eventuality, so that the management routine doesn't fail.

- *Vomiting:* Vomiting should be seen to with a minimum of fuss. The child and bedding should be changed quickly and calmly. No further drink, etc. should be offered.
- *Breath holding:* If possible, talk to the parents about their management of this during the day, and help them to maintain the same non-attention principles during the night.
- *Sweating/puffy eyes/sobbing,* etc. This sort of thing needs to be carefully discussed with parents, so if possible, you reduce anxiety by the accep-

tance that these things *may* happen but are not damaging to the child.

When is morning?

It is helpful to discuss with parents a time that they feel is acceptable for their child to wake in the morning. This prevents the possibility of a child sleeping through the night, but then waking progressively earlier and earlier, as the parents are unsure of the limit they should set. For instance if a child wakes at 5.30 a.m., parents may decide to treat this as night (night waking procedure is followed), but if the child wakes at 6.30 a.m., this is morning. The child is then given the appropriate cue, lifted out of the cot and taken downstairs for breakfast.

'Reward' systems

If you feel it would be helpful to offer an older child (3–5 years) a reward for staying in their room all night, by all means negotiate this with parents. Stickers or stars tend *not* to work well with younger children. A small gift from a 'lucky dip', or special sweet/toy/treat can be magic – and should be given to the child immediately in the morning after a successful night, together with great joy and praise.

Night toileting

If a child is toilet trained by night, you will need to allow the child to get up and go to the toilet. This will need to be discussed with parents. A potty provided in the child's room could be an option. It is important that the child just goes to the toilet then returns to bed with minimal conversation or attention.

Nightmares

Young children have nightmares, but until the child can speak and explain what it is, parents are unaware of the cause of the nightmare. A child may wake screaming, and may be frightened to return to sleep in case the nightmare recurs. Nightmares usually occur in the lightest stages of sleep and are most common in the three to four year age range. By a detailed assessment and baseline recording, the differences between a nightmare and habit waking becomes apparent.

Nightmares can be triggered by something frightening seen on video or TV. The child may also become anxious if there is family disharmony, rows, shouting, and so on. Parents may report a change to the usual good sleeping pattern, and it may be

possible, again, by careful history taking to find a probable cause. It is helpful if parents can explore the child's fears in the daytime, and reassure the child concerning reality, and what is true and 'real' compared to the more frightening fantasy world.

Night terrors

The child is unaware of having a 'terror'. The child is not fully awake, but looks as if they are having a terrifying experience. In the morning, the child is unaware, and does not remember the incident. A night terror usually occurs in older children (5–12 years) and is more common in boys than girls. There may be a familial link (Anders & Weinstein 1972). The night terror occurs usually within the first few hours and occurs in deep sleep. It generally gives way to calm sleep. Waking a child in the initial hours of sleep may prevent a night terror by disrupting the sleep cycle.

Headbanging and rocking

This is part of a rhythmical movement that children will use to soothe themselves, provide a comfort and consequently help them fall asleep (Sallustro & Atwell 1978). Consequently, it can develop to become part of the child's settling routine, and, once established, it can be very difficult to change. Children usually do not hurt themselves although for parents it may be irritating or provoke anxiety. Problems can arise if parents become worried and bring the child downstairs. The child could then learn to be quite coercive, and may escalate the headbanging so that bruising may occur. The child then uses the headbanging as a method of gaining control. The headbanging is then not a comfort mechanism, but an expression of frustration, of gaining parental attention, and part of a 'battle situation'.

Crying babies

The majority of parents describe a 'crying baby' as being a cause of acute anxiety and stress. The baby is described as 'windy' or 'colicky'. As a health professional it can be a temptation to become drawn into this anxiety, and suggest a change of milk, possibly as an 'instant' solution. The lack of evidence behind this approach has been discussed in Chapter 8. However, a full assessment needs to be made that includes the infant's feeding, sleeping, and crying periods and the use of a diary is again essential. Often the infant shows unstable routines, both with feeding and sleeping.

This can result in a cycle of poor feeding as the baby is overtired, and then the baby tends to wake frequently because the need for food has not been met (Pritchard 1986).

Self-help services

Crysis (telephone: 0171 404 5011) is a self-help organisation for parents with babies who cry excessively. They do not differentiate between babies who cry a lot and those that have a sleep problem. As far as the author is aware, there are no self-help groups specifically for those with sleeping problems. A self-help guide for parents can be helpful. *The Good Sleep Guide for You and Your Baby* by Angela Henderson (1997) provides advice for babies from birth to 18 months and it has an inbuilt sleep 'diary'.

14.6 CONCLUSION

From this overview it will be seen that sleeping in the pre-school child is a complex topic and one where disruption and distress can spread throughout the family. A careful, non-judgemental history taking and realistic interventions based on planning manageable goals set in partnership are the most likely ways in which community health nurses can help.

REFERENCES

Anders, T.F. & Weinstein, P. (1972) Sleep disorders in infants and children. *Pediatrics*, **50**, 312–24.

Blurton-Jones, N., Rossietti Terreira, N.C., Farquhar Brown, M. & MacDonald, L. (1978) The association between perinatal factors and later night waking. *Dev.Med.Child Neurol*, **20**, 427–34.

Butler, N.R. & Golding, J. (eds) (1986) *From Birth to Five: A Study of Health and Behaviour of Britain's Five Year Olds*. Pergamon, London.

Brazelton, T. Berry (1984) *To Listen to a Child*. Addison Wesley, Reading, Mass.

Douglas, J. & Richman, N. (1984) *My Child Won't Sleep*. Penguin, Harmondsworth.

Douglas, J. (1989) *Behaviour Problems in Young Children*. Tavistock/Routledge, London.

Eaton Evans, J. & Dugdale, J. (1988) Sleep patterns of infants in the first year of childhood. *Archives of Diseases in Childhood*, **63**, 647–9.

Ferber, R. (1986) *Solve Your Child's Sleep Problems*. Dorling Kindersley, London.

Flower, P. & Tufnell, G. (1994) Sleep problems in children. *Maternal and Child Health*, **19** (1), 6–9.

Henderson, A. (1997) *The Good Sleep Guide for You and Your Baby*, ABC Health Guides.

Jenkins, S., Bax, M. & Hart, H. (1980) Behaviour problems in pre-school children. *Journal of Child Psychology: Psychiatry*, **21**, 5–19.

Leach, P. (1989) *Baby and Child: From Birth to Five*. Joseph, London.

Minde, K., Popiel, K., Leos, N., Falkner, S., Parker, K. & Handley-Derry, M. (1993) The evaluation and treatment of sleep disturbances in young children. *Journal of Child Psychology: Psychiatry*, **34** (4), 521–533.

Parmelee, A. H., Weiner, N.H. & Scultz, H.R. (1964) Infant sleep patterns from birth to 16 weeks of age. *Journal of Paediatrics*, **65**, 576–82.

Pritchard, A.A. & Appleton, P. (1988) Management of sleep problems in pre-school children. *Early Child Development & Care*, **34**, 227–240.

Pritchard, P.F. (1986) An infant crying clinic. *Health Visitor*, **59**, 375–7.

Richman, N., Douglas, J., Hunt, H., Lansdown, R. & Levere, R. (1985) Behavioural methods in the treatment of sleep disorders: a pilot study. *Journal of Child Psychology: Psychiatry* **26**, 581–90.

Richman, N., Stevenson, J., Graham, P.J. (1975) Prevalence and patterns of psychological disturbance in children of primary age. *Journal of Child Psychology*, **6**, 101–13.

Richman, N., Stevenson, J. & Graham, P.J. (1982) *Pre-school to School: A Behavioural Study*. Academic Press, London.

Richman, N. (1987) A community survey of characteristics of 1–2 year olds with sleep disruptions. *American Academy of Child Psychiatry*, **20**, 281–91.

Sallustro, F. & Atwell, C.W. (1978) Body rocking, head-banging, and head-rolling in normal children. *Journal of Paediatrics*, **93**, 704–8.

Weissbluth, M. (1987) *Healthy Sleep Habits, Happy Child*. Fawcett Columbine, New York.

White, B. (1978) The First Three Years of Life. W. H. Allen, London.

15

Toilet Training and Related Issues: Anticipatory Help for Parents and Families

Karen Chalmers

15.1 INTRODUCTION

Achieving bowel and bladder control is a major developmental milestone for both children and their parents, yet little research has been done on the topic since the early 1960s (Hauck 1991). The theory and recommendations for toilet training since 1900 have 'traced a pendulum's path' from systematic control to passive permissiveness (Luxem & Christophersen 1994). Since the mid century the trend has been towards delayed potty training, usually between the second and third year. Community health nurses and other primary health care practitioners are in a unique position to offer anticipatory guidance to parents on toilet training, and to provide additional assistance as needed. The purpose of this chapter is to analyse the research literature on toilet training and related issues, to provide a basis for assessment, anticipatory guidance, health teaching, and, referral for additional assistance if needed.

15.2 RESEARCH ON TOILET TRAINING

There is considerable variation reported in the literature as to when children acquire bowel and bladder control and when lack of control signals a condition which may need further follow-up. The differences found in the literature relate to many factors, including:

- the type of sample studied (e.g. clinical versus community samples);
- the prevailing societal and professional context surrounding toilet training when the data were collected;
- variation in the 'starting point' for toilet training (e.g. the time when the child was first dressed in underpants or training pants, put on the potty, or some other less defined point);
- variation in the end points used to indicate the completion of training (i.e. whether toilet training has been achieved when children can carry out all components of the toileting process independently, signal their caregivers about their need to use the toilet, or respond to their caregivers' questions about toileting needs); and
- variation in the definition of successful toilet training.

Earlier reports indicated that children generally acquire bowel control before bladder control (MacFarlane *et al.* 1954). However, a more recent study found that the majority of children studied (75%) achieved bladder control first (Hauck 1988). The literature consistently reports the majority of children achieve daytime dryness prior to night time dryness (Hauck 1988); however, some children have been found to achieve night time dryness first, or both day and nighttime dryness at the same time (19% each) (Hauck 1988).

Most children achieve bowel and bladder control by their fourth birthday. Berk and Friman's (1990) extensive review of the epidemiological literature on day and night time bladder control over the past 40 years indicated that bladder control was usually achieved between 24 and 48 months of age. In a recent study of over 1100 children, toilet training ages ranged from 9 months to 5 years with a mean of 2.4 years (Bloom *et al.* 1993). Differences between boys and girls are frequently reported in the popular literature and anecdotal reports, with boys considered to take longer to train. In empirical studies boys have been found to be slightly older when their toilet training started (Martin *et al.* 1984) and when they achieved bowel or bladder control (Brazelton 1962, Martin *et al.* 1984). The duration of potty training for boys is reported to take longer; however, these results have not been consistently found (Hauck 1988). Most of the research on toilet training has used middle-class American, British or European samples. There is little readily available research on new immigrants or other social classes.

Managing potty training

Theoretical perspectives

Parents' views on potty training in this century have been heavily influenced by the professional community and the lay literature of the period. The term 'training' reflects the behaviourist perspective of the 1920s and 1930s and is the terminology still widely in use (Hauck 1988). Adoption of conditioning strategies led to early, rigid and frequently harsh training practices. One expert recommended conditioning begin at three to five weeks after birth and that parents be 'unremitting' in their training routines (Watson 1928). Sigmund Freud's psychoanalytic theories linked toilet training with anxiety and inhibition.

If parents failed to train their children the 'right way' at the 'right time', the child would suffer long lasting effects on his or her personality (Hauck 1988). Some clinicians still view problems with urination and defecation from this psychoanalytic perspective (Josephs 1989).

Maturation

The maturational perspective considers that toilet training depends on physiological and cognitive maturation of the child. Proponents of this more recent view, such as Gesell (1943) and Brazelton (1962), used empirical data to establish 'norms' of toilet training milestones. Brazelton identified the pre-requisites to toileting as:

(1) control of the reflex sphincter muscles at about 9 months;
(2) voluntary co-operation in the toileting process at 12–15 months; and
(3) completion of myelinisation of the pyramidal tracts at 12–18 months (p. 14).

Current perspectives on toilet training tend to use maturational 'readiness' (physical, cognitive, and psychosocial) as the guide to begin toilet training, rather than prescriptively define age and time frames (Hauck 1988).

Processes involved in toilet training

There is little current research on toilet training; most empirical literature focuses on problems children experience (e.g. bedwetting or soiling). Also, there is little study of parents' approaches to toilet training. The existing literature suggests that children may best learn independence in toileting using a consistent, supportive approach.

Hauck (1988) interviewed 80 first-time parents of toddlers randomly selected from a health care centre to identify processes involved in toilet training. Parental strategies for potty training varied from the highly structured and parent-directed to child initiated approaches. Parents also considered that they used modelling and praise most frequently, and that these approaches were the most effective in helping their children achieve toileting success. In another American study, Seim (1989) surveyed parents of 266 children about the processes they used to train their first-born children. The largest number of children (43%) were 24–29 months old when training began. Parents reported that their children learned the training process from 'intuition', from themselves (parents), and from friends with small children. Most children were put on the potty chair and praised when successful.

Successful potty training appears to entail both physiological and cognitive readiness on the part of the child, as well as knowledge and skills (Hauck 1988). Three research measures have been developed to assess readiness and toilet practices:

(1) Parental Readiness Inventory;
(2) Child Readiness Profile, and
(3) Toileting Behaviour Report (Hauck 1988).

The items in these questionnaires were developed

from an extensive review of the literature and pilot tested with parents prior to use (see Appendix 15.1).

The Parental Readiness Inventory consists of 13 items addressing thoughts, behaviours, and feelings which parents may have experienced prior to beginning toilet training (e.g. reading about potty training; feeling that people were pressuring them to train their child). The Child Readiness Profile consists of 16 questions about readiness of the child for training (e.g. having bowel movements at predicted times; having a word, symbol or gesture indicating he or she wanted to use the toilet). The final questionnaire is a Toilet Behaviour Report. It consists of 14 items identified from the literature as observable toileting behaviours of varying complexity. Children who are more independent in their toilet behaviour demonstrate more behaviours than children who are less independent. Examples of these behaviours include: undresses all by him or herself before getting on to the toilet; wipes him or herself without any help. Although these questionnaires were developed for research purposes, they are useful for practitioners in assessing readiness for toilet training and mastery of the numerous skills in the process.

Difficulties achieving bowel and bladder control

Most children achieve bowel and bladder independence in the pre-school period. However, difficulties in achieving potty training raise questions in parents and health practitioners as to whether the child's behaviour is 'normal', and whether additional resources or referral are needed. Parents' frustration with potty training also signals the need for the health care professional to intervene sensitively in order to gather further information and provide helping interventions. Frustration over their children's inability to control toileting behaviour has been documented as an important antecedent of physical and verbal abuse (Hauck 1988; Warzak 1993).

15.3 ENURESIS

Enuresis refers to the involuntary passage of urine into the bedclothes or undergarments (Hay *et al.*

1995) which may occur during the day, **diurnal enuresis**, or more commonly during the night, **nocturnal enuresis** or 'bedwetting'. The definition of nocturnal enuresis varies from precise frequencies of wet nights, – such as at least one wet night in three months (Mattson 1994) – to more general statements of bedwetting. Enuresis can be primary or secondary. **Primary enuresis** refers to wetting in children who have never had sustained periods of dryness. **Secondary enuresis** develops after a child has had a sustained period of bladder control (Hay *et al.* 1995).

At least 90% of children who wet the bed have primary nocturnal enuresis (i.e. they wet only at night during sleep and they have never had a sustained period of dryness). Daytime wetting and secondary enuresis are much less common (Hay *et al.* 1995). The incidence of bedwetting is outlined in Table 15.1. Approximately 7% of children between 5 and 16 years of age suffer from nocturnal enuresis (Dobson 1994) with younger children more likely to experience bedwetting than older children. Nocturnal enuresis is reported to be approximately 40% at age 3 decreasing to about 3% at age 12, and 1% by age 18 (Schmitt 1982).

Table 15.1 Percentage of nocturnal enuresis by age.

Age	Percentage of children
3	40
4	30
5	15–20
6	10
7	7
8	6
10	3–5
12	2–3
14	1
18	1

(Compiled from: Schmitt 1982, Wille *et al.* 1994, Hay *et al.* 1995)

Common assumptions often held about children with nocturnal enuresis

There are many assumptions commonly held by parents and health professionals as to why children wet the bed. Each of these is examined and current research reported.

(1) 'Runs in the family'

There is now increasing evidence of a significant genetic component to the causes underpinning bed-wetting (Birch & Miller 1995). Enuresis has been found to be three times more common in families of children with enuresis than in families of non-enuretic peers (Wille 1994a). In a large community study of children with enuresis and controls, a prior history of enuresis was found in 65% of families of the enuretics compared to 25% in controls (Wille 1994b).

(2) Sound sleepers

Children are frequently reported by their parents to be 'heavy' or very sound sleepers. In empirical investigations using a 'wake-up' test, children who wet the bed were found to be more difficult to arouse at night compared to controls (Wille 1994b). Failure to wake up when the bladder is full, ('arousal failure'), has been found in other studies as well (Kirk *et al.* 1996). However, sleep studies have found children to be normal sleepers (Norgaard & Djurhuus 1993). Enuresis can take place at any time in the sleep cycle but usually occurs when the bladder is at full capacity (Norgaard & Djurhuus 1993).

(3) More boys wet the bed than girls at the same age

The incidence of bedwetting is more common in boys, it has been reported to be two to three times as high in boys as girls (Schmitt 1982; Hamburger 1993; Miller 1993; Hay *et al.* 1995).

(4) Most children will 'out-grow bedwetting'

The research confirms that most children do stop bedwetting, with or without any treatment. By age 18 only 1% of children wet the bed (Schmitt 1982).

(5) Behavioural or psychological disturbances

Children who wet the bed have been studied to identify other behavioural or psychological problems. In the majority of cases, there were no abnormalities found. No significant differences in common psychosomatic complaints have been identified in children who were enuretic compared to controls (Wille *et al.* 1994). Although primary nocturnal enuresis can have a wide range of negative experiences which can affect self-esteem, it is not associated with psychiatric or behavioural difficulties (Warzak & Friman 1994).

There is some evidence, though, if bedwetting continues into adolescence, that children may experience some, although slight, difficulties. In a New Zealand longitudinal study (over 15 years), the relationship between nocturnal enuresis in childhood and measures of behavioural adjustment in adolescence was studied. The analysis showed that children who were bedwetting after the age of 10 years showed slight increases in rates of conduct problems and attention deficit behaviours up to the age of 13 years. They also showed increased rates of anxiety/withdrawal up to the age of 15 years (Fergusson & Horwood 1994).

(6) Drinking at bedtime

A common assumption about a contributing factor in enuresis is drinking before bedtime. There is some evidence that this may contribute to bedwetting. In one study, enuresis was elicited in half of a sample of children who had no history of enuresis when they drank water before bedtime (Kirk *et al.* 1996). However, in a Swedish study, no differences were found in fluid intake between those children who wet the bed and those who did not (Mattsson 1994).

(7) 'Lazy' or 'doesn't care' attitude

There is no evidence that children who wet the bed are 'lazy' or unconcerned about their bedwetting. However, children who relapse after successful treatment for bedwetting have been found to express a lack of concern about their bedwetting (Butler *et al.* 1990a).

(8) 'Weak', small or abnormal bladder

There is some evidence that children who wet the bed have altered bladder functioning; however, this does not appear to be related to abnormalities in the structure or mechanical functioning of the bladder in the majority of cases. Enuretic children have been found to have normal bladder capacity (Norgaard & Djurhuus 1993; Wille 1994b). Bladder instability is also not considered to be related to enuresis (Norgaard & Djurhuus 1993). Enuretic children have normal calcium-creatinine quota in the urine (Wille 1994b). However, enuretic children have been found to have a significantly lower morning plasma level of the antidiuretic hormone, vasopressin, than non-enuretic children (Wille *et al.* 1994). Production of night time urine in these children has been found to be up to four times the usual volume, hence the need for bladder emptying (Norgaard & Djurhuus 1993).

(9) Stress or environmental assaults

There have been few studies which have examined environmental stressors and their link to bedwetting. Being bullied has been found to be associated with bedwetting in a large UK study (Williams *et al.* 1996). Sexual abuse should also be considered as a possible cause or contributing factor in persistent bedwetting.

Current thinking

Nocturnal enuresis is currently seen as a biobehavioural problem. Two physiological parameters are thought to be involved:

(1) deficient circadian release of antidiuretic hormone (ADH) (Eggert & Kuhn 1995); and
(2) deficient spontaneous inhibitory muscular responses (Houts 1991).

Children who wet the bed have been found to have a deficiency in ADH, resulting in an increase in urine production during the night (nocturnal polyuria) (Kirk *et al.* 1996). In addition, studies suggest immaturity in the central nervous system of the inhibition of micturition reflex during sleep (Robert *et al.* 1993). This combined, with the lack of arousal to the increasingly full bladder, leads to spontaneous muscle contraction and bladder emptying.

Assessment of enuresis

No clinical guidelines have been identified to guide community health nurses and other practitioners in assessment and referral practices. However, until such guidelines are available, the following practices may be helpful. These recommendations are based on the existing literature:

Assessment of the child's voiding pattern

Is the child dry during the day or wet during the day as well during the night?
Was the child dry at night in the past three months, but now bedwets (secondary enuresis)?

Assessment of the parents' potty training practices

How did/does the parent(s) approach potty training?
Is there a supportive environment for learning?

Assessment of the child's general growth and development

Is the child growing and developing normally, for example physical, social, emotional growth and development?
Are there any clues that there may be other stressors facing this child, that is physical or sexual abuse, or neglect?

Assessment of the parents' reaction to the bedwetting

What is the parent(s)' reaction to the bedwetting?
What does bedwetting mean to the parent(s)?
Was bedwetting a problem in the parent's family of origin?
If so, how was it handled, and how has this influenced the parent in relation to her/his own child's bedwetting?
Does the family have the material resources to cope with the bedwetting, for example a washing machine, extra linens, etc.?
Is the bedwetting being blamed for other issues or problems in the family/marriage, for example is the child being scapegoated?

Assessment of the child's reaction to the bedwetting

How does the child respond, that is feel ashamed, visibly upset, ignores/denies the bedwetting?
Does the child take responsibility for changing his/her bed, putting the sheets in the wash, etc. (if age appropriate)?

Medical assessment

Medical studies of children with enuresis and no further symptoms have found few abnormalities in these children. Medical assessment in persistent bedwetters, though, is important to rule out urinary tract infections, metabolic or nephrologic disorders (Rushton 1993a). Investigation includes taking a careful history to identify any associated problems such as diurnal enuresis, constipation or behavioural problems. Medical examination includes inspection of the external genitalia and lower back, and palpation of the abdomen, as well as urine and blood examination (Schulpen *et al.* 1996). Screening ultrasound is frequently used to rule out birth defects (Maizels *et al.* 1993).

Treatments for enuresis

Several treatments for bedwetting have been proposed over the years. Some remain in current practice. The following is a brief summary of the treatment and empirical support:

(1) Alarms

Alarms are one of the most commonly recommended treatments. Alarms work by conditioning the child to wake up when they void. The early alarms used a pad and bell which required the pad to become wet before triggering the alarm. Today's alarms are activated by a small probe anchored in the child's undergarment or pyjamas, with a cord running from the alarm to the child's wrist. The alarm is triggered as the child begins to release urine. Alarms are considered to be more effective compared to medication use (Maizels *et al.* 1993; Moffat *et al.* 1993). More children in clinical studies have been found to improve using the alarms rather than pharmacological treatments, and these benefits are more likely to be sustained when treatment is discontinued (Christophersen & Edwards 1991, Houts *et al.* 1994). The success rate reported in the literature is variable, but may be as high as 70% (Shapiro 1985), but relapse after discontinuing the alarm is common.

Medications

Pharmacological treatments include tricyclic antidepressants, anticholinergics and antidiuretics. Desmopressin acetate introduced in the 1990s has response rates similar to the older treatments (imipramines and other tricyclics) but without the side effects (Rushton 1993b). When medication treatment alone is given, amitriptyline has been found to be more effective than desmopressin, and the combination of desmopressin and amitriptyline did not confer any additional benefit (Burke *et al.* 1995). Desmopressin has been found to be effective in children with a functional bladder capacity greater than 70% (Rushton *et al.* 1996). Wille *et al.* (1994) in a Swedish study of enuretic children and matched controls (age and sex) found that secretion plasma vasopressin was significantly lower in morning samples in the enuretic children than the controls. This finding may explain why vasopressin substitute therapy is able successfully to treat some children with nocturnal enuresis. They found that desmopressin and the alarm were equally effective in controlling enuresis in enuretic children. Children treated with desmopressin had a more rapid improvement compared with children treated with an alarm; however, the latter had a lower relapse frequency (Wille 1994b).

Other treatments

Other treatments include bladder retention control training, waking schedules, self-monitoring and reinforcement (Warzak & Friman 1994). Biofeedback has been used successfully with children with severe enuresis problems (Mattelaer *et al.* 1995). Retention control training may be more effective in younger children (ages four to five) compared to older children (ages seven and eight) (Ronen & Abraham 1996).

Combinations of treatments

The alarm in combination with desmopressin has been found to be more effective than one single treatment. Combined treatment may be particularly effective for children with severe wetting and those experiencing family and behaviour problems (Bradbury & Meadow 1995). The alarm and dry bed training technique (DBTT) together with enuretic alarm was considered to be more effective than desmopressin alone (Bath *et al.* 1996).

Clinical treatment guidelines

No clinical treatment guidelines have been identified in the UK to assist clinicians in recommending treatment, however, clinical guidelines have been developed by an expert committee in the Netherlands (Schulpen *et al.* 1996). Guidelines for treatment are age specific: up to the age of six years, no medical or psychological intervention is considered to be needed. Between the ages of eight and twelve, an enuresis alarm is prescribed. If that is not successful, medication with desmopressin is recommended for a restricted period of time, and ambulatory dry-bed training in a group setting may follow. For children thirteen years and over, clinical dry bed training according to the Messer/Azrin method is advised. This latter treatment entails waking children each hour throughout the night, and taking them to the toilet in an effort to condition them to wake up when they experience a filling bladder.

The child's perspective

Few studies have sought the child's perspective of the

bedwetting experience. Peer pressure has been found to be associated with successful treatment in some, but not all, studies (Butler *et al.* 1988; Butler *et al.* 1990b). In open-ended interviews, Butler *et al.* (1990b) found that successful treatment was associated with the child's construction of the bedwetting psychologically and being not resistant to change.

15.4 ENCOPRESIS AND SOILING

Encopresis is defined as the passage of stool in an unacceptable place. It may occur either as a failure to establish toilet training (**primary encopresis**), or as a subsequent breakdown in that training (**secondary encopresis**) (Foreman & Thambirajah 1996). It has also been referred to as the involuntary loss of formed, semiformed or liquid stool into the child's underwear in the presence of functional (idiopathic) constipation in a child four years of age or younger (Loening-Baucke 1996). Statistics on encopresis suggest that this problem occurs in approximately 1–1.5% of school children – boys four times as commonly as girls (Hay *et al.* 1995).

Encopresis and constipation are often related. Paediatric constipation/encopresis is thought to be due, in part, to paradoxical constriction of the external anal sphincter muscle during attempted defecation. This inappropriate contraction can lead to delayed, impacted, painful and infrequent bowel movements (Cox *et al.* 1994). Chronic functional constipation is common in childhood (Seth & Heyman 1994). Infants and toddlers with constipation usually have a history of infrequent, hard and painful stools, often accompanied by screaming and stool-holding behaviours. Encopresis is also common in these children. Constipation usually has a functional cause; however, it needs careful assessment to rule out anatomic, endocrinal, metabolic or neurological causes (Loening-Baucke 1994).

Secondary encopresis has been found in cases of sexual assault of children. Children with secondary encopresis who do not respond well to standard treatments may have experienced sexual assault (Boon 1991). Assessment for possible sexual assault is recommended in all cases of secondary encopresis (Feehan 1995).

Encopresis and constipation can be successfully prevented in the community with anticipatory guidance and early dietary intervention (Standtler 1989; Seth & Heyman 1994). Most studies of childhood constipation and encopresis focus on treatment regimens. Parents' and children's views of the problem were sought in one Canadian study (Bernard-Bonnin *et al.* 1993). Parents and children reported that intestinal dysfunction and painful defecation were the most important causes of the encopresis. Treatments including enemas were well accepted by both children and parents. Parents considered that dietary changes were the most useful treatments, while children reported regular toileting was the most effective treatment.

Assessment of constipation/encopresis

Assessment of the child's defecation pattern
Has the child achieved bowel independence in the past? If so, at what age?
What is the quality of the child's stools? For example, soft, hard?
How often does the child have a bowel movement?
Is the passage of stools accompanied by evidence of pain (i.e. screaming, drawing up legs)?
Is there evidence of fecal smearing on the child's underwear or pyjamas?
Does the child 'play' with his or her feces?

Assessment of the child's diet
Is the child's diet lacking in fibre?
Have the parents increased fibre in an attempt to prevent or correct the constipation?

Treatment

Standard medical care involves disimpaction with enemas, followed by laxative therapy and diet modification (increased fibre) to maintain frequent soft stools (Cox *et al.* 1994). Behavioural protocols are also considered important adjuncts to medical treatment. These approaches include the development of a regular toileting schedule, and rewards and sanctions for desired and undesired behaviours (Fireman & Koplewicz 1992). Biofeedback training has been suggested as an effective adjunct therapy for functional constipation and/or encopresis in children; however, findings in controlled studies have been mixed, some reporting success and others no differences (Cox *et al.* 1994; Loening-Baucke 1996). Small group work with children and their parents (focusing on learning to give enemas, increasing fibre, and appropriate toileting techniques) has also been successful in treating encopresis (Stark *et al.* 1990). Complete recovery of encopresis is defined as three or more bowel movements per week with no soiling while off laxatives (Loening-Baucke 1995).

Regression

Loss of bowel and bladder control in children who have previously achieved independence may signal the need for further assessment and intervention. The context in which the regression occurs should signify if additional intervention beyond observation and support is needed. It is widely acknowledged in the nursing and medical literature that young children may regress, particularly with bladder control, during stressful life transitions, such as the arrival of a new baby into the family, or during illness and/or hospitalisation. No empirical literature was located that systematically documented how frequently and in what age groups these behavioural changes occur. Regressive bedwetting is usually intermittent and considered to be transitory. As stated above, though, it is important for community health nurses to remain open to other antecedents of regressive behaviour and act on any suspicions of physical or sexual abuse.

15.5 CONCLUSION

Most children achieve bowel and bladder independence during their early years. Community health nurses and other health professionals can facilitate the process by providing parents with advice and information grounded in empirical knowledge. Difficulties in achieving toileting independence provide a unique opportunity for community health nurses to offer support, assessment and, if needed, referral to other professionals. These interventions provide opportunities to support parents and promote the health of children.

REFERENCES

Bath, R., Morton, R., Uing, A. & Williams, C. (1996) Nocturnal enuresis and the use of desmopressin: is it helpful? *Child Care, Health and Development*, **22** (2), 73–84.

Berk, L. & Friman, P. (1990) Epidemiological aspects of toilet training. *Clinical Paediatrics*, **29** (5), 278–82.

Bernard-Bonnin, A., Haley, N., Belanger, S. & Nadeay, D. (1993) Parental and patient perceptions about encopresis and its treatment. *Journal of Developmental and Behavioural Paediatrics*, **14** (6), 397–400.

Birch, B.R. & Miller, R. A. (1995) Primary nocturnal enuresis: a urodynamic study spanning three generations. *Scandinavian Journal of Urology–Nephrology*, **29** (3), 285–8.

Bloom, D. A., Seeley, W. W., Ritchey, M. L. & McGuire, E. J. (1993) Toilet habits and continence in children: an opportunity sampling in search of normal parameters. *Journal of Urology*, **149** (5), 1087–90.

Boon, F. (1991) Encopresis and sexual assault. *Journal of the American Academy of Child and Adolescent Psychiatry*, **30** (3), 509–10.

Bradbury, M.G. & Meadow, S.R. (1995) Combined treatment with enuresis alarm and desmopressin for nocturnal enuresis. *Acta Paediatrica*, **84** (9), 1014–8.

Brazelton, T. B. (1962) A child-oriented approach to toilet training. *Pediatrics*, **29**, 579–88.

Butler, R., Brewin, C. & Forsythe, W. (1988) A comparison of two approaches to the treatment of nocturnal enuresis and the prediction of effectiveness using pre-treatment variables. *Journal of Child Psychology and Psychiatry*, **29**, 501–9.

Butler, R., Brewin, C. & Forsythe, I. (1990a) Relapse in children for nocturnal enuresis: predictions of response using pre-treatment variables. *Behavioural Psychotherapy*, **18** (1), 65–72.

Butler, R., Redfern, E. & Forsythe, I. (1990b) The child's construing of nocturnal enuresis: a method of inquiry and prediction of outcome. *Journal of Child Psychology and Psychiatry and Allied Disciplines*, **31** (3), 447–54.

Burke, J., Mizusawa, Y., Chan, A. & Webb, K. (1995) A comparison of amitriptyline, vasopressin and amitriptyline with vasopressin in nocturnal enuresis. *Paediatrics Nephrology*, **9** (4), 438–40.

Christophersen, E. & Edwards, K. (1991) Treatment of elimination disorders: state of the art 1991. *Applied and Preventive Psychology*, **1** (1), 15–22.

Cox, D.J., Sutphen, J., Borowitz, S., Dickens, M.N., Singles, J. & Whitehead, W.E. (1994) Simple electromyographic biofeedback treatment for chronic paediatric constipation/encopresis: preliminary report. *Biofeedback Self Regulation*, **19** (1), 41–50.

Dobson, P. (1994) Youthful issues ... nocturnal enuresis. *Nursing Times*, **90** (10), 59–60.

Eggert, P. & Kuhn, B. (1995) Antidiuretic hormone regulation in patients with primary nocturnal enuresis. *Archives of Diseases in Childhood*, **73** (6), 508–11.

Fergusson, D.M. & Horwood, L.J. (1994) Nocturnal enuresis and behavioural problems in adolescence: a 15 year longitudinal study. *Pediatrics*, **94** (5), 662–8.

Feehan, C.J. (1995) Enuresis secondary to sexual assault. *Journal of the American Academy of Child and Adolescent Psychiatry*, **34** (11), 1404.

Fireman, G. & Koplewicz, H. (1992) Short term treatment of children with encopresis. *Journal of Psychotherapy Practice and Research*, (1), 64–71.

Foreman, D.M. & Thambirajah, M.S. (1996) Conduct disorder, enuresis and specific developmental delays in two types of encopresis: a case-note study of 63 boys. *European Child and Adolescent Psychiatry*, **5** (1), 33–7.

Gesell, A. & Ilg, F.F. (1943) *Infant and child in the culture of today*. Harper & Bros., New York.

Hamburger, B. (1993) Treating enuresis. *Canadian Nurse*, **89** (4), 26–8.

Hauck, M.R. (1988) *Factors influencing toileting behaviors in toddlers*. PhD Dissertation. University of Wisconsin, Madison.

Hauck, M.R. (1991) Mothers' descriptions of the toilet-training process: a phenomenological study. *Journal of Paediatric Nursing*, **6** (2), 80–6.

Hay, W., Groothuis, J., Hayward, A. & Levin, M. (1995) *Current Pediatric Diagnosis and Treatment*, Appleton & Lange, Norwalk CON.

Houts, A. (1991) Nocturnal enuresis as a bio-behavioural problem. *Behavioural Therapy*, **22** (2), 133–51.

Houts, A., Berman, J. & Abramson, H. (1994) Effectiveness of psychological and pharmacological treatments for nocturnal enuresis. *Journal of Consulting and Clinical Psychology*, **62** (4), 737–745.

Josephs, L. (1989) The cleaning lady: the fate of an archaic maternal imago. *Psychoanalysis and Psychotherapy*, **7** (2), 116–28.

Kirk, J., Rasmussen, P.V., Rittig, S. & Djurhuus, J.C. (1996) Provoked enuresis-like episodes in healthy children 7 to 12 years old. *Journal of Urology*, **156** (1), 210–213.

Loening-Baucke, V. (1994) Comment: Management of chronic constipation in infants and toddlers. *American Family Physician*, **50** (7), 1465.

Loening-Baucke, V. (1995) Functional constipation. *Seminar in Pediatric Surgery*, **4** (1), 26–34.

Loening-Baucke, V. (1996) Encopresis and soiling. *Pediatric Clinics of North America*, **43** (1), 279–98.

Luxem, M. & Christophersen, E. (1994) Behavioral toilet training in early childhood: research, practice and implications. (review article), *Developmental and Behavioural Paediatrics*, **15** (5), 370–8.

MacFarlane, J.W., Allen, L. & Honzik, M.P. (1954) *A developmental study of the behaviour problems of normal children between twenty-one months and fourteen years*. University of California, Berkeley.

Maizels, M., Gandhi, K., Keating, B. & Rosenbaum, D. (1993) Diagnosis and treatment for children who cannot control urine. *Current Problems in Paediatrics*, **23** (10), 402–450.

Martin, J.A., King, D.R., Macoby, E.E. & Jacklin, C.N. (1984) Secular trends and individual differences in toilet training progress. *Journal of Paediatric Psychology*, **9**, 457–67.

Mattelaer, P., Mersdorf, A., Rohrmann, D., Jung, P. & Jakse, G. (1995) Biofeedback in the treatment of voiding disorders in childhood. *Acta-UrolBelg*, **63** (4), 5–7.

Mattsson, S. (1994) Urinary incontinence and nocturia in healthy school children. *Acta Paediatrica*, **83** (9), 950–4.

Miller, K. (1993) Concomitant nonpharmacologic therapy in the treatment of primary nocturnal enuresis. *Clinical Paediatrics*, Special Edition, July, 32–7.

Moffat, M., Harlos, S., Kirshen, A. & Burd, L. (1993) Desmopressin acetate and nocturnal enuresis: how much do we know? *Paediatrics*, **92** (3), 420–25.

Norgaard, J.P. & Djurhuus, J.C. (1993) The pathophysiology of enuresis in children and young adults. *Clinical Paediatrics*, Special Edition, July, 5–9.

Robert, M., Averous, M., Besset, A., Carlander, B., Billiard, M., Guiter, J. *et al.* (1993) Sleep polygraph studies using cystomanometry in twenty patients with enuresis. *European Urology*, **24** (1), 97–102.

Ronen, T. & Abraham, Y. (1996) Retention control training in the treatment of younger versus older enuretic children, *Nursing Research*, **45** (2), 78–82.

Rushton, H. (1993a) Evaluation of an enuretic child. *Clinical Paediatrics*, Special Edition: treatment of childhood enuresis, July, 14–18.

Rushton, H. (1993b) Older pharmacologic therapy for nocturnal enuresis. *Clinical Paediatrics*, Special edition: treatment of childhood enuresis, July, 10–13.

Rushton, H.G., Belman, A.B., Zaontz, M.R., Skoog, S.J. & Sihelnik, S. (1996) The influence of small functional bladder capacity and other predictors on the response to desmopressin in the management of monosymptomatic nocturnal enuresis. *Journal of Urology*, **156** (Pt 2), 651–5.

Schmitt, B. D. (1982) Nocturnal enuresis: an update on treatment. *Pediatrics Clinics of North America*, **29** (1), 21–36.

Schulpen, T., Hirasing, R., de Jong, T., van der Heyden, A., Dijkstra, R., Sukhai, R. *et al.* (1996) Going Dutch in nocturnal enuresis. *Acta Paediatrica*, **85**, 199–203.

Seim, H.C. (1989) Toilet training first children. *Journal of Family Practice*, **29** (6), 633–6.

Seth, R. & Heyman, M.B. (1994) Management of constipation and encopresis in infants and children. *Gastroenterology Clinics of North America*, **23** (4), 621–36.

Shapiro, S.R. (1985) Enuresis: treatment and over treatment. *Paediatric Nursing*, **9** (3), 203–7.

Standtler, A.C. (1989) Preventing encopresis. *Paediatric Nursing*, **15** (3), 282–4.

Stark, L., Owens-Stively, J., Spirito, A., Lewis, A., & Huevremont D. (1990) Group behavioural treatment of retentive encopresis. *Journal of Paediatric Psychology*, **15** (5), 659–71.

Warzak, W. (1993) Psychosocial implications of nocturnal enuresis. *Clinical Paediatrics*, Special edition: treatment of childhood enuresis, July, 38–40.

Warzak, W. & Friman, P. (1994) Current concepts in paediatric primary enuresis. *Child and Adolescent Social Work Journal*, **11** (6), 507–23.

Watson, J.B. (1928) *Psychological care of infant and child.* W.W. Norton, New York.

Wille, S., Aili, M., Harris, A. & Aronson, S. (1994) Plasma and urinary levels of vasopressin in enuretic and none-nuretic children. *Scandinavian Journal of Urology and Nephrology*, **28** (2), 119–22.

Wille, S. (1994a) Nocturnal enuresis: sleep disturbance and behavioural patterns. *Acta Paediatrica*, **83** (7), 772–4.

Wille, S. (1994b) Primary nocturnal enuresis in children: background and treatment. *Scandinavian Journal of Urology Nephrology Supplement*, **156**, 1–48.

Williams, K., Chambers, M., Logan, S. & Robinson, D. (1996) Association of common health symptoms with bullying in primary school children. *British Medical Journal*, **313** (7048), 17–19.

PARENTAL READINESS INVENTORY

Think back to what it was like BEFORE you started to potty train your child. I am going to read you a list of things you may or may not have done BEFORE you dressed your child in underpants for the first time rather than nappies. Tell me which number best describes what YOU DID on this scale (1 = **never did this, 5 = did this a lot**).

1.	Read about potty training	1	2	3	4	5
2.	Asked people about potty training	1	2	3	4	5
3.	Bought or borrowed things to help with training (potty chair, step stool, underpants, treats)	1	2	3	4	5
4.	Dressed your child in easy to remove clothing	1	2	3	4	5
5.	Planned for TIME needed to train child	1	2	3	4	5

Next are some things that you may or may not have THOUGHT about BEFORE you started potty training your child. Tell me which number best describes how much you THOUGHT about the following things (1 = **never thought about this, 5 = thought about this a lot**).

6.	Made a plan for training your child	1	2	3	4	5
7.	Consider whether or not your child was ready to be trained	1	2	3	4	5
8.	Think about how you would handle accidents	1	2	3	4	5
9.	Think about whether or not you were ready to take your child out of nappies	1	2	3	4	5
10.	Consider how long the process might take	1	2	3	4	5
11.	Think about ways to get your child to cooperate	1	2	3	4	5

Last are some things that you may or may not have FELT before you dressed your child in underpants for the first time. Tell me which number best describes the way you FELT about the following (1 = **never felt this, 5 = thought this a lot**).

12.	Feel that it was time to train your child	1	2	3	4	5
13.	Feel that people were pressuring you to potty train your child	1	2	3	4	5
14.	Total					

CHILD READINESS PROFILE

(1) How old was your child when you first had him or her sit on a toilet or potty chair? (age in months)
_____

(2) How old was your child when you first dressed your child in underpants or training pants rather than nappies? (age in months) _____

Below is a list of behaviours some children do between the ages of about six months and four years of age. Think about when your child did these things in relation to when he/she first wore underpants. Please tell me if your child did the following things BEFORE, within the SAME WEEK, or AFTER the first week, they started wearing underpants. If your child never did the behaviour just indicate that below.

Before = 1   Same week = 2   After = 3   Never = 4   Don't know = 5

A	Walked unsupported?	1	2	3	4	5
B	Stayed dry during the day?	1	2	3	4	5
C	Could release a toy he/she was holding when requested?	1	2	3	4	5
D	Stayed dry for more than 2 hours at a time?	1	2	3	4	5
E	Stayed dry through the night?	1	2	3	4	5
F	Removed own clothing from the lower half of body?	1	2	3	4	5
G	Told you he/she had already 'gone potty' in nappy/pants	1	2	3	4	5
H	Told you he/she had to go to the toilet?	1	2	3	4	5
I	Was able to follow simple directions.	1	2	3	4	5
J	Started having bowel movements (poop, stool) at predictable times?	1	2	3	4	5
K	Usually urinated (pee) when placed on the toilet or potty?	1	2	3	4	5
L	Showed an interest in learning to use the toilet?	1	2	3	4	5
M	Had a word, symbol or gesture indicating he/she needed to use the toilet?	1	2	3	4	5
N	Could sit still for 5 to 10 minutes playing with toys?	1	2	3	4	5
O	Did things to please you? (i.e. picked up toys)	1	2	3	4	5
P	Was willing to sit on a toilet without crying, fussing, or trying to get off?	1	2	3	4	5
Q	Total					

TOILETING BEHAVIOUR REPORT

Below is a list of toileting behaviours that children eventually learn to do all by themselves. Indicate whether your child *currently does these things all by him/herself* on a scale of rarely, sometimes, usually, almost always, or always.

Rarely = 1   Sometimes = 2   Usually = 3   Almost always = 4   Always = 5

(1)	Sits on the toilet or potty seat when placed there without fussing, crying, or attempting to get off.	1	2	3	4	5
(2)	Eliminates into the toilet or potty on a regular basis when seated or placed on the potty.	1	2	3	4	5
(3)	Waits to eliminate until seated on a potty.	1	2	3	4	5
(4)	Lets you know he/she needs to use a toilet or potty.	1	2	3	4	5
(5)	Asks to go to the toilet or goes by him/herself.	1	2	3	4	5
(6)	Helps undress him/herself before getting on to the toilet (with help).	1	2	3	4	5
(7)	Undresses all by him/herself before getting on to the toilet.	1	2	3	4	5
(8)	Climbs on to the full sized toilet by self.	1	2	3	4	5
(9)	Wipes him/herself without any help.	1	2	3	4	5
(10)	Flushes the toilet.	1	2	3	4	5
(11)	Dresses him/herself.	1	2	3	4	5
(12)	Washes his/her hands and dries them on towel.	1	2	3	4	5
(13)	Has bowel movements on the toilet or potty.	1	2	3	4	5
(14)	Stays dry during the night.	1	2	3	4	5

(15)   Total

(16)   How many weeks did it take from the time your child first wore underpants until your child was dry in underpants during the day 80–90% of the time (dry almost always)?
(record in weeks) _____

(17)   How old was your child when he/she was dry in underpants during the day, 80–90% of the time (dry almost always)? Record in months _____

Hauck, M.R. (1988) Factors influencing toilet training behaviors in toddlers. PhD Dissertation. University of Wisconsin. For updated version and further information contact Dr Hauck, e-mail: mhauck1@fairview.org These Appendices are reproduced with the kind permission of the author.

Index